Safe Surgery Guide

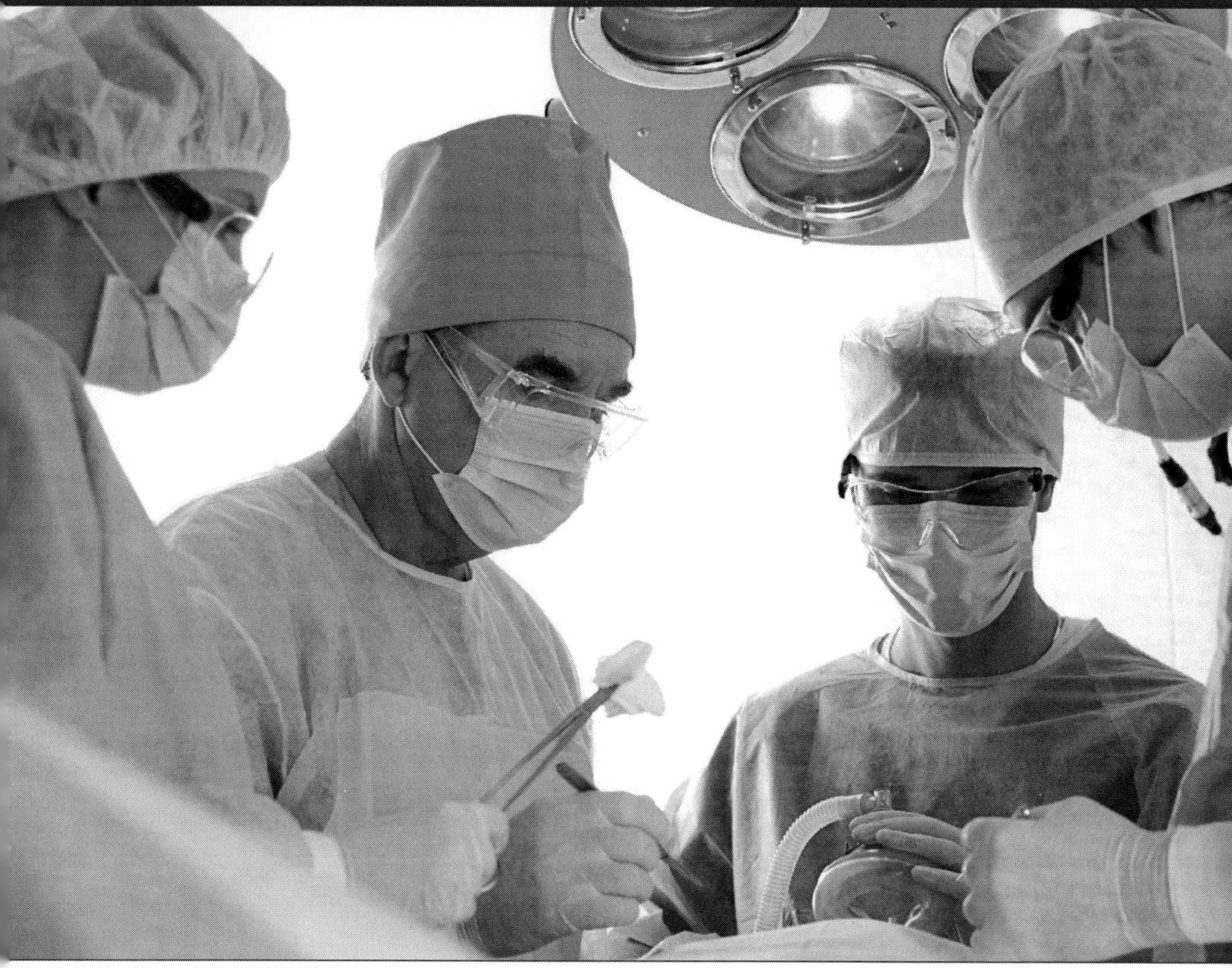

Joint Commission Resources

Joint Commission International

Foreword by
Peter J. Pronovost, M.D., Ph.D.

Senior Editor: Lori Meek Schuldt
Senior Project Manager: Cheryl Firestone
Manager, Publications: Paul Reis
Associate Director, Production: Johanna Harris
Executive Director: Catherine Chopp Hinckley, Ph.D.
Joint Commission/Joint Commission International/Joint Commission Resources Reviewers: Mary Brockway, Kelly Fugate, William J. Kragness, Michael Kulczycki, Joyce Marshall, John Wallin, Joyce Webb

Joint Commission Resources Mission
The mission of Joint Commission Resources (JCR) is to continuously improve the safety and quality of care in the United States and in the international community through the provision of education and consultation services and international accreditation.

Joint Commission International
A division of Joint Commission Resources, Inc.
The mission of Joint Commission International (JCI) is to improve the safety and quality of care in the international community through the provision of education, publications, consultation, and evaluation services.

Printed in the U.S.A. 5 4 3 2 1

Requests for permission to make copies of any part of this work should be mailed to
Permissions Editor
Department of Publications
Joint Commission Resources
One Renaissance Boulevard
Oakbrook Terrace, Illinois 60181 U.S.A.
permissions@jcrinc.com

ISBN: 978-1-59940-407-3
Library of Congress Control Number: 2010934168

For more information about Joint Commission Resources, please visit http://www.jcrinc.com.
For more information about Joint Commission International, please visit http://www.jointcommissioninternational.org.

Contents

Foreword

Patient safety has risen to a level of importance alongside biomedical discoveries that improve upon treatments and therapies. Such heightened awareness has sparked efforts that inched improvements in safety up by 1% annually between 2000 and 2005. Much of this measured improvement came through intense work on increasing the extent to which patients receive recommend therapies, such as appropriate timing of antibiotics for surgery or reducing adverse events from low molecular weight heparin. There is limited evidence that patient outcomes have improved. Nonetheless, progress in patient safety has been slow and stems largely from our inability to measure and track safety effectively. To do so, we must invest more resources in maturing the science of safety and the quality of health care delivery. Effective approaches will require clear goals and measures, the use of evidence-based therapies, local innovation and removal of barriers to safe practice, and a significant culture change to one that values and respects teamwork. In addition, efforts to improve quality will be enhanced through social pressures to make performance transparent, economic pressures to pay more for higher-quality care, and regulatory pressures to ensure that standards are met. All of this hinges on clear goals and valid measures of patient outcomes.

In U.S. efforts to reduce central line–associated bloodstream infections, we have seen that dramatic improvements are possible when health care works collaboratively rather than competitively, when we work interdependently rather than independently, and when we focus on results rather than efforts. Although the epidemiology of preventable harm remains uncertain and imprecise, the available evidence suggests that it is a significant problem. When the sources of harm are added, an estimated 200,000 patients die every year from diagnostic or other medical errors, health care–acquired infections, or not receiving recommended medical care. In large part, this gap stems from minimal research invested in the science of health care delivery. Guidelines are necessary but insufficient. There is a clearinghouse of clinical practice guidelines, with innumerable pages for each guideline, telling practitioners what to do. To make progress, health care organizations must reduce onerous guidelines down to a handful of practices that yield the greatest benefit for patients and are feasible for clinicians to implement. Moreover, we must identify and remove barriers to complying with these practices, we must measure performance, and we must reorganize work to ensure that all patients receive the recommended therapies. All of this requires culture change.

The Joint Commission has taken the lead in advancing the science and meeting these needs. Its *Safe Surgery Guide* provides practical and tested strategies to help improve perioperative safety and quality of care. It takes the systems approach, by breaking down a system—in this case, surgery—into key components and developing strategies to ensure that mission-critical processes are completed. One key component of surgery, for instance, occurs before the procedure begins. Mission-critical processes in this component include communication; hand hygiene; preparing the operating room, patient, and surgical team; and completing the Universal Protocol.

This guide dedicates a chapter to each process and incorporates strategies to improve culture and ensure that the process is completed appropriately. Chapter 1, for example, addresses culture by discussing why communication is necessary in surgery (it engages and educates) and offering structured techniques for constructive conversations. Moreover, Chapter 6 discusses wrong-site surgery and two interventions to prevent it: The Joint Commission's Universal Protocol and the World Health Organization's Surgical Safety Checklist.

By using the tools in this book and continuing to advance the science of health care delivery, surgeons, anesthesiologists, nurses, and others can substantially reduce preventable harm and death of patients.

Peter J. Pronovost, M.D., Ph.D.
Professor, Anesthesiology and Critical Care Medicine, Surgery, Nursing, and Health Policy and Management; Director, Quality and Safety Research Group; Medical Director, Center for Innovations in Quality Patient Care
Johns Hopkins University School of Medicine, Baltimore

Introduction

Every day of every year in every country around the world, patients undergo surgery and other invasive procedures to repair damage, treat illness, and improve the quality of their lives. Some of these procedures are performed in hospitals, while others take place in ambulatory surgery centers of office-based surgery practices. Some are in operating rooms, some are at the bedside, and others are performed in any number of places as situations demand.

Within the United States, surgeons perform more than 50 million operations each year, and Americans undergo an average of 7 operations in their lifetime.[1] Statistics from 2004, reported in 2008, showed that 1 out of every 25 people on the planet undergoes surgery, and that number is probably even higher today.[2] The number of surgeries performed around the world has exceeded global totals for childbirth.[1] The risks associated with surgery have increased as well. Patients are 10 to 100 times more likely to die as a result of a surgical procedure than they are from having a baby.[1]

In the United States, nearly 150,000 people die each year as a result of surgery.[1] For every 100 patients who check into a hospital for surgery, 25 experience complications, and as many as 5 may even die from these complications.[3] Around the world, the risks associated with surgery have left at least seven million people disabled and one million people dead each year—a level of harm that approaches malaria and tuberculosis.[1]

Surgical error is a common type of error in the health care setting. In industrialized countries, nearly half of all adverse events in hospitalized patients are related to surgical care.[3] In the United States, errors related to surgery are second only to medication errors as the most frequent cause of error-related death in health care organizations.[4]

Many organizations have medication safety programs in place to target risks and reduce errors associated with medications. Yet health care organizations are not always as focused on improving safety in the operating environment despite its significant contribution to a health care organization's financial viability. In fact, known principles of surgical safety—such as hand hygiene, sponge counts, and medication labeling on the surgical field—are applied inconsistently even in the most sophisticated settings.[3]

The good news about errors in surgery and other invasive procedures is that they are, for the most part, preventable. However, noticeable and sustained error prevention requires more than talking about the importance of safety. Just as placing a bandage on a surgical incision will not help heal the wound, asking providers to "be safer" or "try harder" will not prevent surgical errors. In fact, there is no single remedy that will improve the safety of the operating environment. Instead, a systematic, collaborative approach that involves all members of the surgical team is necessary. This approach requires the support of leadership and benefits from the direct involvement of the patient and/or patient advocate.

The Purpose of This Book

The *Safe Surgery Guide* is designed to provide a "road map" for organizations to follow to improve safety in the surgical setting. The book's systematic and collaborative approach to improving safety includes evidence-based practices, regulations and guidelines, and strategies from organizations in the field. The process of surgery not only occurs in the operating room but also involves multiple steps to prepare the patient, surgical team, and operating environment; effective postsurgery care to prevent infection or other complications; and interactive discharge planning to prevent unplanned readmissions. Therefore, the book focuses on improving safety not only in procedural and operative areas but also across the entire continuum of the patient's surgical experience. Information in this book applies to a wide range of surgical procedures, from major surgery—the kind that involves an incision, anesthesia, and a significant postoperative recovery—to minimally invasive procedures, such as laproscopic, arthroscopic, or endoscopic surgery.

The book discusses and offers improvement strategies to address some of the most serious adverse events that occur in the surgical setting, including wrong-site, wrong-procedure, wrong-patient surgery; problems with anesthesia or medications; retained foreign objects; and surgical fires.

The book also discusses how to lay the groundwork for safety improvements by establishing a *culture of safety*—in which everyone on a team is focused on working together to provide the safest possible care for the patient—and by embracing systematic improvement methods, such as Lean, Six Sigma, and change management. These methods also are among the elements included in The Joint Commission's Robust Process Improvement™ (RPI), a methodology for improving processes that seeks to continuously increase the quality and efficiency of products and services. Like most aspects of performance improvement, success depends on a culture that values safety and takes a systematic, proactive approach to achieving it.

Although the journey may seem daunting, some organizations already have committed to this path. Improvement strategies to directly address particular risks have helped improve safety in some areas. For example, The Joint Commission's annual report *Improving America's Hospitals: The Joint Commission Report on Quality and Safety 2009* [5] cites improvements in reducing surgical site infections by stopping antibiotics within 24 hours of surgery. Further efforts are under way. The Joint Commission Center for Transforming Healthcare will begin its fourth project on reducing surgical site infections. This project is launched in collaboration with the American College of Surgeons (ACS) and uses data derived from the ACS's National Surgical Quality Improvement Program (NSQIP). NSQIP data on outcomes of surgery are widely regarded as highly reliable, with exemplary risk-adjusted outcomes. Seven of the Center's participating hospitals will be involved in the project. Project results will be available in 2011. In addition, The Joint Commission Center for Transforming Healthcare has been working with hospitals and ambulatory surgery centers to strengthen the safeguards that prevent wrong-site, wrong-side, and wrong-patient surgical procedures. Simply stated, wrong-site surgery should never happen; yet by some estimates, wrong-site, wrong-side, and wrong-patient procedures occur more than 40 times every week in the United States and are the most common type of sentinel event reported to The Joint Commission. The Center project was initiated with two Rhode Island hospitals associated with the Lifespan systems in July 2009. It has expanded to four additional hospitals and three ambulatory surgical centers. Contributing factors and validated solutions will be available by the end of 2010.

Going Beyond the Hospital

In the past, most patients having surgery went to a hospital for the procedure, stayed for one or more days, and were released to their homes almost fully recovered. More recently, many patients go to an outpatient location, such as a physician's office, an ambulatory surgery center, or the day surgery unit of a hospital, and are sent home soon after surgery to complete recovery outside of the health care organization.[6] By 1999, an estimated 75% of all operations in the United States were performed in ambulatory, same-day, or outpatient operating room settings, and that percentage has most likely increased since then.[7] Ambulatory surgery also has become more common outside the United States. In Canada, the proportion of ambulatory surgery tops 80%. Elective surgery is performed as an ambulatory procedure in 55% of cases in Denmark, 50% in Sweden, 48% in Norway, and 37% in Finland.[8]

Although many of the strategies discussed in this publication—for example, using structured communication techniques, engaging in effective hand hygiene, creating a sterile field, preparing the surgical site—apply to ambulatory and office-based surgical settings as well as hospitals, there are some unique challenges faced by these nonhospital settings. Recognizing the importance of safety in both hospital and nonhospital settings, the *Safe Surgery Guide* aims to provide information that is applicable to the shared and unique needs of each setting.

Although not every suggestion or strategy in the book will apply to every organization, the book addresses many of the critical issues present in the surgical environment and will help organizations pursue the goal of safe surgery. Joint Commission and Joint Commission International (JCI) requirements related to surgery and other invasive procedures are similar but different. Consult your Joint Commission or JCI accreditation manual for the specific requirements that apply to your health care organization.

Online extras

To see Joint Commission and Joint Commission International requirements related to safe surgery, visit http://www.jcrinc.com/SSW10/Extras/.

A Note About Terminology

In this book, to prevent confusion and ensure consistency, the term *patient* will be used throughout to represent any individual served within or by a health care facility. The term *provider* is used in this book in a broad sense, referring to any health care professional or facility that serves patients. Definitions of many other terms appear in the glossary at the back of the book.

Overview of Contents

The *Safe Surgery Guide* examines each phase along the surgical continuum, assuming that the decision to have a procedure has already been made. (The process for determining whether a procedure is advised is outside the scope of this book.) The book is divided into three parts, addressing considerations *before, during,* and *after* a procedure. Although they are included in Part 1, the key improvement concepts introduced in the first two chapters—communication and hand hygiene—apply to all aspects of surgery and other invasive procedures. These chapters offer tips, strategies, and tools for improving these critical activities throughout the process. The remaining chapters follow the order of a surgical or invasive procedure, starting in the preoperative setting, moving through the procedural area, and finishing with attention to postoperative care and discharge planning. Case studies throughout the book take a closer look at the activities of some organizations that embrace a systematic approach to improving safety in the surgical setting.

Chapter 1: Communication

This chapter explains why effective communication is necessary in surgery and other invasive procedures and how an organization's leadership must support it. The chapter describes structured communication techniques and training that can help organizations improve this vital aspect of patient safety.

Chapter 2: Hand Hygiene

Clean your hands. It seems to be a simple idea, yet it has been difficult for organizations to practice consistently. This chapter outlines hand hygiene guidelines and standards, discusses preparation of the hands for a surgical procedure, and offers solutions for improving hand hygiene throughout the organization. The Joint Commission Center for Transforming Healthcare has played an active role in developing and promoting hand hygiene improvement solutions, as explained in the chapter.

Chapter 3: Preparing the Operating Room or Procedure Area

The operating room is the first of the three key elements that must be properly prepared before a procedure begins. This chapter explores various facets of this preparation: managing the operating room schedule, creating and maintaining a sterile field, getting the instruments ready, preparing anesthesia equipment and other medical equipment, ensuring proper air quality and ventilation, and controlling traffic into and out of the room.

Chapter 4: Preparing the Patient

The patient is the second key element that must be ready for the procedure upon arrival in the room. This chapter describes the part of the presurgical process that focuses directly on the patient, which includes assessing the patient for risk factors, managing medications, and preparing the surgical site.

Chapter 5: Preparing the Surgical Team

The surgical team is the third key element that must be ready before the procedure can begin. As this chapter explains, proper preparation includes not only the obvious aspect of appropriate surgical attire but also the attitudes and behaviors of the personnel involved. The team will be more successful in its endeavor if all its members approach the procedure in a spirit of collaboration and respect.

Chapter 6: Completing the Universal Protocol for Preventing Wrong Site, Wrong Procedure, Wrong Person Surgery™

The foundation of The Joint Commission's ongoing effort to reduce the incidence of surgical errors is its Universal Protocol for Preventing Wrong Site, Wrong Procedure, Wrong Person Surgery. This chapter explains what wrong-site surgery is and how the Universal Protocol addresses it in three basic, easy-to-follow steps. The chapter also introduces and describes the World Health Organization Surgical Safety Checklist.

Chapter 7: Monitoring the Patient

Throughout the procedure, surgical team members must remain aware of the patient's condition. As described in this chapter, they must closely watch anesthesia and sedation levels, medication needs, glucose level, body temperature, and blood use.

Chapter 8: Avoiding Problems in the Operating Room

This chapter examines some of the problems that can occur during the procedure, all of which pose some degree of risk to the patient. These problems include distractions that can divert attention from the procedure, injuries to members of the surgical team from handling sharp instruments, objects inadvertently left behind in the patient's body, and fire breaking out. The chapter discusses ways to avoid such problems.

Chapter 9: Cleanup of the Operating Environment

This chapter highlights what must be done after the procedure is finished and the patient has left the operating environment. It includes proper disposal of medical waste, transportation of contaminated laundry, and post-operative cleanup of the operating area.

Chapter 10: Postoperative Care

This chapter discusses care of the patient following the procedure. Staff members must assess and respond to the patient's mental and physiological status, determine what medications may be needed, and take steps to prevent postoperative infection.

Chapter 11: The Discharge Process

For the procedure to be considered a complete success, attention must be given to what will happen after the patient leaves the organization. This chapter explains what is involved in effective discharge planning, including how to follow up with the patient to check on his or her recuperation and assess for potential surgical site infections.

Online Extras

You will find bonus features related to this book on the JCR Web site. These Online Extras include additional examples and supplemental information. As shown earlier in this introduction, look for the box with the Online Extras icon. The Online Extras for this book are available at http://www.jcrinc.com/SSW10/Extras/.

Acknowledgments

We are extremely grateful to our expert manuscript reviewers:

- Mary Brockway, M.S., R.N., Associate Director, Division of Standards and Survey Methods, The Joint Commission
- Kelly Fugate, N.D., R.N., Associate Project Director, Specialist, Division of Standards and Survey Methods, The Joint Commission
- William J. Kragness, M.D., Surveyor, Joint Commission International
- Michael Kulczycki, M.B.A., Executive Director, Ambulatory Care Accreditation Program, The Joint Commission
- Mondher Letaief, M.D., M.P.H., Monastir, Tunisia, Joint Commission International Editorial Advisory Board
- Rick Morrow, Master Black Belt
- John Wallin, M.S., R.N., Associate Director, Standards Interpretation Group, The Joint Commission

- Joyce Webb, R.N., M.B.A., C.M.P.E., Associate Project Director, Division of Standards and Survey Methods, The Joint Commission

We also greatly appreciate the additional assistance of the following people in developing key parts of the book:

- Anne Marie Benedicto, M.P.P.A., M.P.H., Chief of Staff and Executive Vice President, Support Operations, The Joint Commission
- Laura Caisley, Project Director, High 5s Project, Joint Commission International
- Joyce Marshall, Senior Research Associate, Division of Standards and Survey Methods, The Joint Commission
- Kelly Podgorny, R.N., M.S., C.P.H.Q., Project Director, Division of Standards and Survey Methods, The Joint Commission

Special thanks are extended to patient safety advocate Peter Pronovost, M.D., Ph.D., who wrote the foreword. We also sincerely thank writer Kathleen B. Vega for her excellent work.

References

1. Gawande A.: *The Checklist Manifesto: How to Get Things Right.* New York: Metropolitan Books, 2009.
2. Weiser T., et al.: An estimation of the global volume of surgery: A modelling strategy based on available data. *Lancet* 372:139–144, Jul. 12, 2008.
3. World Alliance for Patient Safety: *The Second Global Patient Safety Challenge: Safe Surgery Saves Lives.* Geneva: World Health Organization, 2008.
4. Schimpff S.: Improving operating room and perioperative safety: Background and specific recommendations. *Surg Innov* 14:127–135, Jun. 2007.
5. The Joint Commission: *Improving America's Hospitals: The Joint Commission's Annual Report on Quality and Safety 2009,* 2009. http://www.jointcommission.org/library/annual_report (accessed Jul. 24, 2010).
6. Agency for Healthcare Research and Quality: *Making Sure Your Surgery Is Safe.* http://www.ahrq.gov/CONSUMER/surgery/surgery6.htm (accessed Jul. 24, 2010).
7. Mangram A., et al.: Guidelines for prevention of surgical site infections, 1999. *Infect Control Hosp Epidemiol* 20:247–278, Apr. 1999.
8. Toftgaard C.: World Wide Day Surgery Activity 2003: IAAS Survey of Ambulatory Surgery. *Ambul Surg* 13:5–24, 2007.

PART 1

Before the Procedure

This part of the book examines key aspects of preparation leading up to a surgical or other invasive procedure. Please note that the first two aspects, communication and hand hygiene—presented in Chapters 1 and 2, respectively—also apply during and after the procedure. Chapters 3, 4, and 5 discuss proper preparation of the operating room, the patient, and the surgical team, respectively. Chapter 6 offers a detailed explanation of The Joint Commission's three-step preprocedure Universal Protocol for Preventing Wrong Site, Wrong Procedure, Wrong Person Surgery™ and a description of the World Health Organization Surgical Safety Checklist.

Chapter 1

Communication

Sending a rocket into space is one of the most complicated processes that occurs today. There are many moving parts, complex technologies, individuals, and variables. Imagine what would happen if the people involved in this complex process did not communicate effectively with each other. For example, what if the chief engineer and the fuel specialist did not speak about potential risks associated with the fuel before the flight? Or what if the pilot and ground control did not consider potential problems with navigation before liftoff? Even to someone who is not familiar with the science of sending a rocket into space, such a lack of communication would seem ridiculous. Of course everyone involved with this complex journey would share information, gather opinions, troubleshoot problems, and work together to handle any unexpected complications. If they did not, the chances are slim that the rocket would reach its destination and return home safely. In fact, teams that send rockets into space are known for their effective communication, collaboration, and problem solving. That is why so many of the space missions throughout the world are successful.

> **Note:** The key improvement concepts introduced in this chapter pertain to *all* aspects of a surgical or other invasive procedure—that is, they may be applied before, during, and after the procedure.

Why Communication Is Necessary in Surgery and Other Invasive Procedures

In some ways, performing surgery is like sending a rocket into space. There are many moving parts, individuals—the surgeon, the nurse, the anesthesiologist or nurse anesthetist, and the patient—and variables. Significant on-time pressures, high work loads, and dependence on properly working equipment can further add to the complexity.[1] In fact, surgery can be even more complex than rocket science because each surgical patient is slightly different and every surgical procedure has its own nuances.

Unlike rocket science, however, the level of communication that is present between individuals involved in a surgical procedure is unfortunately often relatively poor. Communication failure in the operating environment occurs frequently, with one study showing that 30% of surgical team exchanges involved some form of communication failure, and one third of these exchanges resulted in effects that jeopardized patient safety.[2]

Historically, surgery has been thought of as an individual virtuoso performance, with the surgeon acting as the soloist, and the operating room—also known as the operating theatre or the surgical suite—serving as the stage.[3] As patient safety expert Peter Pronovost writes, "Medicine operates like a private club of self-styled deities where the entrance requirement is an M.D. [degree]."[4] The idea of working as a team, valuing multiple inputs, and solving problems collaboratively is not inherent in many providers' way of thinking. Often these providers have not been trained to appreciate the value of effective communication, including the importance of "setting the stage" every time the team comes together, not only to share information but also to create an environment in which everyone knows the plan, feels valued, and has been specifically invited to speak up and voice both suggestions and concerns.[5]

This emphasis on the individual rather than the team has led to some high-profile incidents in the surgical setting: surgeons operating on the wrong limb, anesthesiologists giving the wrong dose of medication, infections developing at the surgical site, and objects such as sutures or sponges being left in the patient's body. When health care professionals do not communicate well, they can overlook, omit, forget, misinterpret, delay, or misdirect critical information. These lapses in communication can lead to inefficiency, tension between providers, delays in care, work-arounds, wasted resources, and patient inconvenience. In the worst cases, these communication lapses can lead to medical errors.[2] One recent study showed that patients operated on by surgical teams that did not communicate well or exhibit other team behaviors—such as performing briefings and sharing information before, during, and after a procedure as well as during transitions of care—were more likely to experience major complications and even death.[6]

No single individual is responsible for the entire surgical process, therefore surgical team members must interact and communicate effectively to ensure that the care provided to a patient is appropriate and comprehensive. Fundamentally, effective communication between all members of the surgical team lays the foundation on which all the rest of the components of surgery are built.

Although interactive communication is not necessarily the norm in the surgical suite, in the places where it is occurring, the results are impressive. For example, in one Canadian academic hospital, the use of a structured briefing before surgery helped decrease communication failures that had negative consequences by 64%.[7] Similarly, in United States Department of Veterans Affairs hospitals, the surgical teams that had a low mortality rate were shown to have better communication than those with a higher mortality rate.[8]

Communication Is a Key Element in a Culture of Safety

Improved communication before, during, and after surgery helps establish a culture of safety. A *culture of safety* is a culture in which individuals work together as a team to provide consistent care, to anticipate potential barriers to safe care, and to respond to unexpected events that come up. A culture of safety can exist on a macro (organizationwide) level and on a micro (department or team) level. When a culture of safety exists among surgical teams, all team members are able to acknowledge mistakes, learn from them, and take action to correct the situation. In addition, all team members focus on maintaining excellence in performance and accept personal responsibility for safety and quality of care, treatment, and services.

Improved communication is critical to establishing a culture of safety because everyone on the team knows that the team cannot truly deliver the best care possible unless the team members are constantly communicating with one another and striving to improve outcomes and reduce risks together. In addition, team members use structured communication techniques, and any disruptive behaviors that go against a team philosophy are not tolerated. Establishing a culture of safety at the team level helps foster an organizationwide culture that values communication, safety, and quality.

Communication Helps Create Situational Awareness

In addition to fostering a culture of safety, surgical teams that communicate effectively maintain situational awareness. *Situational awareness* is defined as a shared understanding of "what's going on," "what is likely to happen next," and "what to do if what is supposed to happen doesn't."[9] Situational awareness occurs when all team members agree about a procedure or process under way, recognize potential problem areas, and know the plans to address those areas. Maintaining situational awareness is important because it helps providers quickly identify when things are not going according to plan and address potential problems early before they become unmanageable. An ongoing dialogue between team members is required to maintain situational awareness. If situational awareness is lost, communication can break down and mistakes can occur. (More information on maintaining situational awareness can be found in Chapter 8.)

Although acknowledging that effective communication creates an environment conducive to safe surgery may be easy, achieving that level of communication can present some challenges for an organization, depending on its current culture and the commitment of leadership, physicians, and frontline staff to improve communication at all levels. The following sections provide some suggestions on how to navigate the challenging process of improving communication. Many of these topics will be addressed in further detail in subsequent chapters of the book. The purpose of this chapter is to introduce the concepts in the context of laying the foundation for safe surgery.

Leadership Support of Communication

Committed leadership is an essential component of any effort to improve communication, and it is particularly important in improving communication in the surgical suite. Without visible, active, dynamic leaders who require, support, establish, and drive improvement, communication efforts will most certainly stall.

To drive communication efforts, leaders must first and foremost be a visible presence. Given that health care organization executives must put on appropriate surgical attire when entering the surgical suite, it is not surprising that few members of upper management visit the operating room, even if they acknowledge it is the center of the organization's economic enterprise.[10] By visiting the surgical area, actively participating in initiatives to improve communication in that area, incorporating effective communication strategies into policies and procedures, and specifically training professionals—including surgeons, anesthesiologists, surgical technicians, nurses, and unit support staff—in better communication techniques, leaders, particularly at the unit level, can help improve communication and foster the creation and maintenance of teams. To sustain this level of teamwork and communication, leaders must also hold everyone—including themselves—accountable for such behaviors.[5]

Health care providers are extremely tuned in to messages from leadership, and it is important that messages about communication and teamwork be more than rhetoric.[9] In particular, leaders must do the following:

- Require cooperation, teamwork, collaboration, and respect
- Flatten hierarchies and power differences
- Break down communication barriers between groups, such as nurses and surgeons
- Effectively communicate with providers about organizational goals, performance requirements, and quality expectations
- Encourage different disciplines to work together
- Measure behavior and manage to these measures

Another way to lay the foundation for communication is to examine the organization's mission and values. To achieve a culture based on teamwork and communication at both the macro and micro levels, organizations must have a mission that reflects an emphasis on patient safety and links effective communication and teamwork with patient safety efforts. With leadership support from the highest level, leaders at the local level can carry out processes that are consistent with the organization's mission.

When framing conversations about communication and teamwork, it is important to discuss the consequences of these behaviors or a lack of these behaviors. If health care providers see concrete, justifiable reasons behind the effort to improve communication and can understand the harmful consequences of poor communication in terms of poor-quality care, patient safety, risk management, and malpractice, then cultural change will gain more support. If everyone has a common understanding of the importance of teamwork and communication, and the message is continually reinforced, then health care providers will begin to incorporate the concept of effective, interactive communication into their day-to-day activities.

Leadership at all levels, and particularly on a unit level for the operating environment, must set the tone for how communication will be carried out in an organization, and specifically within the surgical area, otherwise health care providers will be left to individually determine their own methods of communicating. Under those circumstances, hierarchical differences, power struggles, personality clashes, and conflicting goals can come into play and hamper effective communication.

Evaluate the Culture of Safety in the Surgical Setting

As a precursor to implementing initiatives to improve communication, organization leadership should consider assessing the current culture of both the organization and the surgical area to see how providers value and incorporate communication into daily activities. As previously mentioned, every organization and health care team within the organization has a culture. Assessing and reassessing the presence of a safety culture allows an organization to get a multidimensional profile of the cultural strengths and weaknesses of the organization and/or specific area of the organization, such as the surgical suite. It can also build awareness among health care providers—including surgeons, anesthesiologists, and nurses—about the importance of safety, teamwork, and quality improvement opportunities.

Specifically, a cultural assessment can establish a baseline picture of a group, make a data-driven case for change, help in selecting interventions that are most appropriate for improving communication and safety, measure the success of any interventions, and track changes in communication, safety, and quality over time.

Some members of a surgical team may balk at the idea of a cultural assessment. "The culture in my operating room is just fine!" they may say. However, if other members of the team are asked, they may offer a different perspective. One landmark study of more than 1,000 operating room staff members from hospitals in five countries—the United States, Germany, Israel, Italy, and Switzerland—found that although 64% of surgeons rated their operations as having high levels of teamwork, other members of the operating team had a different perspective. In fact, only 39% of anesthesiologists, 28% of nurses, and 10% of anesthesiology residents thought the operating environment had high levels of teamwork.[11]

The best way to measure a culture of safety is through a valid and reliable cultural assessment tool. Using such a tool is important because it ensures a standardized, structured, and consistent approach to culture measurement and helps draw out critical information. It allows individuals to "see themselves" and gain insight into relationships that people often do not feel safe discussing openly. It depersonalizes conversations about communication, safety risks, and quality issues and bases discussions on norms and empirical data, rather than "he said/she said" anecdotes.[12]

What constitutes "valid and reliable" will depend on the organization. A simple questionnaire, focus groups, or other tools can be helpful. Or an organization can turn to tools created by other groups for assessment (*see* Sidebar 1-1 on page 7). No matter what tool an organization chooses, some things to consider when selecting a tool include the tool's versatility in measuring different populations and settings, its reliability as validated by statistical analysis techniques, the benchmarking capability of the tool, and its ease of use.[12] Before selecting an assessment/survey instrument, organizations should know the instrument's capabilities, strengths, and weaknesses, and factor those into the selection and implementation process.

A critical component of the safety assessment process is responding to the data gleaned from the survey. If organization leaders do not respond and take advantage of a critical opportunity to discuss and improve organizationwide performance, they have wasted critical time and resources in completing an exercise that has no meaning. In addition to being wasteful, such lack of follow-through may discourage further provider participation in other safety efforts.[12]

Leaders should share survey results with health care providers in the areas assessed, including surgeons, anesthesiologists, and nurses. Based on the results of the survey, organizations may choose to provide enhanced education on teamwork and communication, revise policies that address cultural issues such as disruptive behavior, launch initiatives to improve teamwork and communication, and so on. Regular reassessments can help determine the success of any initiatives, including education efforts, and identify further areas of improvement.

Define Communication Expectations

Communication is one of those terms that people can have trouble grasping. What does it mean to communicate effectively? Is it being nice to someone? Is it being overly detailed? Is it asking a lot of questions? To help health care providers—specifically members of the surgical team—communicate more effectively, organization leaders must define what they mean by "communicating effectively." Such definition can be done formally or informally within meetings, interactions, and training. Leaders should define by example as well as by expectation. Although different leaders will want different things, following are some points to get across to providers about effectively communicating:

- *Perception is reality.* A fundamental mantra for effective communication is: "What I say is not

Sidebar 1-1: Tools for Assessing Culture

Although there are many tools available for assessing culture, the following is a brief description of some well-known instruments.

Agency for Healthcare Research and Quality's Surveys on Patient Safety Culture
The Agency for Healthcare Research and Quality (AHRQ) offers a free comprehensive assessment tool to help health care organizations conduct a safety assessment. The 51-item survey places an emphasis on safety issues, error, and event reporting. It measures both unit-level and organizationwide aspects of a culture of safety.

The survey takes about 10 minutes to complete, and most of the items use "Agree/Disagree" or "Never/Always" response categories. There is room for written comments at the end of the survey. The AHRQ survey does allow for benchmarking with other organizations that complete the survey. More information on the AHRQ survey can be found at http://www.ahrq.gov/qual/patientsafetyculture/.

Safety Attitudes Questionnaire
The Safety Attitudes Questionnaire is a valid instrument for capturing health care provider assessments of teamwork, patient safety, trust in management, and so on. Survey items in the questionnaire were determined based on attitudinal surveys in aviation, observations of providers at work, focus groups with providers, a review of the literature, and roundtable discussions with subject-matter experts.

The survey is two pages long, with 63 questions addressing a variety of topics, including communication, teamwork climate, safety climate, working conditions, and other topics related to safety culture. In addition, the survey has demographic questions that request information such as job position, gender, years of experience, and the respondent's specialty. Respondents answer questions using a five-point Likert Scale (disagree strongly, disagree slightly, neutral, agree slightly, agree strongly), and "not applicable" is also an option. The survey takes approximately five to seven minutes to complete. Organizations using the Safety Attitudes Questionnaire can benchmark their data against other organizations that use the survey. More information about the Safety Attitudes Questionnaire can be found at http://www.uth.tmc.edu/schools/med/imed/patient_safety/questionnaires/SAQBibliography.html.

Recently, Makary et al. developed a surgery-specific Safety Attitudes Questionnaire, which addresses the issues of handling medical errors, knowledge of reporting systems, and perceptions of safety in the operating room. The tool was tested among nearly 3,000 caregivers across 60 hospitals to ensure validity and reliability. More information on this tool can be found at http://www.ncbi.nlm.nih.gov/pubmed/16632997.

Pathways for Patient Safety
"Assessing Where You Stand" is a free online tool in the *Pathways for Patient Safety* series released in partnership by the Health Research and Educational Trust, the Institute for Safe Medication Practices, and the Medical Group Management Association. The tool is a physician-centered safety culture survey designed for group practices in outpatient settings. It takes a step-by-step approach to help practice leaders assess current patient safety procedures, address the culture in their practice, and set goals for improvement. More information on this and other tools in the series can be found at http://www.pathwaysforpatientsafety.org.

Medical Team Training Questionnaire
The U.S. Department of Veterans Affairs (VA), as part of a national program to improve communication in the health care environment, created the Medical Team Training questionnaire. This tool is used to assess organizational culture, communication, teamwork, and awareness of human factors. After pilot testing the questionnaire, the VA administered it to a group of nearly 400 surgical staff members in six facilities. The questionnaire was helpful in identifying hidden problems with communication and focusing efforts to improve communication and teamwork, specifically in the operating room. Although organizations may not be able to use the exact Medical Team Training questionnaire in assessing their own operating room cultures, they can reference it as a starting point for developing their own survey instrument. More information about the Medical Team Training questionnaire and the VA's program can be found at http://www4.va.gov/ncps/MTT/index.html.

Sources

Agency for Healthcare Quality and Research: *Patient Safety Culture Surveys.* http://www.ahrq.gov/qual/patientsafetyculture/ (accessed Jul. 20, 2010).

Makary M., et al.: Patient safety in surgery. *Ann Surg* 243:628–632, May 2006.

Mills P., Neily J., Dunn E.: Teamwork and communication in surgical teams: Implications for patient safety. *J Am Coll Surg* 206:107–112, Jan. 2008.

Sexton J., et al.: The Safety Attitudes Questionnaire: Psychometric properties, benchmarking data, and emerging research. *BMC Health Serv Res* 6:44, Apr. 3, 2006.

important. The only thing that matters is what other people hear." An individual is not his or her own audience. Real communication is contingent on the person who is receiving the message understanding it. Consequently, effective communication requires speaking at the listener's level and making the listener's need the uppermost focus. Doing so involves avoiding jargon, using clear language, using analogies and relevant stories, avoiding abstract concepts, and checking one's body language to ensure that it shows caring, competence, and compassion. For example, when a surgeon speaks with a nurse during a procedure, the surgeon's tone of voice, eye contact, and body language can often communicate something different than what is being said. Consequently, the nurse's perception may be different than the surgeon's intention. By being aware of how information is communicated, surgical team members can ensure that both sender and receiver are in accord.

- *Good communication does not lessen authority.* Just because a person—such as a surgeon, anesthesiologist, or nurse in the operating environment—values others' opinions, seeks feedback, and speaks at a listener's level, it does not mean that he or she is not an expert. Good communication can help improve anyone's abilities, even the most talented, smart, experienced professionals. By taking time to speak cordially with colleagues and address their priorities, both the speaker and the receiver will benefit.
- *Good communication involves empathizing with others.* Acknowledging the opinions of others—even if one disagrees with them—is paramount to achieving good communication. After a surgical team member recognizes and affirms another's point of view, the conversation can move past opinions to explanations, explorations, and other options. This communication is then without judgment or influence and rather is an act of respectful information exchange.
- *Communication should be SAFER.* This acronym represents an overall approach to improving communication that surgical team members should keep in mind. The different elements of this mnemonic are as follows[13]:
  - **S***afe:* Communication reduces morbidity and mortality.
  - **A***ccessible:* Communication skills can be demonstrated by all team members.
  - **F***easible:* Communication can be achieved with practice but without difficulty.
  - **E***ffective:* Communication improves team functioning.
  - **R***ight:* Communication saves lives, time, and money.

Using Structured Communication Techniques

Most health care providers have not been systematically taught how to effectively communicate. Medical and nursing schools, for example, typically focus on clinical information and scientific knowledge but do not have a central focus on how to effectively interact with and respond to peers, patients, and other providers. This lack of a standardized approach in the various educational disciplines means that different disciplines enter the surgical environment with different styles, their own jargon, and little knowledge about the inherent value in standardized and clear communication.[5]

To compensate for health care providers' lack of communication skills, it is helpful to use certain strategies and tools to foster teamwork, communication, and collaboration. Such strategies and tools can be effectively applied across the continuum of surgery and can yield not only better communication but also earlier error detection, proactive risk reduction, and improved satisfaction for both providers and patients. Such tools can also be useful in helping staff in operating rooms speak up when they see a potential problem that could lead to patient harm. This is something that many staff members find intimidating and difficult. By offering specific, easy-to-use tools, organizations can help encourage more collaboration and reduce hierarchy and power differences. Following is a discussion of some of these strategies and tools.

Briefings

Briefings are a critical element in team effectiveness and can determine whether people work together as a cohesive team or as a group of individuals with different ideas and goals sharing the same space. Briefings involve short discussions between team members that aim to place all members of the team at the same starting point. Briefings can create a framework during which health care providers can identify any risk points in a procedure, plan for contingencies, avoid surprises, promote a sense of collaboration, and set the tone for open communication. Briefings can be used at any point along the continuum of surgery. They can be particularly helpful just prior to starting a procedure and during a procedure to help maintain situational awareness.

The Joint Commission's Universal Protocol for Preventing Wrong Site, Wrong Procedure, Wrong Person Surgery™ requires surgical teams to conduct a specific type of preprocedure briefing—typically called a *time-out*—in which the correct site, procedure, and patient are verified. This briefing is also an opportunity to address other issues such as antibiotic administration, medications, allergies, access to critical equipment, anticipated problems, and other salient issues. (*See* Chapter 6 for more information on the Universal Protocol.)

When done effectively, briefings can establish predictability, reduce interruptions, prevent delays, build social relationships, and create capital for future interactions.[14] Briefings have been shown to improve communication and enhance patient safety in the surgical suite. A study from Johns Hopkins Hospital found that operating room teams that participated in two-minute briefings before the surgical incision noted improved teamwork. Team members also perceived the risk of wrong-site surgery to be lower.[15] A Canadian study showed that specific types of briefings, including huddles and surgical time-outs, could change the notion of individual advocacy to one of teamwork and proactive risk reduction.[16] Another study from the United Kingdom showed that a briefing and debriefing improved team members' perception of communication in cardiac surgery.[17]

Briefings also can improve efficiency. Another study from Johns Hopkins Hospital showed that a standardized preoperative briefing could decrease unexpected delay by 36%.[18]

Successful briefings have many distinct characteristics, including the following:

- *Brevity.* For briefings to add value, they have to be seen as providing a positive return for the time spent. Meaningful information is communicated quickly, enhancing operational efficiency, not hindering it.
- *Involvement of all team members.* Briefings involve multidirectional conversations. Engaging team members and explicitly asking them for their input and suggestions brings more expertise to the issue at hand. This interactivity also offers an opportunity to assess people's comfort level and prior experience relative to a particular procedure or task within the procedure. Having team members participate enhances team formation and clarifies that everyone has a responsibility to ensure safe care and to speak up if they perceive something to be unsafe.
- *Use of first names.* Familiarity is a key factor in the willingness of people to speak up when they perceive a problem. A prime indicator of familiarity is the use of first names, or given names. Taking a minute for introductions can allow the team to greet each other and show the importance of teamwork. In one study, researchers observed that when nurses were given a chance to say their names and mention concerns at the beginning of a case, they were more likely to note problems and offer solutions. The use of names seemed to "activate" their desire to participate and responsibility to speak up.[3]
- *Eye contact.* Acknowledging others and paying attention to what they say sends a positive message, thus reinforcing the idea that their contributions have value and importance. Eye contact should be practiced when working with individuals who culturally are comfortable with it. Some cultures view direct eye contact as a threat, and thus it should

TIP Anticipate and Plan

In addition to a preprocedure briefing, team members should consider spending a few minutes at the beginning of the day to look across the schedule, anticipate equipment and supply needs, and plan for contingencies. Doing so allows each preprocedural briefing to be shorter, can prevent delays in starting procedures, and can minimize interruptions during procedures. Such planning also can minimize the need for the circulating nurse to leave the operating room to retrieve necessary equipment and supplies during a procedure.

be avoided in situations in which a team member is uncomfortable with it.

- *Use of questions to act as prompts for the briefing.* Some organizations find it helpful to use a checklist to help structure the briefing process. Case Study 1-1 below shows how one organization used a checklist to structure its briefing. More information on checklists appears on pages 14–15.

Fostering collaboration through briefing is not inherent to many physicians, including surgeons. In some cases, it goes against the very fiber of their being. However, the surgeon's participation in and leadership of briefings is critical in the operating room. To gain surgeon support, organizations may want to present the briefing concept in terms that the surgeon values. Consider the following statements[5]:

"Dr. Smith, if you conduct briefings, your day will run smoother. You will have the equipment you need, when you need it, and everyone will be working together to achieve common goals."

"Dr. Jones, if you conduct briefings, patients will be safer and so will you. Because of the structured communication involved in briefings and the effective communication that results from briefings, patient harm is less likely, continuous learning can be achieved, and malpractice risk is reduced."

Case Study 1-1: Memorial Health System

About the Organization: Located in Colorado Springs, Colorado, Memorial Health System is a community-based health care organization with 650 beds. The organization's 25 operating rooms across two campuses host approximately 18,000 surgeries each year.

Purpose of the Project: To improve the functioning of the operating room through the use of human factors training and a structured preprocedure briefing.

In the early 2000s, Memorial Health System embarked on a journey to improve safety in the operating room (OR) and enhance the care provided to patients. After receiving a grant from the Association for periOperative Registered Nurses (AORN) and the Kimberly-Clark corporation, the organization began a physician- and nursing-led initiative to introduce human factors training, a tool used in aviation to improve teamwork and communication, into the operating room. Leaders in the organization saw many parallels between the airline industry and the operating room and thus decided to use an aviation-based approach in addressing communication failures.

Initially, Memorial Health System contracted an outside company to provide four-hour training sessions on human factors. The training was mandatory for operating room staff but voluntary for surgeons. Physicians and staff were trained together to emphasize the team concept. About 30% of the organization's surgeons across all surgical fields participated in the training.

The fundamental concept included in the training was the idea of a preoperative briefing. Memorial Health developed a structured briefing that is customized to its particular characteristics and needs. The hospital used the World Health Organization Surgical Safety Checklist (*see* Chapter 6) as a guide for its preprocedure briefing but modified it for its own environment. During the training, participants were trained on how to use the structured briefing and on the benefits of the tool.

In general, nursing and other operating room staff received the training program well; however physician response was mixed. Generally, the physicians who participated in the training program thought that it was worthwhile. Most of the other surgeons who did not participate thought the exercise was at best unnecessary and at worst a waste of time.

After the training program, voluntary use of briefings in the operating room increased. Before the training, two physicians regularly conducted preprocedure briefings. After the training, that number rose to 20. Unfortunately, most of the surgeons who participated in the training saw value in the briefing process but did not change their own operative routine. There was a perception that such a briefing would steal precious minutes away from a case.

For the next two years, Memorial Health relied on peer influence and word of mouth to convince physicians to use a preoperative briefing. As participation rates stalled, the organization decided to become more aggressive in its efforts to engage physicians. To do so, Memorial Health used

(continued on page 11)

Case Study 1-1: Memorial Health System *(continued)*

a three-pronged approach. First, the organization invited a well-respected cardiothoracic surgeon from the Mayo Clinic to give a presentation on how preoperative briefings affected his practice.

Second, the organization began to study miscommunication events in the operating room as well as operating room efficiency. Based on this study, Memorial Health found a positive difference in the rooms that performed a preoperative briefing. These briefings decreased the number of times the circulating nurse left the operating room and decreased communication failures among surgical teams that resulted in patient issues, equipment issues, or procedural issues. During this time, the organization also conducted cultural surveys of the operating room using the Agency for Healthcare Research and Quality cultural assessment survey. The use of the preprocedure briefing was associated with greater staff perceptions of teamwork and openness and fewer punitive reactions to errors. *(See* Figure 1-1 below.)

Finally, Memorial Health hired a retired pediatric surgeon for three months to help coach surgeons on how to conduct a briefing. This individual circulated among the operating rooms observing cases. She interacted with surgeons individually and provided guidance and advice on how to effectively conduct the briefing. Her presence not only reminded surgeons to conduct the briefing but also helped surgeons identify the most efficient use of the briefing.

The combination of these three actions increased the number of surgeons performing the briefing by more than 50%. By showing surgeons the positive effects of conducting a briefing using organization-specific data, Memorial Health was able to remove some of the skepticism associated with the process. In addition, providing surgeon-driven analysis and mentoring helped show surgeons how they could use the briefing in their own practice.

Source: Hurlbert S., Garrett J.: Improving operating room safety. *Patient Saf Surg* 3:25, Nov. 20, 2009.

Figure 1-1: Cultural Survey Results

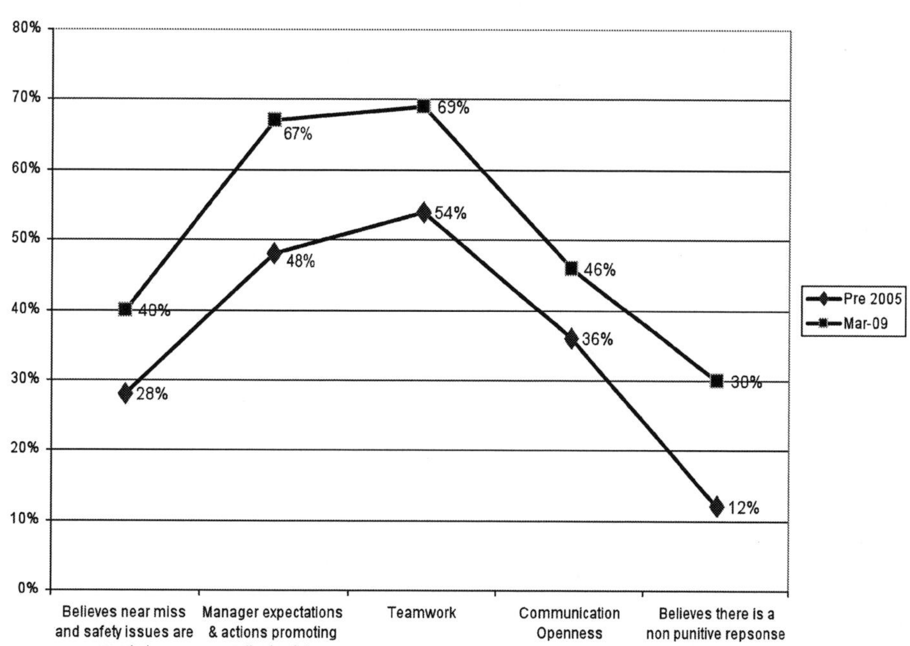

This figure shows some of the data on teamwork that the organization collected.

Source: Memorial Health System. Used with permission.

Situation–Background–Assessment–Recommendation (SBAR) Technique

When structuring communication during briefings, or any time critical information must be shared between two parties, organizations may want to use the Situation–Background–Assessment–Recommendation (SBAR) structured communication technique. This technique is used to standardize communication between two or more people.[19] It is an easy-to-remember, concrete mechanism useful for framing any conversation, particularly critical ones requiring a health care provider's immediate attention and action.[20] It helps set the expectation within a conversation that specific, relevant, and critical informational elements will be communicated every time a patient is discussed.

The SBAR model is particularly helpful in situations in which a nurse–physician encounter must occur. SBAR sets the expectation that critical thinking associated with defining the patient's problem and formulating a solution occur before the conversation takes place. Thus, both parties know that the conversation will include the assessment and recommendation for care that is relevant to the patient's current status.

The following is a description of the steps involved in SBAR:

- *Situation.* This is the part of the mechanism in which the two parties communicating establish the topic of which they are going to speak. In the case of a clinically related interaction, such as a communication between a nurse and an anesthesiologist in the preoperative setting, the individual initiating the SBAR should describe the problem in a simple and straightforward manner, offering a factual and concise description of the situation.[21] It should take no longer than 10 seconds.[22]
- *Background.* This is any information needed to make an informed decision for the patient. Depending on the situation, this information may vary. Some common types of information shared include the time of surgery, list of current medications, any allergies present, most recent vital signs, and other clinical information.

  Any vital sign or other assessment finding should be current within 30 minutes of the conversation. It is important to note here that information should be relevant to the conversation and not include a full history of events since the patient entered the health care organization.
- *Assessment.* The individual initiating the SBAR should state his or her assessment of the situation and the patient's status. If the situation is unclear, the speaker should try to isolate the problem that may be involved and state how severe the problem appears to be. If the problem is life threatening, this should be stated clearly. This aspect of the SBAR interaction may be the most challenging because it involves critical thinking skills and tapping into knowledge as well as experience.
- *Recommendation.* The individual initiating the SBAR should offer a recommendation of what to do next and when it should happen. Depending on the situation, the recommendation may include medication administration, cardiac monitoring, physician evaluation, or other action. If physician evaluation is needed—such as during a preoperative evaluation—the individual initiating the SBAR should ask for the physician to come to the patient, give a clear description of the location, and ask when the physician will be on site.[21]

  By using SBAR to structure interactions, team members can ensure that relevant, important information is communicated quickly and concisely, thus fostering effective decision making that promotes quality patient care.

Callouts

Callouts involve clearly spoken phrases that indicate a phase of a process. They are used to help establish situational awareness and keep everyone focused in the same direction. This technique is often used in the operating room at two points—the start of a procedure and the closing. Surgical teams also may use the callout technique at other times, such as to say the sponge count is correct or the patient is coming off bypass. Further examples of callouts include the following[9]:

- "We're closing."
- "I'm going to need x-ray in about 20 minutes."
- "We'll be done in 30 minutes."
- "We're bleeding more than I like—we may need to open—we'll decide within 5 minutes."

When using the callout technique, participants should speak clearly and loudly so all team members can hear.

Closed Communication Loops

A closed communication loop helps improve the reliability of communication by having the person receiving the communication restate what the sender has said to confirm understanding. One specific type of closed-loop communication is repeat-back. This technique involves the following four steps:

1. The "sender" concisely states information to the "receiver."
2. The receiver repeats back what he or she heard.
3. The sender acknowledges that the repeat-back was correct or makes a correction.
4. The process continues until a shared understanding is verified. Within this model, responding to a message with an "OK" or an "uh-huh" is not sufficient to close the communication loop. The message must be explicitly restated and acknowledged.

This type of communication can be helpful during surgery and other invasive procedures to confirm sponge count, verify any patient allergies, or confirm the correct site, procedure, and patient during the Universal Protocol. For example, the circulating nurse can state, "The patient is allergic to penicillin," and the anesthesiologist can close the communication loop by repeating back, "I understand that the patient is allergic to penicillin."

Closed-loop communication is particularly helpful during times when communication must be reliable and effective. It can help smooth the communication process and ensure that no critical information is lost. If team members practice this type of communication during routine circumstances, then they will be well prepared to use it during acute instances when time pressure and urgency play a role.[23]

Critical Language

During a stressful situation, such as within a complex surgical procedure, not everyone will immediately think of the most appropriate way to attract a colleague's attention and communicate information effectively. This is particularly true if the person needing to get people's attention is hesitant to speak up due to hierarchy issues, his or her cultural background, or a fear of negative consequences for speaking up.

Often providers, such as physicians, may not be aware of a situation, and indirect language may not be strong enough to signal a problem. For this reason, it can be helpful to empower team members with critical language.[5] When spoken, critical language indicates to other team members that work should cease and all attention be focused on the speaker.[9] Such language may include a neutral phrase such as, "I need a little clarity." When this request is made, all providers know that what is meant is, "We need to take a minute and make sure we are doing the right thing." Teams that respond to critical language know there is a concern that needs to be immediately addressed, and all work should cease until that situation is resolved.

Following is an example of the use of critical language and how it can prevent an error in the operating room:

> A surgical team is preparing to perform orthopedic surgery on a 45-year-old runner. Although the surgeon has verified the medical record, she is distracted and tired—this is her third knee surgery of the day, and there have been other issues with this patient that have diverted her attention. As she prepares to operate on the knee, a nurse in the room notices the surgeon's scalpel hovering over the incorrect knee. The nurse is concerned about bringing up an issue to the hospital's most prominent orthopedic surgeon, but the hospital's provision of critical language helps give the nurse the courage to speak up. The nurse clears her throat and says, "Excuse me, doctor, but I need some clarity about the knee on which you are going to operate." The physician, along with everyone else in the room, knows that this is a cue to stop, brief about the situation, and ensure that everyone is comfortable. As she stops, the surgeon realizes her error and moves to the correct knee. The team performs a quick verification of the correct patient, site, and side and proceeds with the operation. The surgeon thanks the nurse for requesting clarification.

Each organization must determine its own critical language that takes into account the culture of the organization. Different phrases may work better in different organizations. When determining appropriate critical language, organizations should keep in mind that such language should be neutral, help staff members focus on doing the right thing, and foster a situation in which no one feels like his or her competence or expertise is being questioned. It is important to stress that seeking clarification is not a challenge to an individual's expertise, it is a justifiable action that is meant to protect patients, who are at their most vulnerable in the surgical setting.[24]

Red Rules

Red Rules, which were first used in the nuclear power industry, are nonnegotiable rules that, except in rare, urgent situations, should always be followed.[25] Red Rules can be designed for many other fields as well. For example, a Red Rule in construction is "Always wear a hard hat on the job site." A Red Rule in transportation safety is "Always have children wear seat belts when riding in a car." Red Rules in surgery are "Always conduct a time-out to verify the correct patient, procedure, and site before surgery," and "If there is any indication we are missing something, never leave the operating room without an x-ray."

Establishing Red Rules is important because it communicates to everyone involved in a process how important that process is and how the organization values the performance of that process. Establishing and enforcing Red Rules can help ensure that the proper care is given 100% of the time and thus can improve patient safety.

To be effective in the surgical setting, Red Rules must be agreed on by everyone in the organization, from the board of directors down to the frontline surgical staff. The rules must be developed collaboratively and enforced consistently. There should be no ambiguity about the rule and its necessity. Everyone who works in the surgical setting should know that complying with the rule is not a judgment call but rather an absolute, nonnegotiable requirement. If an individual, such as a surgeon or physician, ignores a Red Rule, there should be immediate, observable consequences. There is no excuse for doing something that is consciously unsafe.

An organization should have only one or two Red Rules in the surgical area, so that it is clear that these rules are inviolate and must be followed 100% of the time. If there are too many Red Rules, then the importance of each Red Rule is lessened, and compliance with each Red Rule will decrease.

Another key aspect to the success of Red Rules is education. Everyone involved in the process to which a Red Rule applies must be educated in a variety of ways on what the Red Rule is, why it is important, and what the consequences will be if the rule is not followed.

Checklists

One of the most useful structured communication tools is one that can be found not only in the health care arena but in multiple industries and even in everyday life. This tool can build on the knowledge and experience of people involved in a process while making up for their inevitable human inadequacies, such as poor memory, the propensity to be distracted, and the tendency to skip critical steps in a process when stressed out or in a hurry.[3] What is this tool?

The checklist.

According to Dr. Atul Gawande, an international patient safety expert, "Checklists remind us of the minimum necessary steps and make them explicit. They not only offer the possibility of verification but also instill a kind of discipline of higher performance."[3]

Some health care providers are skeptical about the idea of using checklists in the surgical environment. Their perception is that a checklist minimizes their expertise, questions their ability to respond to difficult situations, and promotes "cookbook" medicine, not the craft or art of medicine.

However, many industries that have just as specialized and highly trained professionals as medicine use checklists with great success. Remember the rocket science example from the beginning of the chapter? Aerospace engineers use a variety of checklists to ensure that they perform key steps before, during, and after sending a rocket into space.

Checklists also can foster communication. Consider US Airways Flight 1549, which took off from La Guardia Airport in New York City on January 15, 2009. The captain and first officer completed a variety of preflight checklists before takeoff and had quickly briefed about the flight. A few minutes after takeoff, the plane struck a large flock of Canada geese, lost both engines, and was forced to land in the icy Hudson River. Although Captain Chesley B. "Sully" Sullenberger was in charge of the flight, he did not rely solely on his 20,000 hours of flight experience to navigate and land the plane safely. He turned to the emergency checklist and worked collaboratively with the rest of the flight crew to assess the problem, identify options, guide the plane in a controlled glide into the water, and evacuate passengers safely.[26] The checklists used during this emergency not only helped ensure that no critical steps in the preflight preparations were missed but also fostered interactive communication and problem solving between the captain, first officer, and other members of the flight crew.

If designed appropriately, checklists can ensure that individuals with a variety of expertise and perspectives engage in critical conversations during key points of a process, such as at the beginning of a surgical procedure, when patient conditions change, and before closing up the patient. They ensure that the main components of a process are not overlooked and also create the opportunity for people to talk, coordinate, and manage the nuances of unpredictability in a situation.[3]

Despite some health care providers' reticence to use them, checklists in the surgical setting have been shown to work. For example, Dr. Pronovost reported that one year after Johns Hopkins Hospital implemented a checklist in its surgical intensive care unit, infection rates had dropped nearly to zero, saving eight patients' lives and $2 million.[4]

At Kaiser Permanente in Southern California, researchers tested the use of a checklist in the operating room for 3,500 operations. During that time, staff's average rating of the teamwork climate improved, employee satisfaction increased, the rate of operating room nursing turnover dropped, and the checklist appeared to catch numerous errors, including one instance in which a dose of potentially lethal medication was about to be administered to a patient.[27]

Similar to Kaiser's work, the World Health Organization (WHO) released a 19-step surgical checklist that has also shown improvement in communication and safety within the organizations that have implemented it.[3] (*See* Chapter 6 for more information on the WHO Surgical Safety Checklist.)

Despite their success in some situations, not all checklists are valuable. For example, those that are vague, too long, difficult to use, and impractical may actually cause more harm than good. However, those that are precise, efficient, practical, relevant, and developed by the individuals involved in a process can be quite effective. Checklists must balance a variety of virtues: freedom and discipline, craft and protocol, specialized ability and group collaboration.[3] Other features of effective checklists include the following[3]:

- Has a specific "pause point" or moment where it is logical for the checklist to be used, such as just prior to incision.
- Is brief and easy to complete. After about 60 to 90 seconds, a checklist becomes onerous and may even yield work-arounds and shortcutting.
- Involves simple, straightforward terminology. Wording on a checklist should be simple, exact, and able to fit on one page.
- Is tested for applicability and usefulness. Before use in the field, checklists must be tested in the environment in which they will be used to ensure that they are realistic, helpful, and practical.

Individuals using the checklist should receive training on how to complete the checklist and the importance of completing it. Using the checklist should not be optional but a mandatory part of performing a procedure.[3] Depending on the organization, completing a surgical checklist may become a Red Rule for the surgical setting.

Comprehensive Training in Communication and Teamwork

Effective teamwork and communication skills are not necessarily something a person is born with. Such skills can and should be taught, practiced, and reinforced until they become second nature and a critical part of how an individual operates. Teamwork and communication skills have not traditionally been included in the curriculum of medical and nursing schools. And so the responsibility for such education falls on the health care organization.

Training can mold a group into a unified entity that can face problems, identify issues, and work together to achieve better care for the patient. Engaging in formal, evidence-based team training educates health care providers to recognize potential error and provides the skills and practices to trap, manage, and/or mitigate error and impact.[28]

Studies have shown that communication and teamwork training can improve communication among health care professionals. One study in the United Kingdom showed that a communication skills training intervention using behavioral, cognitive, and affective components not only increased potentially beneficial and more effective patient interviewing styles but also altered physician attitudes and beliefs, thus increasing the likelihood that such skills would be used in a clinical setting.[29] Another study in the United States showed that medical team training using crew resource management principles—a team training approach from aviation—improved communication in the operating room.[30]

Communication and team training should address the value of a team approach to care, how to function as a team, and how to effectively communicate with other team members and patients. Although there are many ways to provide communication and team training, one of the best ways is to bring providers—nurses, surgeons, anesthesiologists, and other specialists—together in multidisciplinary sessions.[5] Specific content for these sessions will vary depending on the organization, but the following are some important aspects to consider including in a communication and team training session:

- *Stories that make points "real."* At the beginning of the training session, to help draw in providers, it may be helpful to use a story to engage their participation and make the topic more relevant.
- *The need for teamwork and communication.* Showing this need can involve providing statistics on how organizations that foster teamwork and communication have better patient outcomes and staff and patient satisfaction than those that do not. Participants should see the direct link between poor communication and error rates, specifically to errors that lead to sentinel events.
- *The nature of team behaviors.* Asking groups to function as teams is not sufficient to change behavior. Training must show participants what team behaviors are. Effective teams exhibit the following behaviors and characteristics:
  — Defined, measurable goals
  — A clear division of labor and well-defined roles
  — Effective leadership and facilitation
  — Effective systems that support team communication and interaction, such as structured communication techniques and strategies to ensure two-way, comprehensive, respectful communication
  — Planned and standardized processes
  — Trust and respect among team members
  — Collaborative problem solving and decision making
  — A preoccupation with safety
  — Trained and oriented team members
- *How to use structured communication techniques.* Many kinds of techniques can be used to help health care providers communicate clearly and effectively. Briefings, SBAR, critical language, and checklists are all examples of structured communication techniques. However, these techniques probably will not come naturally to most providers, and organizations must take the time to train providers on the benefits of such techniques and how to use them in real-world situations. Training should include role playing and simulations so providers can practice using techniques in a safe environment before incorporating them into surgical settings.
- *The importance of nonverbal communication.* Although the spoken word is important, it is not the only way in which messages are conveyed. Tone, eye gaze, stance, facial expression, and hand gestures can communicate their own messages, which may or may not be in sync with the words that are being said. Nonverbal cues can be powerful. For example, if an anesthesia resident asks the attending physician a question, and the physician rolls his eyes before answering, the physician communicates that the resident's question is either not important or not a good question. When educating team members

about communication, organizations should pay special attention to nonverbal communication. In other words, teams must learn that *how* they communicate is just as important as *what* they say.

- *How to resolve conflicts.* Whenever two or more people interact, there is potential for conflict. When power differences, time constraints, and changing patient conditions are added, conflict is even more likely. Health care providers should understand how to resolve conflicts in the operating room, so they can quickly move forward and not derail safe patient care. Training efforts should provide strategies for resolving conflict, including using specific phrases that de-escalate negative situations.

TIP Assign Specific Roles

To be effective, a team must have a structure in which every member of the team has specific tasks and responsibilities. Teams are more likely to function more effectively when there is a clear structure with specific roles.[31] Unclear and ad hoc team structures can lead to confusion, duplication of work, and frustration, which can limit the team's ability to function in rapidly changing, complex, high-stress procedures. Leaders are instrumental in defining team structures and reinforcing the need for specific responsibility designation.

Although providing written and oral education can be helpful in teamwork and communication training, the most beneficial way to provide such training involves giving participants an opportunity to practice their new skills. Role playing and scenarios can help and encourage providers to try out new communication and team behaviors in a controlled setting. Organizations could develop their own scenarios and use mock operating rooms to simulate and train.

Teamwork and communication training should specifically include drills in which team members practice for emergency scenarios to ensure that teamwork behaviors and communication strategies continue during high-stress, emergency situations.

To be successful, teamwork and communication training sessions should have *all* members of the care team present, including physicians. Organizations that are serious about enhancing teamwork and communication make it mandatory for everyone to attend. In organizations where physicians are employees, making teamwork and communication training sessions mandatory is fairly straightforward. Organizations with licensed independent practitioners may have more of a challenge, but creative approaches can help solicit physician participation. For example, one organization offered a stipend for every physician who practices in the hospital to attend communication and team training. Another hospital tied participation in teamwork training to the credentialing process and made it a requirement for physicians to attend.[5]

Although involving physicians in communication and team training can be challenging, if organizations do not involve them, then all the teamwork training in the world will not enhance the dynamics of the care team and improve safety. Licensed independent practitioner involvement is key to the success of any communication training and the subsequent realization of enhanced teamwork.

Measuring Team Performance and Communication Can Help Identify Success

A critical aspect of communication and team training is measuring whether such training is effective at changing team behaviors and improving communication. Careful observations of team characteristics—such as the use of structured communication techniques, respectful discourse, and interactive questioning—can help quantify team performance and highlight areas of improvement.

To effectively observe surgical team performance, organizations must have a systematic process in which trained observers measure performance using standardized definitions. When designing such a process, organizations should keep the following points in mind[32]:

- **How many observations should be done? How frequently?** This will depend on the number of teams an organization is observing and the amount of data necessary.

- **When should observations take place?** It is helpful to assess team performance both before and after communication and team training. Observation efforts before training can highlight differences between team members' perception of their behavior and reality. It can reveal areas of risk and opportunities for improvement. By sharing these differences with team members during communication and team training programs, organizations can clearly illustrate the current picture and where the team needs to improve, which in turn can encourage buy-in and participation in communication and team training as well as awareness of the work that needs to be done. Assessing team performance after communication and team training helps measure the effect of training on the behaviors and efforts of the team. Observing after training can also help identify where posttraining efforts should focus. For example, teams may be conducting briefings and time-outs but few debriefings, in which case this important team behavior can be made a topic for further discussion by the surgical team.
- **What should be observed?** Observers are able to characterize environmental threats; specific team behaviors, such as briefings, read-backs, callouts, time-outs, and SBAR; specific team relationships and attitudes, such as respect and situational awareness; and leadership characteristics, such as motivating the team, seeking input, and resolving conflict. Organizations can observe any or all of these; however, observing too many concepts at one time will generate poor data.
- **How should observation criteria be defined?** How specifically an organization can define and describe what observers should look at makes an impact on how accurate their observations will be. Organizations should make sure items are clearly defined to prevent confusion and problems with consistency.
- **How should observers observe?** One effective way to observe behaviors is to have observers stand in the surgical area and note the performance of team behaviors. They can look for whether the behavior occurs at the required or expected time and give each behavior a grade depending on how well the behavior was performed. To help measure team performance, one organization created a measurement tool for use by a third-party observer in the operating room. For each communication failure observed, the observer used a checklist of options to identify the type of communication failure and any immediate consequences that arose. In addition, the observer recorded the time of the event and documented any relevant observations related to the context of the event.[33]
- **Who will conduct the observations?** The simplest answer to this question is either internal experts or outsiders. Internal experts—those individuals who work in the environment every day—will be more sensitive to the nuances of teamwork and communication behaviors but will be less objective. Consequently, organizations may opt, instead, to bring observers in from outside. Although outside observers are more objective, they will be less sensitive, missing some of the issues and interactions that are more subtle. To overcome the liabilities of both internal experts and others, organizations may choose to use both types of observers, which can help ensure that any observations are accurate. Circulating registered nurses may be the most practical observers. Validate their capability of assessing periodically by using a trainer independent of the operating room team.
- **How will observations be scored?** Defining a consistent scoring system is critical to ensure that observers rate performance reliably. Observers appear to do well when asked to characterize behaviors on a 5-point scale of unacceptable, poor, adequate, good, and excellent.
- **How will observers be trained?** Effective, comprehensive, consistent training is the key to achieving success with this data collection method. Observers must be trained in groups so that they can learn from each other. When possible, use actual operating rooms to train and other areas such as bedside to most realistically practice.
- **How will interrater reliability be assured?** In the context of observation, interrater reliability is the level of agreement between two observers. When interrater reliability is good, two observers will grade team performance in a similar way. When it is not

good, observers will vary in their grading, skewing the results and degrading measurement accuracy. It is important to both establish and maintain interrater reliability. Good training is the key to establishing such reliability.

- **How will the data that were collected during observation be analyzed?** Turning completed observation sheets into simply understandable reports is essential. The two characteristics that can be documented for each observed metric are frequency and quality.

After data have been collected and analyzed, it is critical to share information with the teams being observed. This information sharing prompts buy-in for improvement efforts and encourages consistent participation in communication and teamwork initiatives. Organizations can communicate results by graphically displaying teamwork scores, so team members and organization leaders quickly see the effectiveness of team performance and areas in need of improvement. This visual aid can provide motivation for improvement and reinforce desired behaviors.

Addressing Disruptive Behavior

The majority of health care professionals enter their chosen discipline for altruistic reasons and have a strong interest in caring for and helping other human beings. Most of these individuals carry out their duties in a manner consistent with this idealism and maintain high levels of professionalism. However, the operating room setting inherently attracts people with intense personalities who may be prone to conflict.[34] Unfortunately, intimidating and disruptive behavior in health care organizations does occur,[35] and these behaviors create an unhealthy or even hostile work environment; one that acts as antithesis to team behavior and collaboration.

Disruptive behavior that intimidates or interferes with communication, team performance, or safe care should be addressed promptly, consistently, and appropriately. Such behavior can include, but is not limited to, verbal abuse, harassment, condescending or berating behavior, lack of respect, or physical abuse. Sometimes behavior may not seem overtly disruptive and yet it can quickly derail patient care, such as when an individual deliberately fails to adhere to organizational policies without adequate evidence to support the alternative chosen.[36]

Several surveys have found that most care providers have experienced or witnessed some form of disruptive behavior at some point in their career.[35] These experiences are not limited to one gender and can occur during interactions in and across disciplines.[37, 38] Although most formal research centers on intimidating and disruptive behaviors among physicians and nurses, there is evidence that these behaviors occur among other health care professionals as well, such as pharmacists, therapists, support staff, and administrators.[37]

Consequences of Disruptive Behavior

There are both immediate and long-term consequences to disruptive behavior. After an incident, there is an immediate effect on the individual at the receiving end of the behavior. He or she may feel embarrassed, stressed, frustrated, or angry, and these negative feelings may affect his or her performance in providing patient care. In the long term, disruptive behavior may impede communication, relationship building, and information transfer, which in turn can compromise safety and quality and ultimately contribute to patient mortality.[39] On a personal level, such behavior can lead to job stress, depression, coronary heart disease, absenteeism, and turnover of both the people on the receiving end of disruptive behaviors and those who witness those behaviors.[34] In addition, colleagues may avoid disruptive individuals or may hesitate to speak up for help, for clarification, or to make suggestions about patient care when working with these individuals. Realistically, disruptive behavior can also deflect attention away from the patient, thereby impairing clinical judgment and performance.[40]

Disruptive behavior can not only impede patient safety but also negatively affect patient and family satisfaction. If a patient finds the health care provider's attitude disrespectful or condescending, the patient may choose not to follow treatment or may refuse to return for follow-up visits, which in turn will affect the clinical outcome. In addition, patient dissatisfaction with physician communication has been shown to drive unnecessary litigation. Several studies have linked patient complaints about unprofessional, disruptive behaviors to physicians with high malpractice risk.[41–43]

Disruptive behavior also can impede staff recruitment and retention. If an individual feels disrespected by his or her colleagues, he or she will have less job satisfaction and may seek employment elsewhere. Such staff turnover can affect the quality and safety of the care provided by the organization as well as its financial viability.

Causes of Disruptive Behavior in Health Care

Many of the systemic factors that lead to disruptive behavior stem from the unique health care cultural environment. These systemic factors include increased productivity demands, cost containment requirements, embedded hierarchies, and fear of or stress from litigation. These pressures can be further exacerbated by changes to or differences in the authority, autonomy, empowerment, and roles or values of professionals on the health care team, as well as by the continual flux of daily changes in shifts, rotations, and interdepartmental support staff. This dynamic creates challenges for interprofessional communication and for the development of trust among team members.

Intimidating and disruptive behaviors often go unreported and therefore are not addressed. There are a variety of reasons for this lack of reporting, including fear of retaliation, the stigma associated with "blowing the whistle" or "tattling" on a colleague, and a general reluctance to confront an intimidator. In addition, staff in institutions often perceive that powerful, revenue-generating providers are allowed to behave inappropriately due to the perceived consequences of confronting them.[37]

Tips for Addressing Disruptive Behavior

Although it is easy to say that organizations must deal with disruptive behavior, there is no simple or short-term approach. The following are some specific actions organizations can take to address the topic:

- *Acknowledge the problem.* As with any issue, before an organization addresses disruptive behavior, it must acknowledge that the behavior exists. To help with this effort, organizations should look at their cultural assessment survey, discussed earlier in this chapter, and search for clues about staff perceptions on teamwork and communication and the presence of disruptive behavior.
- *Establish comprehensive policies that address disruptive behavior head-on.* These policies should establish what appropriate behavior in the workforce is and outline a policy of zero tolerance for disruptive behavior, including the organizational response employees can expect if disruptive behavior occurs. In addition, policies should also protect those who report or cooperate in the investigation of intimidating, disruptive, and other unprofessional behavior. Nonretaliation clauses should be included in all policy statements that deal with this issue.
- *Create a surveillance system for disruptive events.* The only way to know if disruptive behavior is occurring in an organization is to collect data on that behavior. A surveillance system allows organizations to gather information on disruptive incidents, analyze that information, and implement an effective response. Such a surveillance system may include disruptive event reports, complaints, or results from satisfaction surveys. As part of the surveillance system, organizations must assign responsibility for receiving event reports and addressing them.
- *Take a proactive approach to education.* The best way to address disruptive behavior is to prevent it in the first place. Organization leaders as well as employees should be trained on the consequences of disruptive behavior and the impact on patients. Proactive skills-based education and training on topics such as teamwork, relationship building, conflict resolution, diversity, and linguistics can help prevent negative situations and further emphasize an organization's commitment to professional behavior.
- *Develop a multifaceted approach to responding to an incident.* A disruptive episode may be a onetime anomaly or the signal of a more significant pattern. Because not all disruptive events are alike, it is important to have varying levels of response and to match the level of intervention with the significance of the event. In some cases, when a disruptive event occurs, simply making an individual aware that he or she was disruptive is enough to address the problem. Taking a process-oriented, nonadverserial, logical approach to this conversation can be helpful.[34] For repeat offenders, organizations may want to consider

requiring training on conflict resolution, anger management classes, and even counseling.

Some organizations choose to define appropriate actions for responding to disruptive behavior in the code of conduct. A *code of conduct* is a document that outlines the core values of an organization and defines what behavior is expected and what behavior is not tolerated. It offers a way to hold people accountable to certain criteria, and everyone in the organization should be familiar with the code, agree to abide by it, and know the consequences of not following it.

Although the human resources department may be the driving force in creating a code of conduct, it is important to gain input from physicians, nurses, and other organization staff about the content. Not only does doing so provide varied perspectives on the issue, but by gathering feedback from multiple disciplines, the organization ensures that no single group can claim the code is irrelevant or not applicable to it.

The code of conduct should be the same for all employees, licensed independent practitioners, patients, families, volunteers, and vendors. Anyone who steps into the health care organization should be expected to comply with the code of conduct. Medical and nursing staff leadership must formally enforce the code and incorporate it into medical staff and organization bylaws and policy.[36]

TIP Build Awareness of the Code of Conduct

To ensure that licensed independent practitioners are aware of the code, organizations may want to have them read through, agree to abide by, and sign off on the code as a requirement for credentialing and privileging.

Consistency Is the Key

The most critical element in effectively addressing disruptive behavior is consistency. All members of the surgical team—from the surgeon, to the nurse, to the housekeeping professional in charge of cleaning the operating room—must know that they will be held accountable for negative behavior and that such behavior will not be tolerated. One of the reasons that both physicians and health care organizations view disruptive behavior policies as ineffective is that such policies are rarely enforced.[37] Commitment to a disruptive behavior program means that senior leadership cannot make any exceptions to the policy, not even if a disruptive individual is a major figure in the organization. For example, if the individual happens to be a surgical specialist, such as a neurosurgeon, who brings in big money for the organization, leaders still must hold that individual accountable for his or her actions.

To ensure consistency, an organization's approach to disruptive behavior must be endorsed by senior leadership and the board and consistently applied to all health care providers and nonclinical staff. The program must have a strong champion—ideally a clinician—who communicates the message that disruptive behavior is absolutely not tolerated.

Communicating with Patients

Although the majority of this chapter has focused on the importance of communication among surgical staff members, one critical member of the team with which surgeons, anesthesiologists, nurses, and other surgical staff must communicate is the patient. Although the scope of this publication does not allow an in-depth discussion of patient communication and education, it is a critical issue that can influence the success of organizations in achieving safe surgery.

When physicians, nurses, and other staff communicate openly and honestly with patients, it sets the tone for care that is positive, informative, and respectful. Communication is a vital component of patient-centered care. If patients and family members feel involved in their care; if their options, wishes, and feelings are acknowledged and respected; and if any decisions are based on thoughtful collaboration among team members, then patients and families are more likely to be satisfied with the patient's care and treatment. Patients and families can also be more relaxed and positive about the care and treatment they receive, which may help patients recover faster and decrease the length of stay. In addition, patients may understand their symptoms better, feel understood by their physician, have greater confidence in their physician's abilities, and be more trusting of their physician.

A key component of patient communication is providing appropriate and comprehensive education to patients about their surgical procedure. Effective patient education helps promote healthy behavior, address anxiety, support recovery, enhance the ability to cope, and involve the patient in decisions about his or her own care. It transfers knowledge and understanding, can change attitudes or perspectives, can help build skills, and ultimately can change behavior. Studies have shown that patient education helps reduce patient stays and improve outcomes and consequently reduces the overall cost of health care.[44]

Patient and family education is a complex process that goes far beyond handing out a pamphlet, describing a procedure, or playing a DVD. Although those are all perfectly acceptable means of sharing information, they must be a part of a larger process that emphasizes the fact that patients and educators must work together to enhance the patient's chances of improving and maintaining health. Patients may think of a health care organization as a place where they go to passively receive treatment that will make them better, but health care professionals know that the patient plays a significant role in ensuring that these interventions have their intended effect.[44]

As part of any effort to educate patients, organizations must encourage them to speak up about questions, concerns, or problems. This encouragement can empower patients to become more involved in their care and help ensure that any care they receive is safe and appropriate (*see* Sidebar 1-2 below).

Providing effective, appropriate, and adequate education is not always easy. Patients in the unfamiliar and oftentimes frightening setting of a health care organization face many learning challenges. Pain, fatigue, and anxiety

Sidebar 1-2: The Joint Commission's Speak Up™ Campaign

In March 2002, The Joint Commission, together with the Centers for Medicare & Medicaid Services, launched Speak Up, a campaign urging patients to help prevent health care errors by becoming active, involved, and informed participants on the health care team. The ongoing campaign includes brochures, posters, and buttons on a variety of patient safety topics. Speak Up encourages the public to do the following:

Speak up if you have questions or concerns. If you still do not understand, ask again. It is your body and you have a right to know.

Pay attention to the care you get. Always make sure you are getting the right treatments and medicines by the right health care professionals. Do not assume anything.

Educate yourself about your illness. Learn about the medical tests you get and your treatment plan.

Ask a trusted family member or friend to be your advocate (adviser or supporter).

Know what medicines you take and why you take them. Medicine errors are the most common health care mistakes.

Use a hospital, clinic, surgery center, or other type of health care organization that has been carefully checked out. For example, The Joint Commission visits hospitals in the United States to see if they are meeting The Joint Commission's quality standards. Joint Commission International (JCI) visits hospitals in other parts of the world to see if they are meeting JCI standards.

Participate in all decisions about your treatment. You are the center of the health care team.

As part of the Speak Up campaign, The Joint Commission has developed the following patient education materials:

- Help Prevent Errors in Your Care
- Help Avoid Mistakes in Your Surgery
- Information for Living Organ Donors
- Five Things You Can Do to Prevent Infection
- Help Avoid Mistakes with Your Medicines
- What You Should Know About Research Studies
- Planning Your Follow-up Care
- Help Prevent Medical Test Mistakes
- Know Your Rights
- Understanding Your Doctors and Other Caregivers
- What You Should Know About Pain Management
- Prevent Errors in Your Child's Care
- Stay Well and Keep Others Well (a coloring book for children)
- Tips for Your Doctor's Visit

can all impede learning. Some patients may speak another language or be functionally illiterate. Others may be intimidated or overwhelmed by their conditions, believing that there is nothing they can do to get better.

As with other types of communication, health care providers should be trained on how to communicate effectively with patients and provide effective education. Such training may involve role playing and input from patients and families to ensure that providers truly understand the information needs and expectations of their patients.

References

1. Hurlbert S., Garrett J.: Improving operating room safety. *Patient Saf Surg* 3:25, Nov. 20, 2009.
2. Lingard L., et al.: Communication failures in the operating room: An observational classification of recurrent types and effects. *Qual Saf Health Care* 13:330–334, Oct. 2004.
3. Gawande A.: *The Checklist Manifesto: How to Get Things Right.* New York: Metropolitan Books, 2009.
4. Pronovost P., Vohr E.: *Safe Patients, Smart Hospitals: How One Doctor's Checklist Can Help Us Change Health Care from the Inside Out.* New York: Hudson Street Press, 2010.
5. Leonard M., Frankel A., Simmonds T.: Effective teamwork and communication. In Frankel A., et al. (eds.): *The Essential Guide for Patient Safety Officers.* Oak Brook, IL: Joint Commission Resources, 2009, pp. 49–60.
6. Mazzocco K., et al.: Surgical team behaviors and patient outcomes. *Am J Surg* 197:678–685, May 2009.
7. Lingard L., et al.: Evaluation of a preoperative checklist and team briefing among surgeons, nurses, and anesthesiologists to reduce failures in communication. *Arch Surg* 143:12–17, Jan. 2008.
8. Mills P., Neily J., Dunn E.: Teamwork and communication in surgical teams: Implications for patient safety. *J Am Coll Surg* 206:107–112, Jan. 2008.
9. Leonard M., Frankel A., Simmonds T.: *Achieving Safe and Reliable Healthcare: Strategies and Solutions.* Chicago: Health Administration Press, 2004.
10. Schimpff S.: Improving operating room and perioperative safety: Background and specific recommendations. *Surg Innov* 14:127–135, Jun. 2007.
11. Sexton J., Thomas E., Helmreich R.: Error, stress, and teamwork in medicine and aviation: Cross sectional surveys. *BMJ* 320:745–749, Mar. 2000.
12. Sexton J., et al.: Assessing and improving safety culture. In Frankel A., et al. (eds.): *The Essential Guide for Patient Safety Officers.* Oak Brook, IL: Joint Commission Resources, 2009, pp. 11–19.
13. Davies J.: Team communication in the operating room. *Acta Anaesthesiol Scand* 49:898–901, Aug. 2005.
14. Makary M., et al.: Operating room briefings: Working on the same page. *Jt Comm J Qual Patient Saf* 32:351–355, Jun. 2006.
15. Preop briefings gain momentum as a strategy for patient safety. *OR Manager* 23:1, 9, Mar. 2007.
16. Khoshbin A., et al.: Evaluation of preoperative and perioperative operating room briefings at the Hospital for Sick Children. *Can J Surg* 52:309–315, Aug. 2009.
17. Papaspyros S., et al.: Briefing and debriefing in the cardiac operating room: Analysis of impact on theatre team attitude and patient safety. *Interact Cardiovasc Thorac Surg* 10:43–47, Jan. 2010.
18. Nundy S., et al.: Impact of preoperative briefings on operating room delays: A preliminary report. *Arch Surg* 143:1068–1072, Nov. 2008.
19. Haig K., Sutton S., Whittington J.: SBAR: A shared mental model for improving communication between clinicians. *Jt Comm J Qual Patient Saf* 32:167–175, Mar. 2006.
20. Kaiser Permanente of Colorado: *SBAR Technique for Communication: A Situational Briefing Model.* Institute for Healthcare Improvement. http://www.ihi.org/IHI/Topics/PatientSafety/SafetyGeneral/Tools/SBARTechniqueforCommunicationASituationalBriefingModel.htm (accessed Jul. 24, 2010).
21. Doucette J.: View from the cockpit: What the airline industry can teach us about patient safety. *Nursing* 36:50–53, Nov. 2006.
22. Pope B., Rodzen L., Spross G.: Raising the SBAR: How better communication improves patient outcomes. *Nursing* 38:41–43, Mar. 2008.
23. Mound T., Brown J.: Closing the communication loop: Using readback/hearback to support patient safety. *Jt Comm J Qual Saf* 30:460–464, Aug. 2004.
24. Hendrickson T.: Verbal medication orders in the OR. *AORN J* 86:626–629, Oct. 2007.
25. Yates G., et al.: Sentara Norfolk General Hospital: Accelerating improvement by focusing on building a culture of safety. *Jt Comm J Qual Saf* 30:534–542, Oct. 2004.
26. Phillips M.: Sully, Flight 1549 crew receive keys to New York City. *The Middle Seat Terminal*, blog, *Wall Street Journal*, Feb. 9, 2009. http://blogs.wsj.com/middleseat/2009/02/09/sully-sullenberger-keys-to-city/ (accessed Jul. 24, 2010).
27. "Preflight checklist" builds safety culture, reduces nurse turnover. *OR Manager* 19:1, 8–10, Dec. 2003.
28. Agency for Healthcare Research and Quality: *TeamSTEPPS: Strategies and Tools to Enhance Performance and Patient Safety.* 2006. http://www.psnet.ahrq.gov/resource.aspx?resourceID=4574 (accessed Jul. 29, 2010).
29. Jenkins V., Fallowfield L.: Can communication skills training alter physicians' beliefs and behavior in clinics? *J Clin Oncol* 20:765–769, Feb. 2002.
30. Awad S., et al.: Bridging the communication gap in the operating room with medical team training. *Am J Surg* 190:770–774, Nov. 2005.

31. Healy A., Vincent C.: The systems of surgery. *Theoretical Issues in Ergonomics Science* 8:429–443, Sep.–Oct. 2007.
32. Frankel A., Knight A.: Using direct observation and feedback to monitor team performance. In Frankel A., et al. (eds.): *The Essential Guide for Patient Safety Officers.* Oak Brook, IL: Joint Commission Resources, 2009, pp. 61–68.
33. Lingard L., et al.: A theory-based instrument to evaluate team communication in the operating room: Balancing measurement authenticity and reliability. *Qual Saf Health Care* 15:422–426, Dec. 2006.
34. Retzlaff K.: Does your facility have an alpha hotel rule? *AORN Management,* Mar. 2010. http://www.aorn.org/News/Managers/March2010Issue/ALPHA (accessed Jul. 24, 2010).
35. The Joint Commission: Behaviors that undermine a culture of safety. *Sentinel Event Alert* 40, Jul. 9, 2008.
36. Porto G., Lauve R.: Disruptive clinician behavior: A persistent threat to patient safety. *Patient Safety & Quality Healthcare* 3:16–24, Jul.–Aug. 2006.
37. Rosenstein A., O'Daniel M.: Disruptive behavior and clinical outcomes: Perceptions of nurses and physicians. *Am J Nurs* 105:54–64, Jan. 2005.
38. Gerardi D.: The emerging culture of health care: Improving end-of-life care through collaboration and conflict engagement among health care professionals. *Ohio State Journal on Dispute Resolution* 23:105–142, 2007.
39. Rosenstein A., O'Daniel M.: A survey of the impact of disruptive behaviors and communication defects on patient safety. *Jt Comm J Qual Patient Saf* 34:464–471, Aug. 2008.
40. Leape L., Fromson J.: Problem doctors: Is there a system-level solution? *Ann Intern Med* 144:107–115, Jan. 17, 2006.
41. Hickson G., et al.: Patient complaints and malpractice risk. *JAMA* 287:2951–2957, Jun. 12, 2002.
42. Hickson G., et al.: Patient complaints and malpractice risk in a regional healthcare center. *South Med J* 100:791–796, Aug. 2007.
43. Stelfox H., et al.: The relation of patient satisfaction with complaints against physicians and malpractice lawsuits. *Am J Med* 118:1126–1133, Oct. 2005.
44. Gaynor S., Patyk M.: Putting the pieces in place: The patient education puzzle. *J Nurs Care Qual* 12:64–68, Feb. 1998.

Chapter 2

Hand Hygiene

The importance of cleaning one's hands is something almost everyone has grown up knowing. Ever since the advent of soap, mothers and fathers around the world have directed their children to wash their hands—before meals, after playing outside, when hands are dirty, and in countless other situations. And yet, somewhere between childhood and adulthood, people (even health care providers) seem to forget—or at the very least dismiss the importance of—this critical lesson.

> **Note:** The key improvement concepts introduced in this chapter pertain to all aspects of a surgical or other invasive procedure—that is, they may be applied before, during, and after the procedure.

Both in and out of the health care setting, unclean hands are the main culprit in the spread of infection. For patients in a health care organization, unclean hands can be particularly problematic because compromised immune systems, comorbid conditions, and the close interaction with infected persons, providers, and surfaces make their risk of developing an infection even greater than that of the average person.

Health care–associated infections—those infections developed as a result of a visit to a health care organization—are a significant cause of morbidity and mortality among patients worldwide. In the United States alone, for example, such infections affect nearly two million hospital patients annually and are responsible for approximately 100,000 deaths each year.[1] The World Health Organization estimates that between 5% and 12% of all patients in developed countries—including those seeking treatment in ambulatory care settings—acquire a health care–associated infection, and the number of critically ill patients in developing countries who acquire such an infection is at least twice as high as in the United States.[2] Although it is not known specifically how many of these infections are caused by poor hand hygiene, studies have shown that by improving hand hygiene, the rate of infection goes down.[3] Because of the significant role unclean hands play in the spread of infection, clean hands—those thoroughly washed with soap and water, sanitized with an alcohol-based hand rub, or scrubbed according to protocol before a procedure—can help limit the spread of infection. In fact, effective hand hygiene has long been considered one of the most important infection control measures for preventing health care–associated infections.

And yet, despite the importance of hand hygiene, health care providers across the spectrum do not clean their hands as often as they should. Studies have shown that regular hand washing is done less than 50% of the time it should be.[4,5] This statistic is disconcerting because hand hygiene plays such an important role in reducing infection transmission.

In the surgical setting, hand hygiene is particularly important. Think about how many processes within the surgical continuum rely on health care providers' hands—not only the surgeon's hands that make the incision and perform the surgery but also the hands of the receptionist or clerk greeting the patient, the residents assisting with surgery, the nurses taking vital signs and handling instruments, the anesthesiologists administering medications, the patient transfer professionals moving the patient, and others. In the past, hand antisepsis in the operating environment has been held up as the epitome of how consistent and standardized hand hygiene processes can reduce infections. Yet some organizations have found that compliance issues still exist in the surgical suite. For example, surgical staff may not scrub for as long as they should, may avoid aspects of the hand antisepsis process, or may skip hand hygiene altogether. One study showed that a significant portion of the surgical staff members who used the toilet in the changing room of the operating room failed to wash their hands afterward.[6]

Why Is Hand Hygiene So Difficult?

Although it may be easy to blame poor hand hygiene rates solely on providers, the issue is more complicated than that. In fact, there are many reasons why health care providers do not clean their hands. For example, the environment of care can present many barriers to hand hygiene. Often, poor design of facilities inhibits proper hand hygiene techniques, including the lack of easy access to or usability of sinks, alcohol-based hand rub dispensers, gloves, and waste receptacles.[7] This lack of "user friendliness" can act as a deterrent to hand hygiene.

A lack of support for proper hand hygiene and accountability for poor hand hygiene can also present barriers to the process. In organizations with high hand hygiene compliance rates, leadership has established and continually supports a culture that requires and expects proper hand hygiene at every opportunity. In such a culture, it is unacceptable or uncomfortable for providers *not* to clean their hands appropriately.

Lack of education is also a factor in low compliance rates. Although most providers theoretically understand the importance of hand hygiene, they may not grasp the true importance of this task in preserving their patients' safety as well as their own. For example, providers sometimes think the use of gloves eliminates the need for hand hygiene or that a quick rinse under warm water should be sufficient.

Finally, the nature of health care itself can present a barrier. Multiple priorities and distractions along with time pressures can cause providers to forget to clean their hands or, if they do remember, to shorten the process in the interest of time. In some cases, the environment does not make it easy for a provider to practice hand hygiene. Consider a nurse whose hands are full of medications and other supplies. When this individual needs to wash his hands, he has to find a place to put the items in his hands while he cleans them. If a patient is in desperate need for the supplies the nurse is holding, he may decide to skip hand washing. "After all," he thinks, "what are the chances of me passing an infection to this patient this one time? My hands look pretty clean." The patient should not be exposed to this risk. (*See* Sidebar 2-1 on page 27.)

Hand Hygiene Guidelines and Standards

Both the U.S. Centers for Disease Control and Prevention (U.S. CDC) and the World Health Organization (WHO) have guidelines that address proper hand hygiene in the health care setting. The Joint Commission requires organizations to comply with either of these sets of regulations. Joint Commission International requires organizations to adopt hand hygiene guidelines from an authoritative source and considers both the U.S. CDC and the WHO guidelines internationally acceptable. Following is a brief overview of the two sets of guidelines.

U.S. CDC Hand Hygiene Guidelines

The U.S. CDC defines hand hygiene as both handwashing, with either plain or antiseptic-containing soap and water, and the use of alcohol-based products (gels, rinses, and foams) that do not require the use of water.[8] The U.S. CDC guidelines are designed to improve hand hygiene practices of health care providers and reduce the transmission of pathogenic microorganisms to patients, residents, and personnel in health care settings.[3] The current U.S. CDC hand hygiene guidelines were published in 2002 and can be found at http://www.cdc.gov/mmwr/preview/mmwrhtml/rr5116a1.htm. The guidelines address the following topics:

- *When to decontaminate hands.* This includes before patient contact, before putting on gloves, before invasive procedures, and after contact with patients (*see* Sidebar 2-2 on page 28 for a more complete listing.)
- *Whether to use soap and water or an alcohol-based hand rub.* The guidelines require staff to use soap and water to wash hands when they are visibly dirty, contaminated with proteinaceous material, or visibly soiled with blood or other body fluids. If hands are not visibly soiled, health care providers may use an alcohol-based hand rub or soap and water for routine hand decontamination.

Sidebar 2-1: Joint Commission Center for Transforming Healthcare Addresses Hand Hygiene

The Joint Commission Center for Transforming Healthcare aims to solve health care's most critical safety and quality problems by working with leading health care organizations in the United States to use a proven, systematic approach to analyze specific breakdowns in patient care and discover their underlying causes to develop targeted solutions that solve these complex problems. There is no one-size-fits-all solution to every problem. The solution will depend on the cause. As causes differ from site to site—or even from unit to unit—solutions or practices that may have worked for one organization may not be so successful in another setting.

In December 2008, the Center began work on its first improvement project: addressing failures in hand hygiene. The Hand Hygiene Project focuses on improving and sustaining hand hygiene compliance. Hand hygiene solutions were developed by eight leading, highly respected organizations, which have a great deal of experience using Robust Process Improvement™ tools such as Lean Six Sigma and change management processes (*see* Sidebar 2-5 on page 35). Their initial work demonstrated that random observation was an unreliable measure of hand hygiene compliance. When baseline performance was measured using a common measurement system, the aggregate baseline compliance rate among the eight participating hospitals was less than 50%. It is believed that the high compliance rate that many organizations report is probably not accurate. After establishing a measurement baseline, the Center identified and analyzed the underlying causes of hand hygiene failure. Solutions that target these specific causes of failure are currently being rigorously tested. Following that, the Center provided a package of proven interventions customized to address those underlying root causes. The next phase of this project is for the Center to create easy-to-use assessment tools that will guide organizations in measuring the scope of the problem and assessing root causes specific to the particular organization's facilities and staff. A poster summarizing the recommendations of the organizations to date can be found in Figure 2-3 on page 33. More information on the work of the Center can be found at http://www.centerfortransforminghealthcare.org/projects/display.aspx?projectid=5.

Source: Joint Commission Center for Transforming Healthcare.

- *Hand hygiene technique.* Technique includes the process for effectively decontaminating hands when using either an alcohol-based hand rub or soap and water (*see* Sidebar 2-3 on page 28.)
- *Surgical hand antisepsis.* The guidelines offer a specific process that should be used to clean hands before surgery.
- *Selection of specific types of hand hygiene agents.* The guidelines offer suggestions on selecting appropriate cleaning agents for use in the organization.
- *Skin care.* The guidelines offer tips to protect the skin of health care providers, including providing lotions or creams.
- *Other aspects of hand hygiene,* including prohibiting artificial nails and the use of gloves, are discussed. (*See* Sidebar 2-4 on page 28.)
- *Education.* The guidelines recommend that organizations provide education and monitor adherence with hand hygiene practices.
- *Administrative measures.* The guidelines recommend that organizations develop a hand hygiene program and offer readily accessible alcohol-based hand rubs.

Although the guidelines outline the appropriate use of alcohol-based hand rubs and require health care organizations to make such hand rubs available for use by health care providers, individuals are not required to use hand rubs. However, if a health care provider chooses not to use an alcohol-based hand rub, then he or she must use soap and water instead. Towelettes are not a substitute for hand washing with an antimicrobial soap or alcohol-based hand rub because towelettes are not as effective at reducing bacterial counts on the hands of health care workers.[3]

World Health Organization Guidelines on Hand Hygiene

In 2005 the World Health Organization developed the *Guidelines on Hand Hygiene in Health Care*[9] to provide organizations with scientific evidence and recommendations to

Sidebar 2-2: Indications for Handwashing and Hand Antisepsis

The U.S. Centers for Disease Control and Prevention recommends the following indications for hand hygiene:

- When hands are visibly dirty or contaminated with proteinaceous material or are visibly soiled with blood or other body fluids
- Before having direct contact with patients
- Before donning sterile gloves when inserting a central intravascular catheter
- Before inserting indwelling urinary catheters, peripheral vascular catheters, or other invasive devices that do not require a surgical procedure
- After contact with a patient's intact skin (for example, when taking a pulse or blood pressure or when lifting a patient)
- After contact with body fluids or excretions, mucous membranes, nonintact skin, and wound dressings if hands are not visibly soiled
- If moving from a contaminated-body site to a clean-body site during patient care
- After contact with inanimate objects (including medical equipment) in the immediate vicinity of the patient
- After removing gloves
- Before eating and after using a rest room
- If exposure to *Bacillus anthracis* is suspected or proven

Source: Boyce J., Pittet D.: Guideline for hand hygiene in health-care settings. *MMWR Recomm Rep* 51(RR16), Oct. 25, 2002. http://www.cdc.gov/mmwr/preview/mmwrhtml/rr5116a1.htm (accessed Aug. 21, 2010).

Sidebar 2-3: Methods for Hand Hygiene

A critical aspect of hand hygiene is the method an individual uses to decontaminate and clean his or her hands. There are two types of hand hygiene: hand washing and hand antisepsis. According to the U.S. Centers for Disease Control and Prevention (U.S. CDC), effective hand washing involves the following steps:

1. Wet hands. Water temperature should be comfortable, but not too hot as it may lead to dermatitis.
2. Apply soap, and rub hands vigorously together for at least 15 seconds, covering all surfaces of hands and fingers. Wetting the hands prior to applying soap reduces skin irritation.
3. Rinse hands with water.
4. Dry thoroughly with a disposable towel.
5. Turn off the faucet using the towel.

The steps for hand antisepsis with an alcohol-based hand rub are as follows:

1. Apply a palmful of product.
2. Rub hands vigorously, covering all surfaces of hands and fingers.
3. Rub until hands are dry. The entire procedure should take approximately 20 to 30 seconds.

A simple Web tutorial about hand hygiene practice is available on the U.S. CDC's Web site at http://www.cdc.gov/handhygiene/training/interactiveEducation.

Sidebar 2-4: Refrain from Wearing Jewelry and Artificial Nails

According to the U.S. Centers for Disease Control and Prevention (U.S. CDC), it is not advisable for health care providers to wear jewelry—such as rings, bracelets, and watches—because of the increased likelihood that bacteria will congregate under and around these items, and these items may not be effectively cleaned by hand washing. Sometimes, these items can even impede the proper hand hygiene of the rest of the hand. One recent study showed an increased frequency of potential pathogens among nurses who wore at least one ring, and even higher frequency among nurses who wore more than one ring.

In addition to jewelry, artificial nails can harbor bacteria and also damage natural nails, resulting in fungal or bacterial infections of the nail bed. Health care providers should not wear artificial nails and should keep their natural nails shorter than one-quarter inch or one centimeter in length.

Sources: Alp E., Voss A.: Hand hygiene among laboratory workers. *Infect Control and Hosp Epidemiol* 27:978–980, Sep. 2006.

Winslow E., Jacobson A.: Can a fashion statement harm the patient? Long and artificial nails may cause nosocomial infections. *Am J Nurs* 100:63–65, Sep. 2000.

reduce infections by improving hand hygiene. Just like the U.S. CDC hand hygiene guidelines, the WHO hand hygiene guidelines provide a comprehensive review of scientific data on hand hygiene rationale and practices in health care settings. This extensive review is designed to support training materials and help plan implementation strategies. The WHO *Guidelines for Hand Hygiene in Health Care* can be accessed online at http://whqlibdoc.who.int/publications/2009/9789241597906_eng.pdf.

Just as the U.S. CDC has recommendations on how specifically to clean hands with soap and water and an alcohol-based hand rub, the WHO also provides recommendations. Figures 2-1 and 2-2 on pages 30 and 31 illustrate the WHO recommendations for cleaning hands.

Although both the U.S. CDC and WHO guidelines address the topic of hand hygiene and are similar in many ways, there are a few differences. Since the WHO guidelines were released after the U.S. CDC guidelines, they expand on many areas of the U.S. CDC guidelines and provide more clarity in certain situations. While the U.S. CDC guidelines are U.S.-based and designed for health care providers, the WHO guidelines are applicable to the global community, the public, patients, and small, local health care settings, as well as larger health care systems.

Surgical Hand Preparation

The U.S. CDC, the WHO, and the Association of periOperative Registered Nurses (AORN) have specific guidelines for cleaning hands before surgery. These involve not only cleaning the hands with soap and water if they are visibly soiled but also removing dirt and debris from underneath fingernails and sanitizing the hands. These guidelines include the following steps[9,10]:

- Remove rings, watches, and bracelets before beginning surgical preparation.
- Don a surgical mask. If other individuals are at the scrub sink, the mask should be worn in the presence of hand-scrubbing activity.
- Wash hands and forearms with soap and running water immediately before beginning the surgical scrub.
- Remove dirt and debris from underneath fingernails using a nail cleaner, preferably a disposable one. Ideally this should be done under running water. To facilitate this process, fingernails must be kept short and clean at all times.
- Rinse hands and forearms under running water.
- Dry hands and forearms with a disposable paper towel.
- Use antimicrobial soap or an alcohol-based hand rub to sanitize the hands, according to the manufacturer's instructions. In the United States, a surgical hand antiseptic that is compliant with U.S. Food and Drug Administration (FDA) regulations should be used for all surgical hand antisepsis.
- If quality of water is not assured in the operating room, perform surgical hand antisepsis using an alcohol-based hand rub before donning sterile gloves.
- When performing surgical hand antisepsis using alcohol-based surgical hand preparation, dispense the manufacturer-recommended amount of product and rub thoroughly until completely dry.
- When performing surgical hand antisepsis using an antimicrobial soap, apply the antimicrobial agent to wet hands and forearms using a soft, abrasive sponge. Scrub hands and forearms for the length of time recommended by the manufacturer, typically from 2 to 5 minutes. Long scrub times, such as 10 minutes or more, are not necessary. During scrubbing, visualize each finger, hand, and arm as having four sides. Wash all sides effectively, keeping the hand elevated. This process should be done for both hands. Rinse hands and arms in one direction from fingertips to elbows. Avoid splashing surgical attire and turn off water when it is not directly in use. Discard used sponges or other cleaning material in appropriate containers. Once cleaned, hold hands higher than elbows and away from surgical attire. Dry hands and arms with a sterile towel.
- Do not combine surgical hand scrub and surgical hand rub with alcohol-based products one after another.
- After cleaning hands with either an antimicrobial soap or an alcohol-based hand rub, don a sterile surgical gown and gloves.

According to AORN, a surgical hand scrub should occur before donning sterile gloves for surgical or other invasive procedures. To facilitate surgical scrubbing, organizations should consider locating a multiuser sink near the entrance to the procedure room.[10]

Figure 2-1: WHO Handwashing Technique with Soap and Water

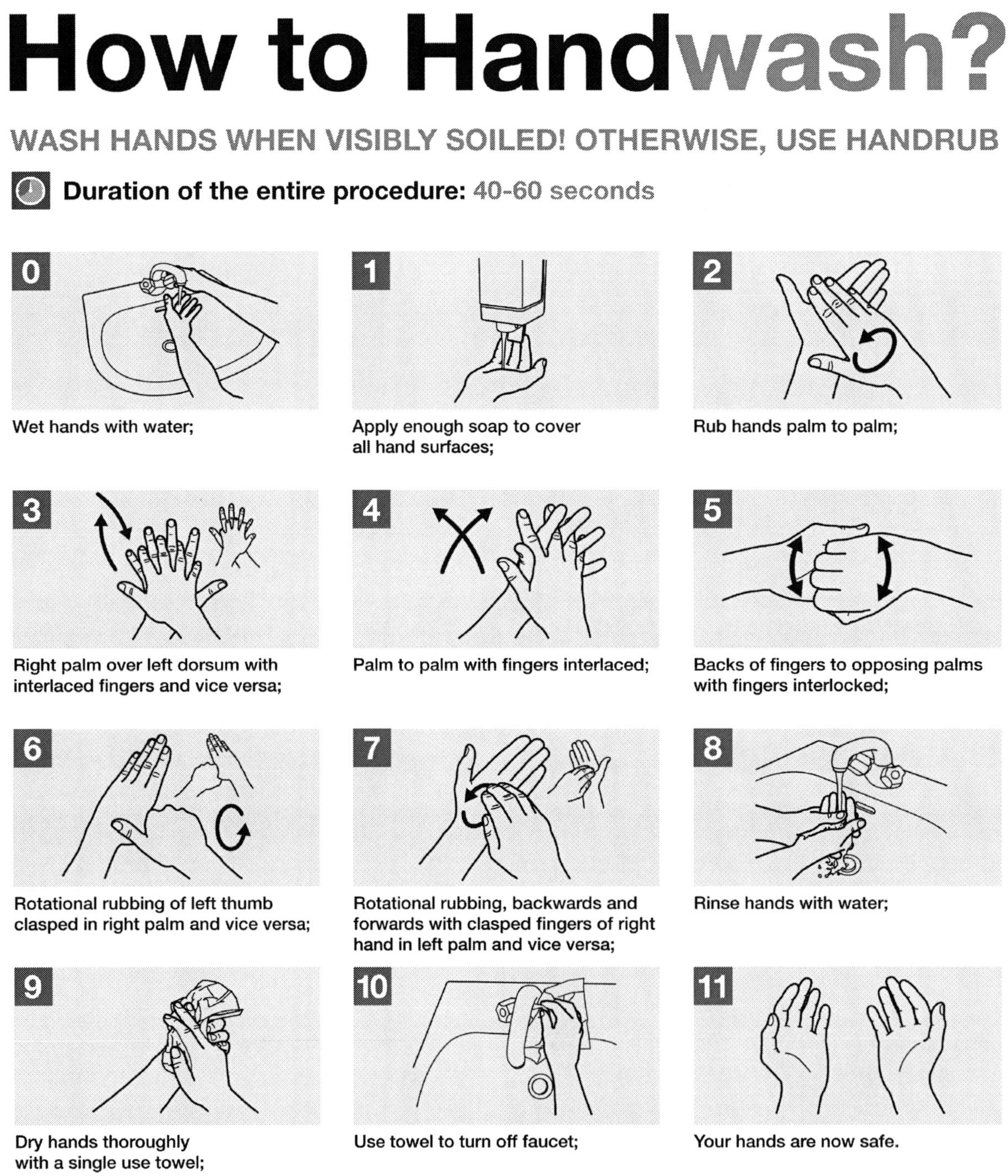

This figure shows the World Health Organization technique for cleaning hands with soap and water.

Source: World Health Organization, http://www.who.int/gpsc/5may/How_To_HandWash_Poster.pdf. © World Health Organization 2009. Used with permission.

Figure 2-2: WHO Hand Hygiene Technique with Alcohol-Based Formulation

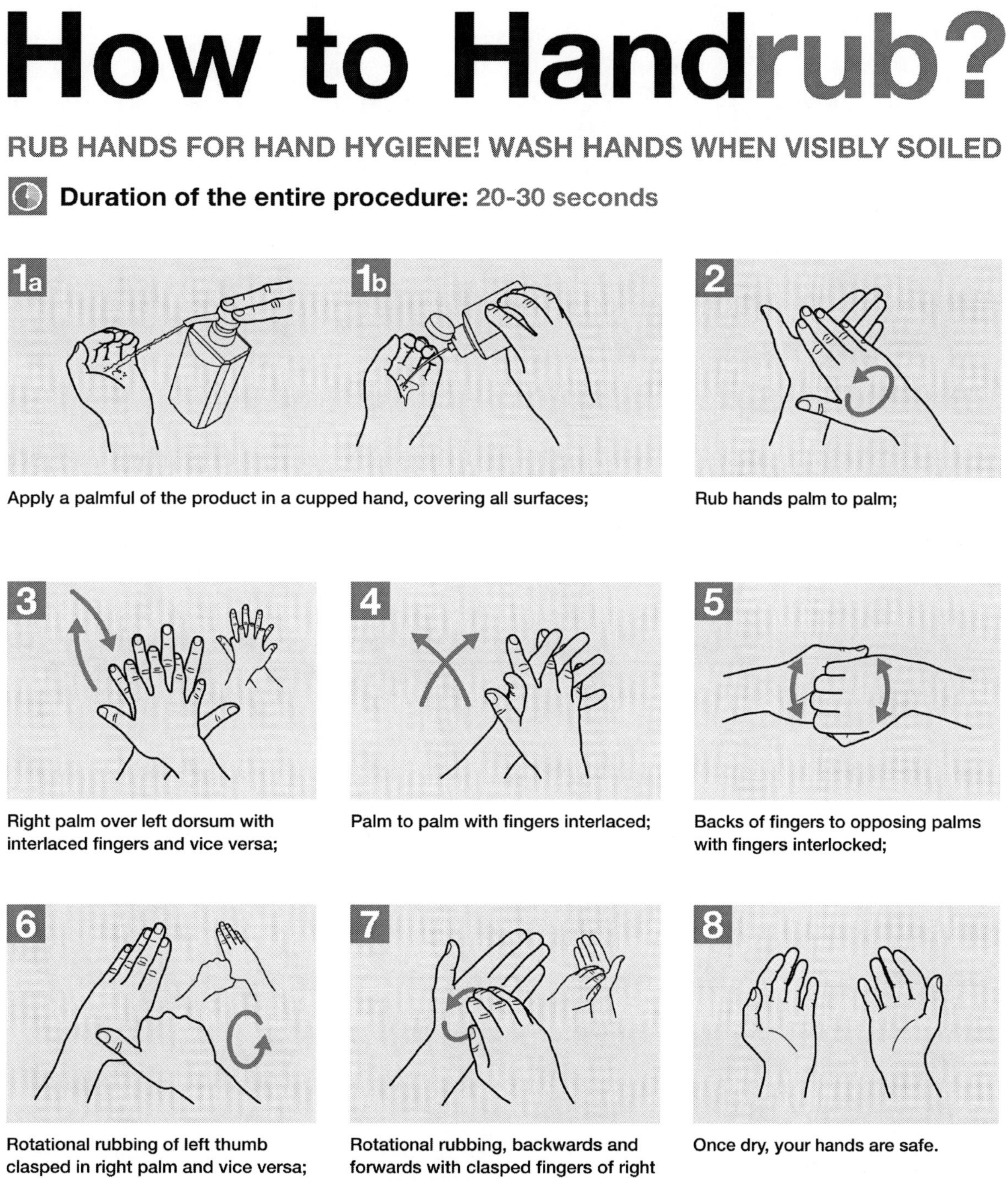

This figure illustrates the World Health Organization technique for hand sanitation with an alcohol-based hand rub.

Source: World Health Organization, http://www.who.int/gpsc/5may/How_To_HandRub_Poster.pdf. © World Health Organization 2009. Used with permission.

Organizations should also standardize the procedure for surgical scrubbing as well as the antiseptic products used throughout the organization. The following section takes a brief look at some points to consider when selecting an antiseptic product.

Antiseptic Product Options

Antiseptics used for surgical hand antisepsis should be fast acting and long lasting. They should remove dead skin, reduce microorganisms on intact skin, provide persistent protection against bacteria, and be effective against a wide variety of microorganisms. In addition, they should be nonirritating to prevent skin reactions.

There are many different options available for antiseptic hand hygiene, including povidone iodine solutions, chlorhexidine, and antimicrobial soap. The different options have different benefits. For example, using antimicrobial soap is a more traditional approach to hand hygiene, and the staff may be familiar and comfortable with its use. The downside is that such soap may dry out skin and cause irritation that can lead to bacteria growth and infection. In addition, antisepsis using antimicrobial soap can take more time, use more water, use more laundry or disposable towels, and cost more money.

Alcohol has bacteria-fighting properties that help eliminate bacteria faster than soap can. In addition, bacteria take longer to reappear on skin after the use of an alcohol-based rub. A 60% to 95% alcohol preparation provides the most rapid and effective reduction of microorganisms on the skin. However, this type of product does not have a long-lasting effect. Using an alcohol-based hand rub that has an antimicrobial agent in it, such as chlorhexidine, may be preferable for some organizations,[11] as this combination has been shown to be effective in reducing bacteria and does not cause negative skin reactions.[12] It also has more residual effect than alcohol alone.[3]

Yet another study showed that preoperative hand decontamination with povidone iodine constituted sufficient cleaning, provided it was conducted for at least three minutes. This brushless method was effective for shorter surgeries.[13]

Which products an organization selects will depend a lot on the organization, provider preferences, budget considerations, and other factors. For hospitals, for example, it is recommended that the hospital form a multidisciplinary committee to give input on the selection process. Different disciplines will have different perspectives on the issue, and everyone's opinion should be considered.

In addition to gathering opinions, U.S. organizations should research the Food and Drug Administration (FDA) guidelines governing antiseptic agents, including alcohol-based hand rubs, and ensure that any possible candidates comply with these guidelines. Organizations outside the United States should consult their own country's or locality's regulations.

Providers should also read labels and understand the technical information associated with a potential product. One way to do this is to talk with the sales representative from the company selling the product and obtain the written technical information supporting the product's claims.

Solutions for Improving Hand Hygiene

The key to improving hand hygiene in the health care setting, and specifically within the surgical suite, is to take what is known about the importance of hand hygiene and how to effectively clean hands, and translate that knowledge into action. This cannot be done with a simple slogan or snazzy campaign. Similarly, merely demanding that health care providers try harder is not the answer. Comprehensive, systematic, and sustainable change is the only solution.[4] The following sections discuss some components of a systematic approach to improving hand hygiene.

Study the Problem Before Acting

Improving hand hygiene in a health care organization is fundamentally a performance improvement activity. Like any such activity, implementing initiatives without understanding whether those initiatives will adequately address the issue under consideration is an exercise in frustration and possibly a waste of time. Using a systematic process to examine the issue can help identify specific risk points and areas of improvement and target initiatives so they have the most success. One such systematic process is Robust Process Improvement™ (RPI). This is The Joint Commission's methodology for improving processes, which seeks to continuously increase the quality and efficiency of products and services. The successful adoption of RPI techniques can produce substantial improvements in the quality of processes, such as hand hygiene.

The Center for Transforming Healthcare is working with leading health care organizations throughout the United States to use RPI to improve hand hygiene compliance and reduce the chance of infection. Figure 2-3 below and Figure 2-4 on page 34 show the preliminary information generated from this work. Many of the solutions discussed within these posters are further addressed in subsequent sections of this chapter.

A well-known systematic improvement methodology used in an RPI-driven initiative is called Lean Six Sigma (*see* Sidebar 2-5 on page 35). Although using a formalized improvement strategy is not required when engaging in hand hygiene improvement, a methodology such as Lean Six Sigma can help organizations focus their implementation efforts and ensure an efficient, effective, and appropriate process that results in improved safety and quality.

Figure 2-3: Identifying Causes, Targeting Solutions

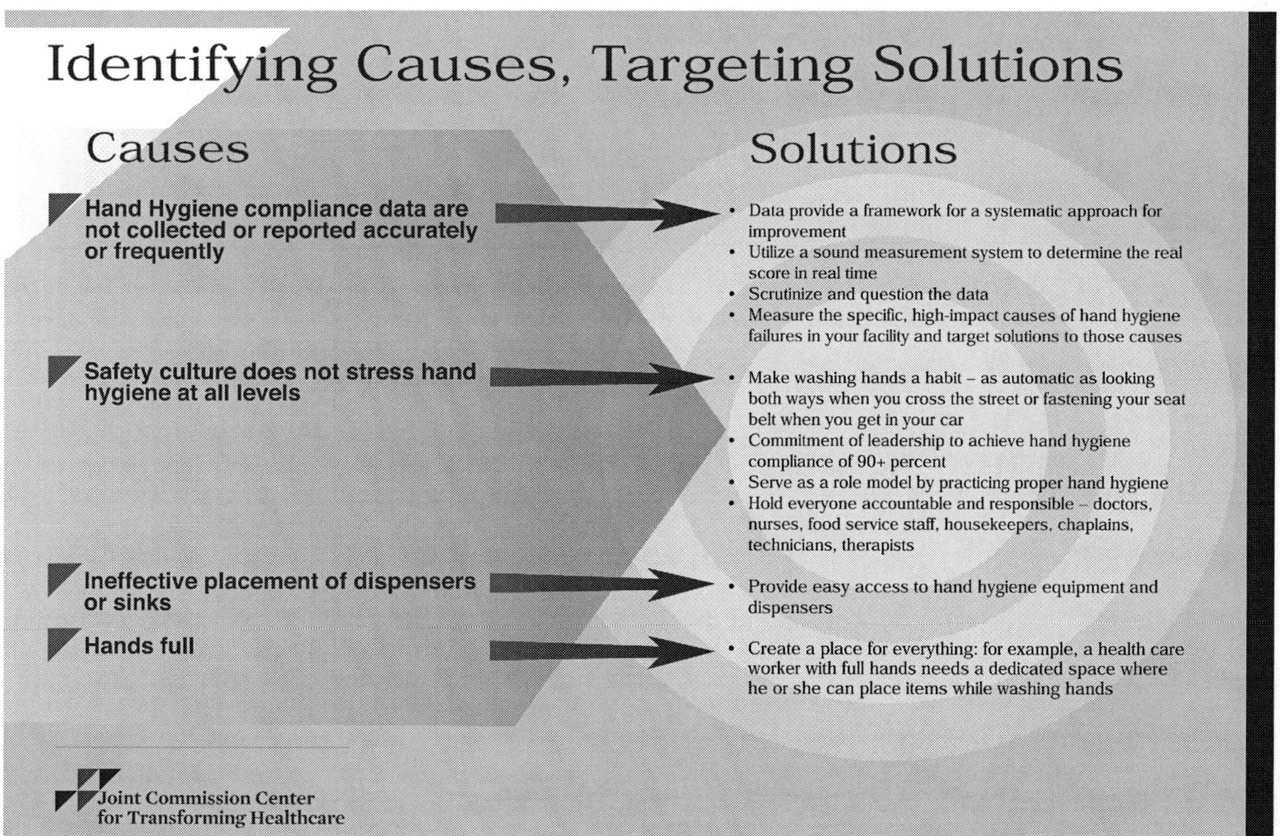

This poster summarizes possible causes of poor hand hygiene compliance and offers solutions to help address the issue.

Source: Joint Commission Center for Transforming Healthcare; http://www.centerfortransforminghealthcare.org/UserFiles/file/hand_hygiene_storyboard.pdf.

Figure 2-4: Effective Hygiene is in Our HANDS

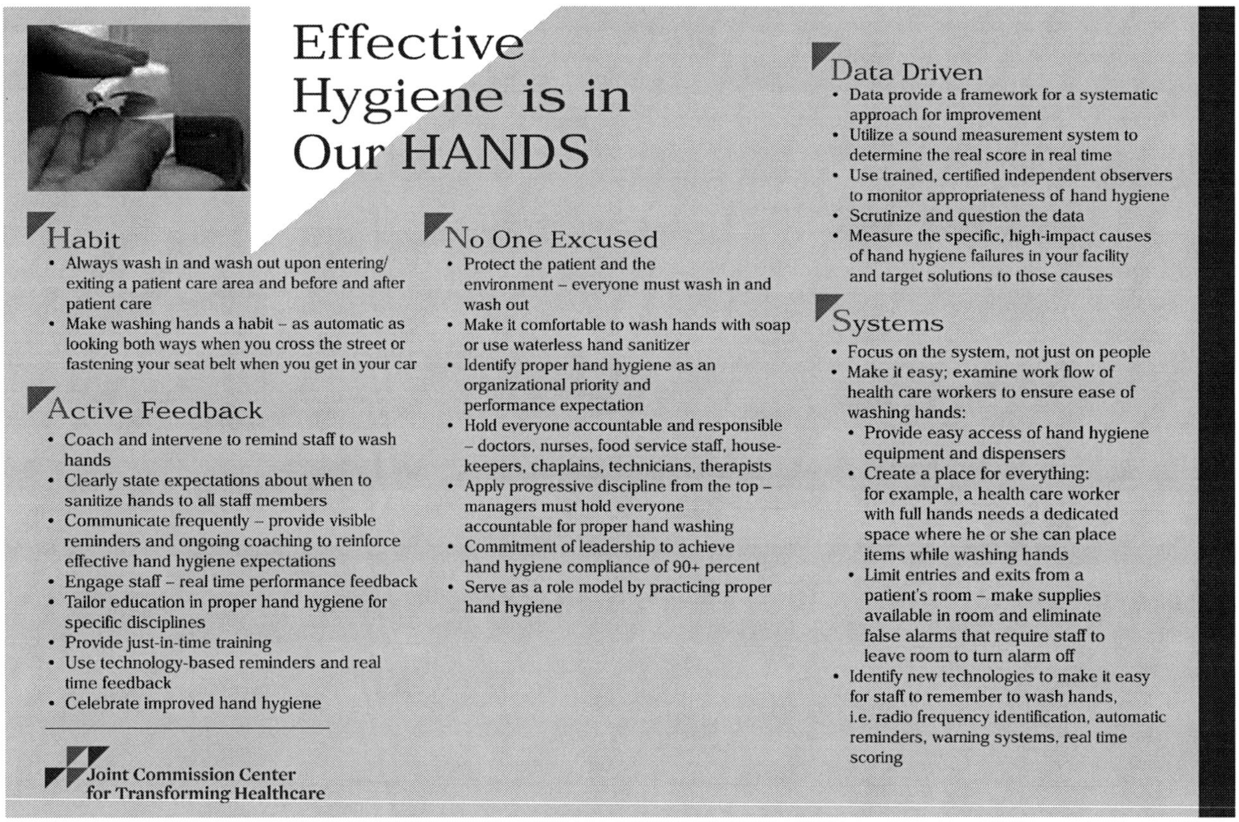

This poster summarizes the recommendations of the Joint Commission Center for Transforming Healthcare's hand hygiene project.

Source: Joint Commission Center for Transforming Healthcare; http://www.centerfortransforminghealthcare.org/UserFiles/file/hand_hygiene_storyboard.pdf.

Systematic improvement methodologies, such as Lean Six Sigma, are strengthened and reinforced by change management methods. Change management increases an initiative's likelihood of success. Using a systematic improvement methodology can also help create and reinforce a culture of safety, in which organizations are transparent about issues and actively work to proactively reduce risk.

Many Joint Commission–accredited hospitals use the plan-do-study-act (PDSA) process as a performance improvement method (*see* Sidebar 2-6 on page 36).

Address Environmental Barriers to Effective Hand Hygiene

According to the Joint Commission Center for Transforming Healthcare and other organizations focused on improving hand hygiene compliance, there are several environmental barriers to good hand hygiene in health care organizations, including the location of hand-washing stations and the availability of hand-washing supplies. Addressing these environmental barriers can help improve hand hygiene compliance across an organization and specifically within the surgical suite.

Sidebar 2-5: Lean Six Sigma

Sometimes it is difficult for an organization to select the most appropriate quality improvement and implementation method for its needs. The Joint Commission with its Robust Process Improvement™ (RPI), as well as many health care organizations, deciding that a combination of methods may be the most suitable, have adopted a methodology called Lean Six Sigma to help achieve rapid service improvement and better quality of care. Lean thinking aims for zero waste—that is, elimination of any activity that uses resources but creates no value to the patient. Lean encourages improvement as the outcome of a broad horizontal process directed by an empowered staff at all levels, from management to frontline team members. Six Sigma aims for zero defects, or errors. Six Sigma focuses on high-quality production and depends heavily on statistical data to measure success. *DMAIC* is an acronym for *define, measure, analyze, improve,* and *control.* It is the core of Six Sigma methodology and describes its problem-solving sequence. The DMAIC process is an improvement system for existing processes that do not meet specifications and therefore need modification. DMAIC also guides development of processes. Derivative acronyms used by some organizations include *DMADV—define, measure, analyze, design, verify.*

An additional benefit of Lean Six Sigma is that the methods overlap. Lean's ongoing efforts to eliminate waste contribute to Six Sigma's need to reduce variations. In addition, just as Six Sigma strives for zero defects, Lean, too, tries to prevent errors. The skills of both Lean and Six Sigma are necessary to achieve high reliability. Combining the two methods results in a process improvement methodology that can be more effective than either method alone. For example, Morton Plant Hospital in Clearwater, Florida, used a combination Lean Six Sigma approach to redesigning processes, and it improved patient satisfaction more than 50%, reduced emergency department length of service by 21%, and saved more than $4 million.

Recognizing the complementary nature of the two methodologies, many companies have used Lean and Six Sigma concurrently, utilizing different pieces of both methodologies to address specific improvement problems along a value stream. This practice of combining different tool sets and playing to strengths is sometimes referred to as a *blended approach.* RPI's blended approach includes Lean Six Sigma and change management methods.

Sources:

American Society for Quality: *Lean Six Sigma in Healthcare.* http://www.asq.org/healthcaresixsigma/ (accessed Jul. 20, 2010).

Sunyog M.: Lean Management and Six-Sigma yield big gains in hospital's immediate response laboratory: Quality improvement techniques save more than $400,000. *Clin Leadersh Manag Rev* 18:255–258, Sep.–Oct. 2004.

To be effective in improving hand hygiene, sinks and soap dispensers and/or alcohol-based hand rub dispensers should be easily visible upon entry to the surgical area. Organizations should consider installing additional units in changing rooms and possibly at the entrance to the operating room. The U.S. CDC recommends that organizations also conveniently locate alcohol-based hand rub dispensers at the entrance to each patient room, exam room, treatment room, or similar areas. Dispensers may also be located inside rooms near the door or adjacent to each bed.[14] In addition to patient care areas, health care organizations should consider locating dispensers in other high-traffic areas, in easily visible locations, at nursing stations, and on medication carts, and/or supplying portable individual dispensers.[15]

In addition to conveniently locating hand-washing facilities, it is important to ensure that hand hygiene supplies such as hand sanitizer, soap, waste receptacles, and gloves are always readily available. To ensure adequate supplies, an organization should assign responsibility for changing and restocking alcohol-based hand rub and soap dispensers in the organization. This assignment may go to housekeeping or facilities staff. Whoever is assigned the role should make sure all the dispensers are clean and working properly and should ensure that the correct amount of product is available and dispensers are not empty.

Involve Users in Choosing Products

To ensure the regular use of soap and alcohol-based hand rubs and prevent skin reactions and irritations,

Sidebar 2-6: Plan-Do-Study-Act

Perhaps the most famous quality improvement implementation tool is known as the plan-do-study-act (PDSA) cycle. Based on the scientific method, this well-established process for improvement can help guide the implementation process and ensure that any changes are effective and sustained over time. The PDSA cycle (also called the PDCA cycle, with the word *check* replacing the word *study*) is attributed to Walter Shewhart, a quality improvement pioneer with the United States–based company Bell Laboratories in the 1920s and 1930s. The cycle is also widely associated with W. Edwards Deming, student and later colleague of Shewhart.

The PDSA cycle is explained as follows:

- *Plan* refers to first understanding the process, then proposing an improvement, and finally deciding how an improvement action will be tested and how data will be collected to determine what effect the action has on the process.
- *Do* means to test the improvement by implementing the action on a small scale.
- *Study* involves analyzing the effect of the action being tested.
- *Act* means to fully implement the action or reassess the improvement action taken and perhaps then choose another action.

For example, a hospital that is trying a new alcohol-based hand rub can test the new product on a small scale by working with one unit that is willing to participate in the change process. This unit can implement the following PDSA test:

- Plan: Test staff satisfaction and effectiveness of the new hand rub.
- Do: Use the new hand rub for two weeks across the unit.
- Study: Measure staff satisfaction, product usage, and infection rates in that unit for the week.
- Act: Use information from the initial test to plan further tests or to discontinue plans to use the hand rub.

PDSA cycles are meant to test changes on a small scale to see if they result in improvement. Small-scale tests may involve 1 individual or 10 individuals and should never be looked on as successes or failure, merely more opportunities for learning.

When implementing a complicated process, organizations should plan for more than one PDSA cycle, with each cycle focusing on one aspect of the process. Testing changes in this way can help verify that a change will result in improvement, predict how much improvement can be expected from a change, and minimize resistance upon full implementation.

After testing a change on a small scale, learning from each test, and refining the change through several PDSA cycles, organizations can implement the change on a broader scale—for example, for an entire pilot population or on an entire unit.

Source: Simmonds T., Haraden C., Munch D.: Care process improvement. In Frankel A., et al. (eds.): *The Essential Guide for Patient Safety Officers*, Oak Brook, IL: Joint Commission Resources, 2009, pp. 103–112.

organizations must involve health care providers when choosing appropriate hand hygiene products. Some providers will avoid using alcohol-based hand rubs because these hand rubs can irritate their skin. This concern can be addressed by giving providers information about the emollient properties of alcohol-based hand rubs, by providing hand lotions or creams "to minimize the occurrence of irritant contact dermatitis associated with hand antisepsis or handwashing,"[7] and by involving health care providers in selecting the hand rubs.[5] The organization should also take responsibility for providing alternative products for providers with documented dermatitis.

TIP Let Providers Help Choose

Before deciding which hand hygiene product to use in an organization, it is important to provide nurses, physicians, and other surgical staff with the opportunity to evaluate the various products under consideration. By involving these individuals in testing different hand rubs and choosing the most appropriate one, organizations can make sure that providers are comfortable with the product that is chosen and will actually use it.

Engage Leadership

Without a strong leadership commitment to improving hand hygiene compliance, initiatives to improve compliance—no matter how well designed—are destined to fail. Leadership support is critical in this effort as health care providers will pay attention to what organization leadership says and does. Leaders can show their commitment by setting an ambitious but realistic goal for hand hygiene efforts, such as achieving a hand hygiene compliance rate of more than 90%.[4]

Leaders should also serve as role models by practicing proper hand hygiene in their daily work processes. If leaders do not demonstrate good hand hygiene practices, all the talk about improved hand hygiene becomes merely rhetoric to be ignored.

Leaders should also hold everyone accountable and responsible for proper, regular, and consistent hand hygiene. This includes staff in the operating room as well as physicians, surgeons, and other individuals who work in this setting. To help establish accountability, leaders may want to make compliance part of performance evaluations and competency reviews. This shows all health care providers, including the medical staff, that the organization has made hand hygiene a priority.

Identify Role Models

When targeting improved hand hygiene in the perioperative environment, organizations may want to identify individuals in the physician and nursing community who can help improve hand hygiene compliance. By watching a peer thoroughly wash his or her hands or use a hand rub before or after examining a patient, health care providers can be encouraged to improve their hand hygiene habits and speak up if they see someone else not following hand hygiene protocols. Conversely, watching a peer not clean his or her hands can be detrimental to hand hygiene programs. It has been shown that good hand hygiene compliance is significantly lower in groups in which a ranking member of the group does not perform hand hygiene.[16]

Make Cleaning Hands a Habit

To not only improve hand hygiene compliance but also sustain it, cleaning hands must become a habit for everyone who works in the organization. This habit should be as automatic as looking both ways when crossing the street, fastening a seat belt when getting into a car, or saying "thank you" when receiving a gift. There are several ways to make hand hygiene habitual. For example, organizations should establish hand hygiene as a priority from a provider's first day of employment. This can set the expectation for routine hand hygiene as an automatic part of daily operations. Other ways to establish the hand hygiene habit include the following[4]:

- Clearly state expectations about when to sanitize hands to all providers.
- Coach and intervene to remind providers to clean their hands.
- Communicate frequently; provide visible reminders and ongoing coaching to reinforce effective hand hygiene expectations.
- Make it comfortable to wash hands with soap or use waterless hand sanitizer.
- Create a place for everything: For example, a health care provider with full hands needs a dedicated space where he or she can place items while cleaning hands.
- Identify new technologies to make it easy for providers to remember to clean hands, such as radio frequency identification, automatic reminders, warning systems, and real time scoring. (*See* Sidebar 2-7 on page 38.)
- Create scripts that help health care providers when approaching a peer about hand hygiene compliance. A script may involve such statements as the following:
  - "Thank you for washing your hands. It really makes a difference."
  - "Do you need some hand sanitizer? I have some nearby."

> **TIP Make Hand Hygiene Convenient**
>
> Some organizations give out pocket hand sanitizers to all new employees to reinforce the organization's position on hand hygiene.

Provide Comprehensive Education

One key element to sustaining good hand hygiene in the perioperative setting is comprehensive, targeted education. Without a strong education program, hand hygiene efforts

Sidebar 2-7: Using Technology to Improve Hand Hygiene Compliance

There are many automated and computerized tools on the market that may help organizations improve hand hygiene compliance. Some of these technologies include the following:

- Sensor-activated faucets, soap dispensers, and towel dispensers to prevent having to touch the sink or towel dispenser when performing hand washing
- Automated hand dryers that eliminate the need for paper towels
- Radio frequency systems that monitor the use of soap, water, paper towels, and alcohol-based hand rubs. Sometimes these systems are tied into a reminder system. If the system senses that the toilet was used but the sink or alcohol-based hand rub dispenser was not, a prerecorded voice is broadcast over the loudspeaker to remind a health care provider to wash his or her hands.
- Automated hand-wash stations that ensure the proper amount of soap/sanitizer, water, and time for hand hygiene. Within these systems, a user places his or her hands inside the machine and the system administers a step-by-step, time- and temperature-controlled hand hygiene experience. Water automatically stops when the appropriate amount of time has passed. Some of these systems are equipped with a display that walks users through the wash cycle. Sometimes these stations are equipped with reminders that prompt users to wash their hands.

Source: Pyrek K.: Handwashing and cross contamination. *Infection Control Today,* Mar. 2004. http://www.vpico.com/articlemanager/printerfriendly.aspx?article=60167 (accessed Jul. 12, 2010).

will most likely flounder. Education on hand hygiene can increase awareness of its importance and foster compliance with hand hygiene protocols. It can put the action of hand hygiene in the context of daily work activities and underscore the organization's commitment. Before designing education efforts, it may be helpful to survey health care providers, including members of the medical staff, about their awareness of the importance and proper methods of hand hygiene to help focus education efforts and address areas where knowledge is deficient.

Within education efforts, health care providers should be educated about the importance of cleaning their hands, when to clean their hands, and how to clean their hands. Organizations should provide evidence-based information about hand contamination to help address any misperceptions about hand hygiene, how hand hygiene products affect normal skin physiology, and the link between proper hand hygiene practices and the transmission of infection. Education should also discuss the role of gloves, jewelry, and fingernail length in spreading infection. The idea should be reinforced that each health care provider must take personal responsibility for his or her own hand hygiene. Training efforts should also outline current hand hygiene initiatives in the organization and the level of compliance on specific units.[14] For ambulatory surgery centers, the ASC Quality Collaboration offers a Hand Hygiene Toolkit with a variety of resources for organizations' internal improvement and education efforts. Further information is available at http://www.ascquality.org/advancing_asc_quality.cfm.

Education can take many forms, including posters, newsletter articles, one-on-one education, and presentations at staff meetings. Organizations may want to get creative when designing education programs. For example, some organizations have used screen savers with targeted messages; fluorescent dye-based training methods to demonstrate correct hand hygiene techniques to clinical staff;[15] blood agar plates with bacterial growth from a physician, nurse, or organization leader's hands; and voice messages from senior leadership and physician champions about the importance of hand hygiene.

One effective way to provide education is to do just-in-time training. This kind of training involves having an individual who is an expert in hand hygiene monitor health care providers in their daily environment and provide education in real time. In the surgical setting, it may be helpful to have peers educating peers. For example, a surgeon showing another surgeon how to appropriately clean his or her hands before surgery will be more effective than a nurse educating the surgeon. Similarly, a nurse will be a better choice to educate other nurses.

Measure Compliance with Hand Hygiene

To truly understand how effectively and consistently health care providers perform hand hygiene, organizations must assess compliance with hand hygiene protocols. Although there is no universally accepted standard for measuring compliance with proper hand hygiene practices, the following are two commonly used methods for compliance measurement[5]:

- *Direct observation.* This occurs when an individual covertly or overtly observes health care providers cleaning their hands. Direct observation is recommended by the U.S. CDC and WHO and may be the best way to assess compliance with hand hygiene recommendations. Direct observation reliably assesses behavior, provides detailed information, can pinpoint areas of strength or weakness, and can assess adherence with hand hygiene opportunities and techniques. That said, direct observation can also be time-consuming, resource intensive, and costly. In addition, if direct observation is overt, it may lead to changes in behavior because of the observation, otherwise known as the "Hawthorne Effect"—the tendency of people being observed to behave differently from the way they would behave otherwise.[17] As discussed in Chapter 1, direct observation efforts should be planned and use trained observers. This allows consistency in observations. When designing observation efforts in the surgical setting, organizations may want to post observers in scrub areas to unobtrusively monitor hand hygiene practices, including the methods of hand hygiene, the length of time it takes to perform hand antisepsis, and whether recleaning is done periodically. These observations can help indicate whether chosen interventions are appropriate and if further work is necessary.
- *Self-reporting.* In self-reporting, a health care provider self-reports his or her own level of compliance. Self-reports can take the form of a questionnaire, a survey, interviews, logs, and diaries. Although less costly, time-consuming, and resource intensive than observation, this method is not particularly reliable. Health care providers can forget how often they clean their hands or sometimes exaggerate their hand hygiene adherence, thus presenting an overly positive picture. When using self-assessment tools, organizations may want to verify results using another assessment method. For example, organizations can perform a small number of direct observations to corroborate the findings of the self-assessment.

Regardless of the method of data collection an organization uses, the data should provide a framework for a systematic approach to improvement. Organizations should spend time interpreting the data—scrutinizing and questioning them when things do not make sense. Organizations should also consider measuring the specific, high-impact causes of hand hygiene failures in their facilities and target solutions to those causes.

Organizations that emphasize good hand hygiene as part of an overall emphasis on safety can help improve hand hygiene compliance across the surgical continuum. Organizations should foster a culture in which not only is it important to engage in frequent and thorough hand hygiene and antisepsis, but it is unacceptable not to do so. This requires visible leadership support and involvement, repetition, reminders throughout the workplace, monitoring, and feedback. By committing to improved hand hygiene at all levels of the organization, hand hygiene can become part of the organization's culture.

TIP Free Resource on Hand Hygiene

The Joint Commission has published a monograph entitled "Measuring Hand Hygiene Adherence: Overcoming the Challenges." The monograph is the result of a two-year collaboration with major infection prevention and control leadership organizations in the United States and abroad to identify effective approaches for measuring adherence to hand hygiene guidelines in health care organizations. This monograph can be downloaded from The Joint Commission Web site free of charge at http://www.jointcommission.org/PatientSafety/InfectionControl/hh_monograph.htm.

References

1. Centers for Disease Control and Prevention: *Estimates of Healthcare-Associated Infections.* http://www.cdc.gov/ncidod/dhqp/hai.html (accessed Jul. 24, 2010).
2. World Health Organization: *The Burden of Health Care–Associated Infection Worldwide.* http://www.who.int/gpsc/country_work/burden_hcai/en/index.html (accessed Jul. 24, 2010).
3. Boyce J., Pittet D.: Guideline for hand hygiene in health-care settings: Recommendations of the Healthcare Infection Control Practices Advisory Committee and the HICPAC/SHEA/APIC/IDSA Hand Hygiene Task Force. *MMWR Recomm Rep* 51(RR16), 2002. http://www.cdc.gov/mmwr/preview/mmwrhtml/rr5116a1.htm (accessed Jul. 24, 2010).
4. Joint Commission Center for Transforming Healthcare: *Facts About the Hand Hygiene Project.* http://www.centerfortransforminghealthcare.org/projects/about_hand_hygiene_project.aspx (accessed Jul. 24, 2010).
5. Haas J., Larson E.: Compliance with hand hygiene guidelines: Where are we in 2008? *Am J Nurs* 108:40–44, Aug. 2008.
6. Baird C., Nunn T., Gregori A.: Inadequate standards of hygiene in an operating theatre changing room. *J Hosp Infect* 59:268–269, Mar. 2005.
7. Suresh G., Cahill J.: How "user friendly" is the hospital for practicing hand hygiene? An ergonomic evaluation. *Jt Comm J Qual Patient Saf* 33:171–179, Mar. 2007.
8. Siegel J., et al.: *2007 Guideline for Isolation Precautions: Preventing Transmission of Infectious Agents in Healthcare Settings.* Healthcare Infection Control Practices Advisory Committee, 2007. http://www.cdc.gov/hicpac/2007IP/2007isolationPrecautions.html (accessed Jul. 24, 2010).
9. World Health Organization: *WHO Guidelines on Hand Hygiene in Health Care (Advanced Draft): A Summary: Clean Hands Are Safer Hands.* 2005. http://www.who.int/patientsafety/events/05/HH_en.pdf (accessed Jul. 24, 2010).
10. Association of periOperative Registered Nurses (AORN): *Recommended Practices for Surgical Hand Antisepsis/Hand Scrubs.* In *Perioperative Standards and Recommended Practices.* Denver: AORN, 2010, pp. 79–80.
11. Fry D., Burger T.: Hand hygiene compliance: Step up, reach out. *Nurs Manage* 36(suppl.):12–15, Nov. 2005.
12. Grabsch E., et al.: In-use efficacy of a chlorhexidine in alcohol surgical rub: A comparative study. *ANZ J Surg* 74:769–772, Sep. 2004.
13. Aksoy A., et al.: An investigation of the factors that affect surgical hand disinfection with polyvidone iodine. *J Hosp Infect* 61:15–19, Sep. 2005.
14. Underwood M.: Hand hygiene. In *APIC Text of Infection Control and Epidemiology,* 3rd ed. Washington, DC: Association for Professionals in Infection Control and Epidemiology, 2009, pp. 19-1–19-6.
15. Institute for Healthcare Improvement: *How-to Guide: Improving Hand Hygiene.* Apr. 3, 2006. http://www.ihi.org/IHI/Topics/CriticalCare/IntensiveCare/Tools/HowtoGuideImprovingHandHygiene.htm (accessed Jul. 24, 2010).
16. Lankford M., et al.: Influence of role models and hospital design on hand hygiene of health care workers. *Emerg Infect Dis* 9:217–223, Feb. 2003.
17. Eckmans T., et al.: Compliance with antiseptic hand rub use in intensive care units: The Hawthorne Effect. *Infect Control Hosp Epidemiol* 27:931–934, Sep. 2006.

Chapter 3

Preparing the Operating Room or Procedure Area

In every invasive procedure, from the most complex to the most straightforward, there are three elements that must interact effectively and efficiently to achieve a safe outcome. These three elements are (1) the operating room (OR, also known as the operating theatre or surgical suite) or procedure area; (2) the patient; and (3) the surgical team. This chapter and the following two chapters will examine each of these three elements and discuss how organizations can properly prepare them before the surgery or other invasive procedure begins. This chapter focuses specifically on the operating room or procedure area. Chapter 4 describes the part of presurgical process that focuses directly on the patient, and Chapter 5 discusses preparation of the surgical team.

Getting the operating room or procedure area ready for a procedure involves many activities, including managing the operating room or procedure area schedule, creating the sterile field, setting out the surgical instruments, checking anesthesia equipment, ensuring proper ventilation of the operating environment, and controlling traffic. The following sections take a closer look at these activities. (*Note:* Ensuring that the operating room or procedure area is clean is also important. Because the majority of cleaning activities typically take place following a procedure, the topic of cleaning the operating room or procedure area is addressed in Chapter 9.)

Managing the Operating Room or Procedure Area Schedule

As the patient population of health care organizations around the world continues to age[1] and, simultaneously, developments in surgery continue to advance, the demand for operating room facilities and procedure areas continues to grow.[2] These facilities or areas can incur high costs but reap tremendous revenues for an organization. Because of this, the need to manage the operating rooms and procedure areas within an organization is paramount.

A well-managed operating room or procedure area maximizes utilization while minimizing cancellations and use after regular business hours.[3] An efficient operating room or procedure area schedule allows for both urgent and elective procedures of various types and durations, keeping in mind the needs of both patients and health care providers working in the procedure setting.

If an organization manages its operating room or procedure area well, it can reap many benefits, including the following:

- Improved patient care
- Patient satisfaction
- Provider satisfaction, including that of surgeons, anesthesiologists, and nurses
- Optimized revenue

Conversely, if a schedule for an operating room or procedure area is managed poorly, a patient safety issue can result, as well as patients, physicians, and staff becoming frustrated. In addition, when time in the operating room or procedure area is underutilized, revenues can be lost needlessly.

Managing the schedule should be a team effort. Surgeons, anesthesiologists, OR managers, scheduling staff, individuals responsible for cleaning and disinfecting medical equipment, and organization leadership should all work together to balance the organization resources with the needs of the patient. To this end, organizations may want to form a multidisciplinary team to examine the issue of efficiency in the operating room or procedure area, define the problem (if there is one) in the context of the organization, proactively identify areas of improvement, and use systematic methodologies, such as Lean and Six Sigma, to improve performance.

Although there are a variety of ways to effectively manage the schedule for the operating room or procedure area, the following sections offer some strategies for organizations to consider.

Manage Block Time Effectively

Using block time is a common practice in most organizations. It can be thought of as a type of reservation; surgeons know that on a particular day at a particular time, there will be an operating room or procedure area reserved for their use. Within that time frame, a surgeon can conduct elective or urgent procedures, several short procedures, or one long procedure. Block time can be assigned to a particular surgeon, practice, or specialty, depending on organization policy.[4] If a surgeon, practice, or specialty regularly underutilizes its block time, it could lose that time, just as a person who does not show up for a restaurant reservation can lose that reservation.

How block time is managed in an organization is a very sensitive issue. Patient safety, revenue, and surgeon and staff satisfaction can all be significantly affected by how an organization manages its block time. For example, if an organization designates block time in all of its operating rooms or procedure areas, then there may be difficulty in scheduling urgent cases, which can compromise patient safety. Or, if an organization does not reevaluate the block time of a surgeon who regularly underutilizes it, the organization may not be optimizing its revenues. If surgical staff members spend time waiting for surgeons who do not show up for their block time, then staff dissatisfaction can result.

Following are some strategies organizations should consider when managing block time:

- *Set clear rules.* Surgeons should have a complete understanding of an organization's block time policy and what to expect with regard to that policy. They should understand under what conditions their block time could be bumped and how to constructively resolve any conflicts with block time. Rules must be fair and consistently applied and take into consideration the needs of the patient, the surgeon, and the organization.
- *Consider utilization as one guideline in managing block time.* Typically block time is adjusted based on utilization. If a surgeon does not use his or her block time, he or she loses it. Although utilization is a typical way of managing block time, it is not the only way or even, necessarily, the best way. Utilization does not take into consideration variable costs, reimbursement issues, or patient waiting times. Some experts feel it is questionable whether utilization can even be estimated precisely.[5] While utilization should be one consideration for managing block time, some other variables to consider include staffing allocations, operating room efficiency, medical equipment availability, predictability of work hours, patient delays, and the balancing of overutilized and underutilized time.[5]

TIP Set Modest Expectations

It is unrealistic to think that every surgeon in an organization will use 100% of his or her block time every month. When determining utilization goals, organizations may want to set a more modest expectation, such as an average of 80% utilization over three months.[6]

- *Regularly review block time.* Organizations may want to consider collecting and reviewing data on block time monthly. That is not to say that changes should be made monthly, but monthly data can be reviewed to identify utilization, operating room efficiency, medical equipment availability, staffing allocation, and patient delay patterns that need addressing. Organizations that rarely review and tweak the block time schedule may not be aware of the need to revise that schedule and could face significant challenges when it is necessary to make changes. Conversely, organizations that regularly review, adjust, and manage the block time schedule will not meet as much resistance when changes to the schedule need to be made. Surgeons should know how block time will be reviewed, what the criteria are for reducing or increasing block time, and how frequently changes will be made.

- *Add an urgent room.* Many organizations have found it useful to designate an operating room for urgent care use. This operating room is free from block time and is devoted to unscheduled, urgent, add-on cases. The benefits of this type of room are that it can increase overall efficiency and reduce variability in scheduled surgical flow. Organizations that are regularly bumping other cases for urgent ones should consider this strategy. If an organization has regular gaps in its operating room or procedure area schedules, then such a room may not be necessary. Utilization of an urgent room should never be 100% because that would defeat the purpose of having it available as an urgent room. Although capacity will not be maximized, such a room can streamline the scheduling process and prevent other surgeries from being bumped. In the long run, an urgent room can save surgeons time, increase their productivity, and improve the financial strength of the organization. For example, St. John's Hospital, an 866-bed not-for-profit hospital in Springfield, Massachusetts, designated one of its operating rooms for add-on and urgent cases. This initiative resulted in a 5.1% increase in patient throughput. In addition, there was a 4.5% decrease in blocked rooms for surgical cases. This number is significant because the block time decreased while the throughput time increased, showing that the add-on room provided the flexibility necessary to get patients in and out more quickly.[7]
- *Define release times.* Release times define when the guaranteed availability of a surgeon's block time expires before the day of surgery. These can be different for different specialties. For specialties in which cases are booked far in advance, such as joint replacement or cosmetic procedures, release times may be significantly before the surgery date. Conversely, procedures that are not booked far in advance, such as cardiac procedures, may have release times that fall 24 hours before surgery. Varying release times can help an organization add more flexibility into the OR schedule. For example, release times that occur far in advance of surgery can be used to free up time to add more urgent cases.[6] Regardless of the amount of time rooms will be kept open, organizations should have a specific policy that is consistently enforced.[10]

TIP Define Procedures for an Urgent Room

If an organization chooses to create an urgent room, it must specifically define what types of procedures can be done in that room. Some definitions could include the following[8]:

- *Emergent.* These procedures occur when there is a threat to life or limb, and should be done within 30 minutes.
- *Priority.* These cases should be performed within 30 minutes to 4 hours.
- *Urgent.* These cases should be performed within 4 to 24 hours.
- *Nonurgent.* These cases can be performed after 24 hours.

Cases in the first three categories should be considered for the urgent room.[9] To prevent inconsistency in scheduling, operating room schedulers should be educated on what cases can be performed in an urgent room.

Smooth Out the Elective Surgery Schedule

When looking at an organization's surgical schedule, it is not uncommon to see a large percentage of the elective procedures scheduled for the beginning of the week, with few scheduled for later. Unfortunately, if an organization has an elective surgery schedule that is heavy on some days and light on others, these peaks and valleys in demand for resources can cause significant patient flow problems. By smoothing out the variability in the OR schedule, organizations can reduce capacity stress and improve the overall ability of the organization to deal with the inevitable variability in arrivals.[11]

Some organizations may hesitate to take on the process of smoothing out the elective surgery schedule for fear of reducing surgeons' productivity or satisfaction, causing surgeons to take their business elsewhere, such as the ambulatory surgery center down the road. However, by using data to examine the effects of such a schedule shift, organizations can anticipate the increase in productivity and revenue that such a shift might cause. By sharing these data and testing schedule changes on a small scale, organizations can gain buy-in from surgeons for such a shift. Organizations should actively solicit surgeon feedback and encourage surgeons to be involved in the decision-making process. Doing so helps maintain support for the smoothing effort.[12]

TIP Smooth Out the Discharge Schedule

One way to free up beds for incoming patients needing surgery or another invasive procedure, and thus to prevent backups in the operating room or procedure area, is to spread out discharges throughout the day. In many organizations, physicians batch their discharge work, typically to the afternoon. Therefore, patients are not necessarily being discharged when they are clinically ready but when the physician has time. This practice can keep patients in beds longer than necessary. By encouraging physicians to change their rounding habits to spread out discharges throughout the day, organizations can free up beds earlier, leaving them available for the patients who need them. Even switching rounding habits to visit patients who are being discharged first can free up beds sooner.[13] Without this smoothing of the discharge schedule, a backlog of discharges or releases can cause nurses and other providers to rush, leading to a higher risk for errors and increased patient wait times.

TIP Designate Scheduling Staff

To help with consistency in scheduling for the operating room or procedure area, organizations may want to designate particular scheduling staff to the operating room or procedure area. Doing so can help reduce delays in scheduling, cancellations, and booking errors. In addition, organizations should consider locating the scheduling department for the operating room or procedure area *within* the operating room or procedure area. Such a location can provide schedulers with easy access to key staff and allow for more real-time decisions.[14]

Sequence Urgent Cases

Although smoothing out the schedule for elective procedures can help improve patient flow through the operating room or procedure area, there are times that more than one urgent case arises and a decision must be made as to how to order those cases. There are many ways to prioritize urgent cases, but it can be helpful to choose one consistent and systematic approach. One consideration when prioritizing urgent cases is each patient's medical deadline. This is the time window for the best possible care and is a deadline for when the case needs to be started to avoid an increase in morbidity or mortality.[15] For example, the medical deadline for appendicitis in a 13-year-old who has shown symptoms for 36 hours may be 1 hour, as the risk of a perforated appendix is greater among patients having surgery more than 37 hours after the onset of symptoms.[16]

Another factor to consider when prioritizing urgent cases is the estimated case duration. Schedulers can obtain this estimate from surgeons, although these estimates are sometimes inaccurate. Probably the best way to determine case estimates is through historical data on the procedure. Taking an average of all the times such a procedure has been performed can help determine a realistic case estimate.

To further prioritize cases, organizations may want to consider the following four ordered priorities[15]:

1. Safety of the patient
2. Surgeon and patient access to the operating room or procedure area
3. Maximizing operating room efficiency
4. Minimizing the average patient wait time

To ensure consistency with prioritization, leadership should get involved and consider developing, implementing, and enforcing a standardized practice for prioritizing urgent cases.

Use Parallel Processing

Parallel processing is the concept of preparing a patient in another room for a procedure while another procedure is wrapping up in the operating room or procedure area. Such processing typically involves performing anesthesia induction in another room. Using a separate room from the operating room or procedure area for anesthesia induction can shorten the time an operating room or procedure area is not in use and may allow extra cases each day compared with a traditional sequenced induction.[2] One recent study showed that a parallel processing system resulted in an approximately 50% reduction in nonoperative time and an accompanying 12% reduction in operative time, thus allowing the completion of additional procedures in the same staffed interval.[17] Using induction rooms may require additional staff, equipment, and facilities. However, the benefits of increased throughput may outweigh these costs depending on the organization. There are also other ways to employ parallel processing without adding resources, including redesigning workflow processes and reassigning staff tasks.[2] Before pursuing a parallel processing approach, organizations should closely examine the cost-benefit ratio when making the decision.

Use a Preoperative Clinic

A preoperative clinic is a designated area away from the perioperative area in which patients can come to receive information about their surgical visit, receive a presurgery evaluation—including an anesthesia evaluation—and allow providers to create a plan of care for the patient both during and after surgery. Often staffed by anesthesiologists and registered nurses, a preoperative clinic provides a valuable way to centralize medical information and coordinate preoperative care. The benefits of such clinics are many. For example, they can reduce operating room or procedure area delays and cancellations because they optimize a patient's medical condition before surgery.[18] During one study on the efficiency of a preoperative clinic across a three-month period, researchers found that nearly 650 patients needed further information or testing before they were considered ready for surgery. If these patients had not gone through the clinic but waited to be seen on the day of surgery, it is likely their procedure would have been delayed or canceled.[19]

Preoperative clinics can also improve patient satisfaction, reduce unnecessary testing, and decrease the patient length of stay. Fundamentally, a preoperative clinic can help completely identify any necessary information about a patient before the day of surgery, so that knowledge of the patient's status is complete. All these factors can lead to significant cost savings for an organization.[19] One study found that avoiding cancellations alone could save an organization an average of $1,500 per case.[20]

Better Coordinate the Duties of the Procedure Team

If every member of the procedure team has specific, designated tasks and is clear about those tasks, organizations can improve efficiency in the operating room or procedure area. For example, at Community Hospital located in Munster, Indiana, members of the perioperative team are clear on which specific job functions they will be performing before, during, and after surgery. This saves time because the team does not need to have repeated, in-depth discussions on which tasks need to be performed and who will perform them. That is not to say that the team does not communicate before, during, and after the procedure, but repeated assigning of roles and duties is not necessary. This consistency among team members and team members' responsibilities helps smooth the schedule in the operating room or procedure area. Designated perioperative team members double-check all supplies, equipment, and implants needed for the next day's surgical procedures. These individuals locate any missing items and make arrangements for any sterilized medical equipment to be delivered at the appropriate time before surgery. Because of this, no time is wasted between procedures searching for missing supplies or equipment.[21]

Use Technology to Manage the Process

Most organizations use software programs to help manage the schedule for the operating room or procedure area. Such programs are often designed for scheduling, with an ideal system also allowing organizations to track patients and resources and monitor turnaround times and patient wait times.[22] Although many of these systems require some form of manual data entry, wireless patient tracking systems can automatically time-stamp important events, thereby lessening the need for manual data input.[23] Such technological tools as big-screen dashboards, text pagers, or electronic whiteboards can show data about where a patient is in the perioperative process and can help clinicians with optimal decision making about real-time management of the operating room or procedure area.[24] Following is a brief discussion of some helpful forms of technology:

- *Infrared tracking.* This system helps track patients throughout an organization, keep them moving through the perioperative process, and ensure that no patient is misplaced. Often this system uses some sort of tracking badge that is placed on the patient's wrist next to his or her identification bracelet. A unique badge number is assigned to the patient. The tracking badge tracks the patient's location, and the amount of time spent in each location, by emitting infrared signals to sensors mounted throughout the perioperative area. Each time a patient moves to a new area or completes a specific process, such as checking in or completing surgery prep, the system displays that information and records the information in a database. At any given time, any staff member can see where a patient is and how long he or she has been there.[25]
- *Cell phones, or mobile phones.* In these systems, a call button system can be used to text message a nurse's phone whenever the patient arrives in a new location or completes a process. For example, when the patient arrives in the preoperative area and the registrar completes the registration process, the registrar can push a call button to send a text message to the nurse notifying him or her that the patient has been checked in. The call button/ phone text messaging system can be used at a variety of points throughout a patient's surgical experience, including when the patient is prepped for surgery, when the perioperative team is ready for surgery, and when the room is ready for surgery. In addition, housekeeping staff members can be given alphanumeric pagers that let them know when an operating room or procedure area needs to be cleaned. They can then use the nurse–call button system to notify the nurse that the room has been cleaned.[25]
- *Electronic whiteboard.* An electronic whiteboard is like a chalkboard posted on an organization's intranet site. This allows information about patients to be added, subtracted, and supplemented in real time, so that perioperative team members can quickly view a patient's status. An electronic whiteboard can integrate information from the previously described infrared tracking system and nurse–call button system. Electronic medical records can also be integrated, if warranted. To view an electronic whiteboard, organizations may choose to use a Web-based application and display it over monitors strategically located throughout the perioperative environment.[25]

Improve On-Time Starts

If a surgery is late in starting, it can disrupt the operating room or procedure area schedule for the entire day. Patient wait times can spiral, delays in equipment can result, and staff members can either be rushed to complete a procedure or be forced to wait around for the next procedure to start. Patient safety, revenues, and patient and staff satisfaction can all be affected. So, how can organizations ensure an on-time start? There are several actions organizations can take to help procedures begin on time. Following is a discussion of some of those actions.

Estimate time appropriately. When scheduling procedures in the operating room or procedure area, organizations need to consider how long those procedures typically take to complete. Operating room or procedure room managers can obtain this information by speaking with the surgeon about the anticipated time of the procedure or by looking at historical records of such procedures. Some organizations use a computer program to help with scheduling. This program takes into account the average time for particular surgeries and, using modeling, determines how best to schedule certain procedures. No matter what method is used, organizations should make sure this method is accurate. Data collection that compares the projected completion time of a particular surgery with its actual completion time can help determine if estimation methods are accurate.

Move cases later in the day. When an operating room or procedure area is running late, moving scheduled cases to other free operating rooms or procedure areas can reduce late starts. Common among many surgical areas, such an intervention can have a significant impact on tardiness in the surgical setting. For example, one recent study showed that moving cases to other operating rooms reduced tardiness by an average of between 4 and 10 minutes per operating room day depending on the location. For those cases that were moved, late starts were reduced by 59 minutes per case. Thus moving the cases greatly benefited the surgeons and patients whose cases were moved.[26]

Ensure the availability of information. The availability of operating rooms or procedure areas is not the only thing that can cause a procedure to be delayed or canceled. A preoperative process that does not run smoothly can derail an operating room or procedure area schedule as well. A patient safety issue can also arise if all the key information is not available at the appropriate time. For example, if allergy information is not available and a procedure starts without it, medication reactions can occur that cause serious patient harm. Organizations that streamline the preoperative process can help increase the likelihood for on-time starts because all the appropriate information will be available and accessible to the perioperative staff.

To help streamline the preoperative process, some organizations are turning to electronic medical records. Although not required by The Joint Commission or Joint Commission International (JCI), automation can help improve documentation, reduce errors, and save time. For example, organizations can use an electronic medical record that is integrated with a scheduling program to schedule surgery and related appointments, pull lab test results for access in the operating room or procedure area, quickly identify allergies, review medications given, verify medical history, and plan for postoperative care, such as rehabilitation and physical therapy. Some systems can remind clinicians of required steps in the preoperative process. For example, if a nurse is charting in the system preoperatively, a message can pop up to remind the nurse to double-check for any medication allergies and verify the surgical site. Reminders can also be set at scheduling to indicate if a patient needs certain tests, such as an electrocardiogram or a particular blood test. Reminders can be set to various urgencies to highlight issues that must be addressed immediately, such as "the patient is going into surgery in 15 minutes, and the x-rays are not present." The advantage of integration is that after a patient's information is entered into the system, it can be available throughout the surgical episode.[27]

Recalibrate the surgical schedule. There are many ways to tweak the surgical schedule to allow for regular late starts. For example, organizations can add a gap or buffer between cases of different surgeons to reduce the likelihood that the second surgeon's case would start late. Organizations can also recalibrate the schedule based on the average tardiness of the first cases of the day. The downside to recalibrating the OR schedule is that if providers are aware of any buffers added to the schedule, they can factor them in when arriving for surgery. For example, if a surgeon knows the surgical start time is actually 10 minutes later than the posted time, he or she may arrive 10 minutes late to the surgery. Organizations pursuing this approach should be careful to limit the number of people aware of the recalibrated schedule.[26]

Keep physicians on time. If one asks a nurse why surgical procedures do not start on time, the nurse may answer, "Because the surgeons are always late." Although this may or may not be the primary reason for late starts in an organization, it is one that happens frequently in many organizations. A study conducted in one hospital showed that 60% of delayed minutes were caused by a late surgeon.[28] Surgeons have been found to cause delays more frequently than any other member of the surgical team.[2] Furthermore, these delays can be significantly longer than other delays in the surgical schedule.[29] To help improve the timeliness of the start of surgery, organizations should consider improving the promptness of their surgeons. Some ways to do so include the following:

- *Educate surgeons on the importance of being on time.* While this may seem obvious, it is important to set expectations regarding on-time surgery starts. Organizations should outline their expectations and the reasons behind them, including improved patient safety, staff satisfaction, and efficient use of resources. In addition, the cost savings of starting procedures on time should be shared.
- *Share start time data.* By collecting data on the number of times procedures are late in starting and the reasons for this tardiness, organizations can determine whether surgeon tardiness is a factor. Organizations should share these data with their surgeons. If possible, provide each surgeon with his or her on-time record as compared to his or her peers. Making surgeons aware of their relative performance will provide them an opportunity to improve independently, based on factual data.
- *Look at data and improve systems issues for late starts.* Aside from issues related to specific surgeon tardiness, leadership should address any underlying systems-level issues that are found to contribute to

late starts. A root cause analysis can uncover such systems issues.

- *Reward surgeons who are on time.* Some organizations reward their surgeons and anesthesiologists for on-time starts. Organizations that track start times of surgeries can determine whether a surgeon or anesthesiologist has a practice of starting on time. Rewards can take many forms, including financial compensation, first-case time slots, or other incentives.
- *Establish consequences for repeated tardiness.* Some organizations enforce a policy that if a surgeon is late multiple times for surgery, that surgeon loses his or her first-case time slot for a period of time. It is important to note that any penalties for tardiness should be supported by the chief of surgery. The operating room manager cannot enforce tardiness policies without the full and complete support of medical staff leadership. It also is important to note that the organization must insist that operating room staff always be on time so that no surgeon can justify his or her own tardiness by claiming "the operating room is never ready."
- *Gain physician buy-in to scheduling.* When creating the operating room schedule, whether an organization uses block time or not, it is important to involve physicians, including anesthesiologists and surgeons, in the scheduling effort. If the physicians have a say in the process and helped create the schedule, they may be more likely to follow the schedule and start procedures on time when possible. Engage the physicians and the operating room team in sequencing the process to reduce wasted time, such as setup that should already have been completed before the starting time for the procedure.
- *Set the tone up front.* When negotiating physician contracts, organizations should set the tone up front for on-time starts. If the surgeon or anesthesiologist knows it is a priority for the organization and that tardiness will not be tolerated, he or she will be more likely to comply.

Monitor Operating Room or Procedure Area Performance

No matter what methods organizations use to improve efficiency in the operating room or procedure area, they should monitor the success of their initiatives to see if further work is necessary. Useful measures for this effort include amount of time the operating room or procedure area is not in use, operating room or procedure area start times, amount of overtime, cancellation rate, and patient wait times.[2]

There is no perfect way to create a schedule for the operating room or procedure area. Life in the operating room or procedure area is a balancing act with a series of trade-offs and compromises. Surgeons, anesthesiologists, schedulers, managers, and organization leadership must all work together to implement a schedule that is consistent yet flexible, efficient yet malleable, and well considered yet able to change with the specific dynamics present on a particular day.

Before a procedure can begin, health care providers must prepare the area where the procedure takes place, including creating a sterile field, laying out instruments, and checking equipment. The next few sections address these aspects of preparing the operating room or procedure area. Please note that these preparations should be carried out by skilled personnel who have received specialized training. The following sections offer only a general description of the steps involved and should not be considered all-inclusive.

Creating and Maintaining a Sterile Field

When preparing the area where a procedure will take place, health care providers must create a sterile field—also known as a surgical field—by placing sterile towels or surgical drapes around the procedure site and on the stand that will hold sterile instruments and other items needed during the procedure.[30] The individual charged with setting up the surgical field will vary depending on the organization but may be a nurse, technician, or other health care provider. This individual must be properly dressed in sterile surgical attire so that nonsterile attire does not come in contact with the surgical field. (*See* Chapter 5 for more information on sterile attire.) Only sterile objects and personnel may be allowed within the sterile field. If even one nonsterile object or person enters a sterile field, it is considered no longer sterile.

It is important to note that when a sterile field is created around a procedure site, items below the level of the draped patient are considered outside the field and thus do not need to be sterilized.

Cautions to keep in mind to help maintain a sterile field after it is created include the following[30]:

- Do not place sterile items near open doors. Windows should remain closed.
- Place only sterile items within the sterile field.
- Ensure that hands are scrubbed for surgery before handing sterile equipment.
- Do not allow sterile personnel to reach across unsterile areas or to touch unsterile items.
- Do not allow unsterile personnel to reach across the sterile field or to touch sterile items.
- Recognize that the edges of a package containing a sterile item are considered unsterile.
- Recognize that a sterile barrier that has been penetrated (wet, cut, or torn) is considered contaminated.

Health care providers interacting in and around the sterile field must be conscious of where their bodies are at all times and move within or around the sterile field in a way that maintains its sterility status. When in doubt about the sterility of an item or area, providers should consider the item or area to be contaminated.[30]

TIP Transport Laundry Supplies Appropriately

When sterile laundry supplies (such as those needed for creating a sterile field) are taken to the operating room from outside the surgical suite (such as from the laundry department or outside laundry facility), they should be transported on a covered cart. Before entering the operating room or procedure area, supplies should be removed from their outside containers used for shipping and transport.[31]

Getting the Instruments Ready

After the sterile field is established, health care providers must lay out the instruments onto the sterile field. These instruments must be sterile. If not cleaned, decontaminated, and sterilized properly, medical equipment can transmit infections to the patient or health care provider using the equipment.

The entities responsible for cleaning, sterilizing, and disinfecting equipment in a health care organization vary depending on the organization. For example, a hospital may have a sterile processing department or may perform these activities in decentralized locations, such as on particular units where equipment is used. For some hospitals, as well as ambulatory surgical centers and office-based practices, cleaning, disinfecting, and sterilizing may be done through a contracted facility off site. Regardless of where equipment is cleaned and sterilized, members of the perioperative team must establish and maintain good communication with the individuals responsible for cleaning and sterilizing equipment to ensure that instruments are delivered and ready for use during surgery.

What Is Sterilization?

The sterilization process destroys all forms of microbial life, including bacteria, viruses, spores, and fungi. There are several types of sterilization, including steam, ethylene oxide, and ozone sterilization. In recent years, there has been a lack of clarity about sterilization and the appropriate way to clean medical equipment, devices, and supplies. Organizations have historically used the term *flash sterilization* to describe many different approaches to disinfecting medical equipment. Experts in the field agree that although the process of flash sterilization is sound, the term is out of date and does not fully and accurately describe the sterilization cycles currently used in health care organizations. More important, the concept of flash sterilization does not include the critical steps of cleaning, decontamination, and aseptic transport that must accompany any sterilization cycle.

The term *immediate-use steam sterilization* is more appropriate to describe the abbreviated cycle of steam sterilization that is meant to effectively clean, disinfect, and sterilize instruments that will be used immediately. This process involves following the manufacturer's instructions during sterilization and transferring items immediately to the sterile field using aseptic technique.

To help organizations more adequately and appropriately manage the overall process of cleaning, disinfection, and sterilization of medical equipment, devices, and supplies, The Joint Commission has refocused its survey efforts by examining all the critical processes involved in cleaning, disinfection, and sterilization, including the following:

- *Cleaning and decontamination.* This process involves removing any visible soil on the equipment prior to sterilization. Depending on the equipment, the complexity of the cleaning process can vary, from simply brushing the equipment to taking it apart and using special cleaning techniques. When determining how to appropriately clean and decontaminate instruments, manufacturers' instructions should be consulted and followed.
- *Disinfection.* This is a process that eliminates all pathogens except spores. It includes both low-level and high-level disinfection. The disinfection level is determined by the physical nature of the inanimate object and the level of infection risk to the patient. (For example, low-level disinfection is used for blood glucose meters, and high-level disinfection is used for flexible endoscopes.)
- *Sterilization.* Whatever method of sterilization is chosen, The Joint Commission expects U.S. health care organizations to use sterilization equipment approved by the U.S. Food and Drug Administration (FDA) and follow the manufacturers' instructions. Consequently, an organization must know the specifications of its sterilizers and follow those specifications. JCI expects international organizations to ensure adequate equipment cleaning and sterilization by using a coordinated approach that is appropriate for the equipment being cleaned.
- *Storage or return to the sterile field.* To prevent recontamination, every piece of equipment must be carefully protected after it has been sterilized. For full steam sterilization, packs of instruments are wrapped and sealed, and this offers sufficient protection. For other types of sterilization, instruments can be transported in "flash pans" or other covered vessels that are specifically designed to prevent contamination. The goal is to maintain sterility until equipment is used.

Staff involved with cleaning, disinfection, and sterilization must be familiar with these different processes and be competent to perform them appropriately. Organizations are responsible for providing adequate training to ensure this understanding and ability.

Joint Commission International notes that infection risk is minimized with proper cleaning, disinfection, and sterilization processes, such as the cleaning and disinfection of endoscopes and the sterilization of surgical supplies and other invasive or noninvasive patient care equipment. Cleaning, disinfection, and sterilization can take place in a centralized sterilization area or, with proper oversight, in other areas of the organization such as an endoscope clinic. For organizations outside the United States, JCI requires that equipment cleaning and sterilization are appropriate for the type of equipment and that an organization have a coordinated oversight process that ensures all cleaning, disinfection, and sterilization methods are the same throughout the organization.

Types of Sterilization

While organizations can sterilize medical equipment in a variety of ways, there are some advantages and disadvantages to different methods. Following are some of the methods with their advantages and disadvantages.

- *Steam sterilization.* This is the most widely used and dependable form of sterilization in which steam under pressure is the sterilizing agent. Temperatures in steam sterilization should reach least 121°C (250°F). The critical factors in ensuring the reliability of the steam sterilization method are proper temperature and time; and the complete replacement of the air with steam, so there is no entrapment of air.[32] Steam sterilization is not appropriate for all types of equipment, and organizations should consult a manufacturer's guidelines before using steam sterilization on a particular piece of equipment. An often-used type of steam sterilization involves an abbreviated cycle that follows the manufacturer's instructions and uses aseptic technique to transfer the sterilized equipment to the sterile field for immediate use. Formerly called *flash sterilization,* the term *immediate-use steam sterilization* is more appropriate for this activity.
- *Ethylene oxide sterilization.* This is a sterilization process that involves the chemical ethylene oxide (ETO). ETO is a common chemical, and nearly half of all medical devices sterilized are sterilized using

ETO.[33] ETO is very effective at killing microbes in hard-to-reach and hard-to-clean places. It can thoroughly clean an instrument without damaging it. It does require significant aeration time, however, to preserve the safety of both the individuals handling the equipment and patients. Exposure to ETO is extremely harmful to people, and the U.S. Occupational Safety and Health Administration (OSHA) has specific standards that govern its use. (*See* OSHA's Web site at http://www.osha.gov.) At toxic levels, ETO smells like ether. Exposure to ETO in health care settings is usually through inhalation and can cause a variety of symptoms, ranging from eye pain and sore throat to convulsions, nerve damage, and impaired thinking. In addition, health care providers exposed to ETO can have an increased chance of contracting some cancers.[33]

- *Ozone sterilization.* This is a chemical sterilization process that uses ozone—a combination of three atoms of oxygen rather than the normal two. It works by establishing negative pressure in the sterilization chamber. Ozone is produced in the sterilizer itself from the water, oxygen, and electricity. At the end of sterilization, the ozone is converted back to oxygen and water vapor and released into the room. Operationally, it requires electricity, some potable water that has passed through a demineralizing filter, and medical-grade oxygen gas. As with all chemical sterilants, excessive exposure to ozone can cause a serious health hazard. Fortunately, ozone is highly detectable by the human nose, and a staff member would know if ozone was present in the area before it became a health hazard.[34]
- *Gas plasma sterilization.* This method uses a combination of hydrogen peroxide vapor and low-temperature gas plasma to rapidly sterilize medical instruments without leaving toxic residues. This method is particularly suited to heat-sensitive and moisture-sensitive instruments.

Regardless of the sterilization method or methods organizations choose, they should have policies and procedures in place that govern the safe use of these methods. Staff should be familiar with these policies and consistently comply with them and ongoing monitoring.

Maintaining Sterilization

Once cleaned and disinfected or sterilized, surgical equipment must remain sterile until its use. When performing immediate-use steam sterilization, organizations need a process to ensure sterile transport to the sterile field. However, if sterilizing instruments using another form of sterilization and storing the equipment for later use, there are several choices in methods to maintain sterility of surgical instruments, including rigid containers, peel-open pouches, and sterilization wraps. Health care facilities may use a combination of these packaging options. The packaging material must allow penetration of the sterilant, provide protection against contact contamination during handling, provide an effective barrier to microbial penetration, and maintain the sterility of the processed item after sterilization.[35]

Proper physical storage of devices and instruments that have been sterilized is an important part of maintaining sterility. Safe storage times for sterile packs vary with the type of wrapper and storage conditions, such as open versus closed cabinets. Once sterilized, all items should be marked with an expiration date that clearly indicates when instruments will lose their sterility. Any item that has been sterilized should not be used after the expiration date has been exceeded. Sterile items should also not be used if the package becomes wet, soiled, torn, punctured, or in any way tampered with. All items should be assessed for package integrity prior to use.[36]

Considering Single-Use Devices

Single-use devices are designed to be used once and then thrown out. Often, they are manufactured at a lower cost to justify their disposal. There are positives and negatives associated with this type of equipment.

On the positive side, single-use devices are guaranteed clean and free of contaminants and so can eliminate the possibility of spreading protein and bacteria that remain on medical instruments after decontamination and sterilization, such as those that lead to Creutzfeldt-Jakob disease (*see* Sidebar 3-1 on page 52). In addition, because these instruments are used fresh out of the package, they do not suffer from fatigue or wear and tear.

On the negative side, there are concerns among providers about the strength, flexibility, and effectiveness of certain single-use devices. These defects can present risks for patient safety regarding the quality of the instrument and its ability to perform to expectations.[37]

Another concern associated with single-use devices is the tendency of health care organizations to reuse these devices. Although these items were originally meant to be used one time, some organizations are using them multiple times. Approximately 20% to 30% of U.S. hospitals reported that they reuse at least one type of single-use device.[38] Reuse of single-use devices involves regulatory, ethical, medical, legal, and economic issues and has been extremely controversial for more than two decades.[39]

In August 2000, the U.S. FDA released a guidance document on single-use devices. In this guidance document, the FDA states that organizations or third-party reprocessors will be considered "manufacturers" and regulated in the same manner. In other words, a reused single-use device will have to comply with the same regulatory requirements of the device when it was originally manufactured.[40] Most U.S. health care organizations do not realize this and therefore run the risk of noncompliance.

JCI requires international organizations to define the conditions under which single-use devices can be reused when laws and regulations permit. This definition should occur within organization policy and be consistent with national laws and regulations and professional standards. Such a policy should include identification of all of the following:

- Devices and materials that can never be reused
- The maximum number of reuses specific for each device and material that is reused
- The types of wear, cracking, and other deterioration that indicate the device cannot be reused
- The cleaning process for each device that starts immediately after use and follows a clear protocol
- The process for the collection, analysis, and use of infection prevention and control data related to reused devices and materials

Preparing Anesthesia Equipment

In most surgical procedures, the use of anesthesia and sedation is required. Different types of anesthesia medication and equipment will be used depending on the procedure, the patient, and the patient's history and physical.

A critical part of preparing the operating room or procedure area is checking the anesthesia equipment to ensure

Sidebar 3-1: Preventing Creutzfeldt-Jakob Disease

Creutzfeldt-Jakob disease is a rare, fatal, brain disorder. Traditional sterilization methods may not always get rid of any Creutzfeldt-Jakob disease infectious agents known as *prions*. Prions are resistant to a number of standard disinfection and sterilization methods.

An additional concern about Creutzfeldt-Jakob disease is that it may take years to manifest itself and can be definitively diagnosed only by direct examination of brain tissue, usually obtained at autopsy. Consequently, if there is any chance that a patient could have this rare brain disorder, organizations should consider disposing of any surgical instruments used on the patient after use. Organizations should also consider using disposable medical devices for brain surgery. Unfortunately, both of these options can be extremely costly to the institution.

If organizations choose to reprocess devices or if the presumptive diagnosis is made during a neurosurgical procedure, instruments should be cleaned using sodium hydroxide and a high-temperature autoclave, or the instruments should be quarantined until a biopsy confirms that the patient is not infected with Creutzfeldt-Jakob disease. Another advisable cleaning method involves soaking devices in concentrated sodium hydroxide for one hour. It is important to note that sodium hydroxide is extremely corrosive. As always, before using any specific cleaning methods on equipment, organizations should consult with the manufacturer. Further information on cleaning instruments of Creutzfeldt-Jakob disease patients can be found at http://www.who.int/csr/resources/publications/bse/whocdscsraph2003.pdf.

Source: Centers for Disease Control and Prevention: *Guidelines for Environmental Infection Control in Health-Care Facilities.* 2003. http://www.cdc.gov/hicpac/pdf/guidelines/eic_in_HCF_03.pdf (accessed Jul. 24, 2010).

that it is functioning properly. Although anesthesia equipment has changed over the years, its basic function remains the same: to safely put a patient to sleep for a procedure and wake him or her up again after the procedure ends. There are several risks associated with this process, including the risk for equipment failure—which, if it were to occur, could be fatal to the patient. The key to ensuring safety is to proactively address these and other risks.

When working properly, anesthesia machines mix the correct concentrations of gas and drugs for the patient to inhale and exhale, causing the patient to lose consciousness. Anesthetic gas affects the nervous system and numbs the nerve pathways. During an operation, patients who are anesthetized remain unconscious, are immobile, might require breathing support, are free from memory, and have no sensation.[41]

Wall outlets or cylinders supply air, oxygen, and nitrous oxide to anesthesia machines. Pressure regulators reduce the pressures, which are then passed through an oxygen failure alarm. Flowmeters control the flow of gas, which is mixed and passed over a vaporizer containing the anesthetic agent. The gas then goes through a pressure relief valve and backflow valve, then to the common gas outlet, ready to be given to the patient. Expired gas can be stripped of carbon dioxide and recirculated, or "scavenged" out of the room.[41] (*See* Sidebar 3-2 below.)

Sidebar 3-2: Ensuring Health Care Provider Safety Around Anesthesia Equipment

For a number of years, anesthesiologists have been aware that working around anesthetic gases, such as nitrous oxide, can present certain health hazards, such as reproductive issues, liver and kidney disease, and neurological disorders.

When delivering anesthesia to patients, more gas is used than is strictly necessary. Any excess gas is vented from the patient's breathing circuit through a pressure release valve. This prevents pressure from building up within the circuit. Unless this excess gas is removed, it can accumulate in the air of the operating room or procedure area and cause harm.

The process of removing excess anesthesia gases from the procedure environment is called *scavenging.* The primary objective of scavenging is to capture the excess gases released from the pressure relief valve and direct them to a waste gas evacuation system. Once in the system, they are then exhausted outside the building.

A scavenging system has three major components: a gas-capturing assembly that traps the gas for disposal, a disposal system that vents the gas outside, and an interface between the gas-capturing assembly and the disposal system. There are many different varieties of scavenging systems. Organizations should review the different types and select which kind best serves the needs of the organization.

Even an effective scavenging system does not dispose of all anesthetic gases present in the operating room or procedure area. Excess gases can come from leaks, inappropriate use of the anesthesia equipment, and from other equipment, such as a mass spectrometer. Excess gas from these sources cannot be captured by a scavenging system. Consequently, additional measures should be taken to ensure the most healthful environment possible. These measures can include the following:

- Routine servicing and preventive maintenance of the equipment
- Purchasing low-leakage anesthetic equipment
- Using low-leakage anesthetic techniques. This includes turning on the nitrous oxide only after the face mask has been applied to the face of the patient.
- Conducting regular leak testing. This can be done in a variety of ways, such as by using an infrared nitrous oxide analyzer or by submerging the suspected leak site in water. If submersion is not possible, application of an 80% water and 20% liquid soap solution will expose any leaks.
- Regularly monitoring trace gases. This can be done through air sampling and testing or through the use of infrared analyzers.

Employees working in the operating room or procedure area should be regularly informed about the risks and possible toxic effects of exposure to anesthetics. In addition, in the preemployment physical, organizations should document the worker's baseline health, including any abnormal pregnancies. All records of this information should be maintained.

Source: Blanks S., et al.: Scavenging of waste anesthetic gases. PTSM Series 1987, pp. 27–33.

Before a procedure, members of the perioperative team should check the gas connections to the anesthesia machine to be sure all connections are appropriate, are secure, and deliver the right amount of pressure.[42] Designated team members who are trained and competent in this activity should be responsible for its completion. Also, such staff should work with the department in charge of maintaining the equipment—possibly the biomedical department or other medical equipment maintenance area—to make sure the equipment is kept in good working order. Consistent upkeep and testing reduces anesthetic gas leaks, maintains optimal performance of scavenging equipment, and ensures that the appropriate percentage of anesthetic is being delivered.[41]

When preparing the anesthesia equipment, health care providers should not only set up the appropriate equipment for the procedure but also gather the right reversal agent for the type of medication being administered. This agent will allow the anesthesiologist to "back out" of the anesthesia during an emergency situation. As with other aspects of the surgery, a checklist can be used to select the proper equipment, medication, and reversal agent for each level of sedation. More information about anesthesia medication and safety issues associated with anesthesia medication can be found in Chapters 4 and 7.

Preparing Other Equipment

In addition to anesthesia equipment, other equipment that should be prepared and checked may include but not be limited to equipment to monitor vital signs, heart rate and oxygenation, respiratory frequency and adequacy of pulmonary ventilation, blood pressure, and cardiac functioning. Resuscitation equipment should also be present. As with anesthesia equipment, the perioperative team must work with individuals charged with maintaining and cleaning medical equipment to ensure that all elements are clean and in proper working order.

Ensuring Proper Air Quality and Ventilation

Heating, ventilation, and air-conditioning (HVAC) systems provide circulating air throughout health care facilities, including in and out of operating rooms or procedure areas. These systems provide temperature and humidity control and filtration of various contaminants. When HVAC systems are not functioning optimally, they can be a source of patient safety and workplace safety hazards. Consequently, verifying the appropriate function of the HVAC system before the start of surgery is recommended.

HVAC systems address the following aspects of ventilation and air quality in the operating room or procedure area:

- *Pressure relationships.* Space pressurization is used to ensure that air movement is directed from a clean space into a less-clean space. Positive-pressure operating rooms or procedure areas can ensure clean air in the room at all times.
- *Air exchange rates.* This is how many times the air is replaced in the room. The more clean air that is circulated into a space, the less the impact of any contaminants.
- *Filtration efficiencies.* Filtration is the primary defense against fungi in ventilation systems. It can take a variety of forms but could include HEPA filters or prefilters that work to remove particles from the air.

If any of these areas are not functioning properly, then an infection risk is present in the operating room or procedure area. Conversely, if these areas are all working at optimal functioning, the risks of infection can be severely limited.

To ensure proper ventilation of the surgical environment, operating rooms or procedure areas should be held at positive pressure so that air travels out of the room into adjacent areas.[43] Air should come into the room through ceiling vents high on the walls and exit the room via air outlet exhaust vents located near the floor, across from the inlet vents.

The U.S. Centers for Disease Control and Prevention developed guidelines regarding infection control and ventilation for operating rooms. Following are some of the suggestions included in these guidelines[38]:

- Maintain positive-pressure ventilation with respect to corridors and areas adjacent to the operating room.
- Maintain at least 15 air changes per hour, of which at least three should be fresh air.

- Filter all recirculated and fresh air through appropriate filters providing a minimum of 90% efficiency.
- In rooms not engineered for horizontal laminar air flow, introduce air at the ceiling and exhaust near the floor.
- Keep operating room doors closed except for passage of equipment, personnel, and patients, and limit entry to essential personnel.

Organizations should have a backup system that can be used for emergency ventilation in the event that an air ventilation system malfunctions. Such a system could involve portable units for fans or filters. Obviously, backup systems should be used in the short term, while every effort is made to restore the main ventilation system. It is important to note that ventilation systems for the operating room or procedure area should be functioning at all times; this is particularly important for ambulatory surgery centers that may operate only during the week.

One option for organizations to consider regarding ventilation is natural ventilation. This involves the use of building openings—windows, doors, wind towers, and so forth—to allow outdoor air inside and indoor air outside. Natural ventilation can be economic and efficient and may offer better access to natural light. In general, the advantage of natural ventilation is its ability to provide a high air exchange rate at low cost, with a very simple system.

Although it has advantages, natural ventilation also has some disadvantages. For example, natural ventilation is variable and depends on outside climate conditions. It may be difficult to control and may not work as expected. Normal operation may be interrupted for numerous reasons, including windows or doors not opening, equipment failure, utility service interruption, poor design, poor maintenance, or incorrect management. Other possible drawbacks, such as noise, air pollution, insect issues, and security concerns, also exist. Before considering a natural ventilation system, organizations should be familiar with the advantages and disadvantages of such a system and how those will factor into maintaining ventilation to areas where surgery and other invasive procedures are performed.[44]

TIP Establish Schedules for Maintenance and Cleaning

Fans, coils, belts, and filters within a heating, ventilation, and air-conditioning (HVAC) system all require regular maintenance to function properly. Organizations should establish preventive maintenance, cleaning, and inspection schedules for the HVAC system and stick to them. It is also important to keep accurate, up-to-date records of not only routine maintenance but also requested maintenance and quality management activities, including the use of instrumentation to determine appropriate air change, filtration, and pressure parameters for areas requiring special ventilation.

Controlling Traffic

With the many personnel involved in a typical surgery or other invasive procedure, it is easy to see how health care provider "traffic" could be a problem if not controlled. Movement of people into and out of the operating room or procedure area should be kept to a minimum to reduce the amount of bacterial shedding, air turbulence, and accidental contamination of the patient, sterile equipment, and supplies.[31]

To establish good traffic control, health care organizations should designate three specific traffic zones related to the surgical suite, monitor who is allowed in these zones, and clearly define what personal protective equipment they must wear. Following are three recommended traffic zones[31,45]:

- *Unrestricted Zone.* In this zone, individuals in street clothes can be permitted. Only authorized individuals should be allowed in this area.
- *Semirestricted Zone.* This is the area adjacent to the operating room or procedure area that includes areas that support the surgical suite, such as the hallways, offices, and supply rooms of the operating room or procedure area. Scrub attire must be worn in this zone, including a long-sleeved scrub suit, hair cover, and clean shoes or shoe covers.
- *Restricted Zone.* This zone consists of the operating and procedure rooms; the clean core; and scrub and sink areas. Full surgical attire should be required in this zone, including masks. Personnel who are not

scrubbed should wear long-sleeved jackets buttoned closed. Masks are required in rooms with open sterile supplies.

To further prevent unintentional contamination of the operating room or procedure area, the room doors should remain closed except when needed open for equipment, personnel, and patient transport.[31] It is also important to ensure that all equipment and surgical instruments involved in a procedure are present in the operating room or procedure area before the procedure begins so that there will be no unnecessary traffic into and out of the suite.[43]

TIP Use Signs to Limit Traffic Flow

To help ensure limited traffic flow, some organizations have posted procedure-specific signs on the door of the operating room or procedure area (for example, NO ENTRY: JOINT REPLACEMENT IN PROGRESS) to help keep unwanted visitors and infections out.

References

1. World Health Organization: *Our Ageing World.* http://www.who.int/ageing/en/ (accessed Jul. 24, 2010).
2. Marjamaa R., Vakkuri A., Kirvelä O.: Operating room management: Why, how, and by whom? *Acta Anaesthesiol Scand* 52:596–600, May 2008.
3. Pandit J., Westbury S., Pandit M.: The concept of surgical operating list "efficiency": A formula to describe the term. *Anaesthesia* 62:895–903, Sep. 2007.
4. Santibañez P., Begen M., Atkins D.: Surgical block scheduling in a system of hospitals: An application to resource and wait list management in a British Columbia health authority. *Health Care Manag Sci* 10:269–282, Sep. 2007.
5. What's the best way to adjust block time? *OR Manager* 20:11, Nov. 2004.
6. Patterson P.: A few simple rules for managing block time in the operating room. *OR Manager* 20:1, 9–10, 12, Nov. 2004.
7. The Joint Commission: St. John's Regional smooths OR schedule to ease overcrowding. *The Source* 3:8–10, Oct. 2005.
8. Dempsey C., Rudolph M.: Questions managers ask on patient flow. *OR Manager* 21:20–21, Jan. 2005.
9. Boston hospital sees big impact from smoothing elective schedule. *OR Manager* 2:1, 10–11, Dec. 2004.
10. Mazzei W., Blasco T., Patterson P.: What's the best way to manage urgent and emergent OR cases. *OR Manager* 21:1, 10, 12, Mar. 2005.
11. MacLellan D., et al.: Applying clinical process redesign methods to planned arrivals in New South Wales hospitals. *Med J Aust* (suppl. 6)188:S23–S26, Mar. 2008.
12. Saver C.: Ways to break loose from OR holds. *OR Manager* 24:14–15, 2008.
13. Hospital moves to smooth surgery schedule. *OR Manager* 19:11, Nov. 2003.
14. Marr J.: The positive effects of surgical services redesign. *J Nurs Adm* 35:281–282, Jun. 2005.
15. Dexter F.: How do we sequence urgent cases? *OR Manager* 21:12, 14, 16, Mar. 2005.
16. Lau W., et al.: Acute appendicitis in children. *Aust N Z J Surg* 57:927–931, Dec. 1987.
17. Smith M., Sandberg W., Foss J.: High-throughput operating room system for joint arthroplasties durably outperforms routine processes. *Anesthesiology* 109:25–35, Jul. 2008.
18. Ferschl M., et al.: Preoperative clinic visits reduce operating room cancellations and delays. *Anesthesiology* 103:855–859, Oct. 2005.
19. Correll D., et al.: Value of preoperative clinic visits in identifying issues with potential impact on operating room efficiency. *Anesthesiology* 105:1254–1259, Dec. 2006.
20. Dexter F., et al.: Validation of statistical methods to compare cancellation rates on the day of surgery. *Anesth Analg* 101:465–473, Aug. 2005.
21. Olmstead J., et al.: World-class OR turnaround times: Secrets uncovered. *AORN J* 85:942–945, 947–949, May 2007.
22. Marcario A., Vasanawala M.: Technology and computing in the surgical suite: Key features of an OR management information system and opportunities for the future. *Anesth Analg* 95:1120–1121, Oct. 2002.
23. Marjamaa R., et al.: Time accuracy of a radio frequency identification patient tracking system for recording operating room timestamps. *Anesth Analg* 102:1183–1186, Apr. 2006.
24. Dexter F., Willemsen-Dunlap A., Lee J.: Operating room managerial decision-making on the day of surgery with and without computer recommendations and status displays. *Anesth Analg* 105:419–429, Aug. 2007.
25. Bahlman D., Johnson F.: Using technology to improve and support communication and workflow processes. *AORN J* 82:65–73, Jul. 2005.
26. Wachtel R., Dexter F.: Reducing tardiness from scheduled start times by making adjustments to the operating room schedule. *Anesth Analg* 108:1902–1909, Jun. 2009.
27. Patterson P.: Automation eases the preop process. *OR Manager* 21:12–13, Feb. 2005.
28. Data helps ASC conquer late case starts. *OR Manager* 21:25–26, Apr. 2005.

29. Escobar A., et al.: Task analysis of the preincision surgical period: An independent observer-based study of 1558 cases. *Anesth Analg* 103:922–927, Oct. 2006.
30. Engender Health for a Better Life: *Infection Prevention Online Course: Creating and Maintaining a Sterile Field.* 2004. http://www.engenderhealth.org/ip/aseptic/at6.html (accessed Jul. 24, 2010).
31. Church N., Bjerke N.: Surgical services. In *APIC Text of Infection Control and Epidemiology,* 3rd ed. Washington, DC: Association for Professionals in Infection Control and Epidemiology, 2009, pp. 45-1–45-14.
32. Berkeley Lab Environmental Health & Safety Division: *Sterilization.* http://www.lbl.gov/ehs/biosafety/Biosafety_Manual/html/sterilization.shtml (accessed Apr. 29, 2010).
33. Conviser S.: The future of ethylene oxide sterilization. *Infection Control Today,* Jun. 1, 2001. http://www.infectioncontroltoday.com/articles/061feat4.html (accessed Jul. 24, 2009).
34. Reichert M., Schultz J.: Is the new ozone sterilizer right for your OR? *OR Manager* 19:23–24, Nov. 2003.
35. Dunkelberg H., Fleitmann-Glende F.: Measurement of the microbial barrier effectiveness of sterilization containers in terms of the log reduction value for prevention of nosocomial infections. *Am J Infect Control* 34:285–289, Jun. 2006.
36. Centers for Disease Control and Prevention: *Guideline for Disinfection and Sterilization in Healthcare Facilities.* 2008. http://www.cdc.gov/hicpac/pdf/guidelines/Disinfection_Nov_2008.pdf (accessed Jul. 24, 2010).
37. Rowley E., Dingwall R.: The use of single-use devices in anaesthesia: Balancing the risks to patient safety. *Anaesthesia* 62:569–574, Jun. 2007.
38. Centers for Disease Control and Prevention: *Guidelines for Environmental Infection Control in Health-Care Facilities.* 2003. http://www.cdc.gov/hicpac/pdf/guidelines/eic_in_HCF_03.pdf (accessed Jul. 24, 2010).
39. Greene V.: Reuse of disposable devices. In Mayhall C., (ed.): *Hospital Epidemiology and Infection Control,* 2nd ed. Philadelphia: Lippincott Williams & Wilkins, 1999, pp. 1201–1208.
40. Food and Drug Administration (FDA): *Enforcement Priorities for Single-Use Devices Reprocessed by Third Parties and Hospitals.* Rockville, MD: FDA, 2000.
41. Finch L.: Going under—Anesthesia equipment. *24x7,* Jan. 2007. http://www.24x7mag.com/issues/articles/2007-01_06.asp (accessed Jul. 24, 2010).
42. Bowers M.: Safe learning and assessment for anaesthetic apparatus checks. *J Perioper Pract* 18:156–160, Apr. 2008.
43. Roy M.: Operating room. In Wenzel R., Brewer T., Butzler J. (eds.): *A Guide to Infection Control in the Hospital.* Boston: International Society for Infectious Diseases, 2002, pp. 68–71.
44. Atkinson J., et al.: *Natural Ventilation for Infection Control in Health-Care Settings.* World Health Organization, 2009. http://www.who.int/water_sanitation_health/publications/natural_ventilation.pdf (accessed Jul. 24, 2010).
45. Blanchard J., Chobin N.: The operating room. In Jarvis W. (ed.): *Bennett & Brachman's Hospital Infections,* 5th ed. Philadelphia: Lippincott Williams & Wilkins, 2007, pp. 449–460.

Chapter 4

Preparing the Patient

Preparing the patient for surgery or other invasive procedures is a critical step along the surgical continuum. If preparation efforts are done well, procedures can run smoothly and have fewer surprises. Such efforts can reduce the likelihood of errors and ultimately result in positive outcomes for the patient. Conversely, if elements of the patient preparation process are rushed or skipped, there is an increased possibility of unanticipated events, complications, and errors, which can negatively impact patient outcomes, length of stay, and satisfaction, all of which can affect the financial health of the organization.

To effectively and comprehensively prepare a patient for surgical or other invasive procedures, perioperative teams must engage in a variety of multidisciplinary tasks. Some of these tasks include assessing the patient for risk factors, effectively handling the medication management process—including ordering, reconciling, and labeling medications for surgery—and preparing the surgical site. The following sections examine these activities.

Assessing the Patient for Risk Factors

Like all patients, surgical patients have unique characteristics, such as age, size, preexisting conditions, allergies, and medical history, which combine to make each surgical procedure slightly different. Unique patient characteristics are an important predictor of complications in surgery.[1] A comprehensive preprocedural assessment is necessary to consider a patient's unique characteristics and pinpoint any possible risks that could play a factor in the procedure, including those related to anesthesia and sedation.

Prior to surgery or invasive procedures, health care providers, including nurses, surgeons, and anesthesiologists, should participate in the assessment process to identify potential risks and determine appropriate medications. All providers involved in the surgical procedure should be familiar with the content of the assessment and be aware of any risks identified within the process. (*See* Sidebar 4-1 on page 60 and Sidebar 4-2 on page 61).

Like all aspects of the patient preparation process, the presurgical assessment should be thorough and comprehensive. If rushed, a health care provider may miss critical information, such as laboratory data, allergies, the existence and status of preexisting diseases not indicated on the history and physical, and changes in the health of the patient. This lack of information might lead to an inappropriate choice of anesthetic, the decision to use or not use a medication, or the failure to plan appropriately for the postoperative period. For example, if the preoperative assessment is not complete, a provider may fail to recognize that a patient has sleep apnea, which could result in a serious respiratory response to sedation.

Depending on the organization, a presurgical assessment may take place on or before the day of the surgery or procedure. Patients may come to the surgical area for the assessment or to a preprocedure clinic located nearby. Regardless of where and when the assessment takes place, it should be designed to capture all necessary information to ensure a successful patient outcome.

Risks to Watch for Within the Assessment

Some key items to assess for during the presurgical assessment include the following:

- *Allergies.* If anesthesia and sedation are going to be used for a procedure, it is important to identify allergies, such as to eggs or soybeans, as these may preclude the use of certain anesthesia/sedation medications.[2] (*See* Sidebar 4-3 on page 62.)

Sidebar 4-1: The Preadmission Nurse

Some health care organizations have created a staff position whose sole responsibility is the collection of assessment data. This position, which typically is filled by one or several registered nurses, is responsible for orienting a patient to the surgical area, making appropriate referrals for further assessments as necessary, and identifying potential problems that could negatively affect the surgical process. For example, a preadmission nurse in a surgical setting may discover an anesthetic concern with a particular patient during assessment. The nurse can notify the anesthesiologist to evaluate the patient and address that problem before the day of surgery. The nurse can also identify potential cardiac, pulmonary, or renal problems and share that information with the surgeon and anesthesiologist. This type of position may be particularly helpful in outpatient surgery settings, where patients may come in before the day of surgery to be assessed. Some benefits of having a designated preadmission nurse include the following:

- Allows time to thoroughly explore a patient's health history and follow up on potential issues, such as anesthesia problems
- Allows time to gather information from other facilities and physicians before admission
- Allows time to address the needs of patients with emotional or anxiety concerns
- Provides dedicated staff and prevents other nurses from being called away from the care of other patients to perform the assessment
- Allows staff to facilitate the patient's tour of the facility, if necessary, and build trust. This can improve satisfaction.

Source: Mathias J.: Preadmit nurse avoids rushed assessments. *OR Manager* 21:27–28, Jul. 2005.

- *Medical problems.* These problems may include high blood pressure, asthma, and any other cardiac or respiratory issues. Specifically, providers must identify the risks of airway problems because these risks are the most dangerous aspect of general anesthesia.[3] Patients should also be screened for undiagnosed diabetes prior to a procedure because hypoglycemia can increase the risk of surgical site infection. Those patients who are found to have diabetes should be educated about maintaining their blood glucose levels during their postoperative phase.
- *Tobacco use.* Smoking can increase a patient's risk for infection. Patients should be encouraged to quit smoking prior to the procedure.[4]
- *Alcohol and illicit drug use.* Patients who abuse drugs or alcohol and those who are opioid-tolerant may need more medication to achieve the desired level of sedation and analgesia.
- *Previous experiences with sedation and anesthesia.*
- *Weight.* Perioperative teams must accurately obtain patient weight to help with medication dosing. (*See* page 63 for more information.)
- *Current medications,* including prescription, over-the-counter (nonprescription), and herbal medications.[2]
- *Whether or not there are risks for anesthesia and sedation.* These could include advanced age, obesity, pregnancy, sleep apnea, or a history of substance abuse, as well as severe cardiac, respiratory, hepatic, renal, or central nervous system disease.
- *Patient preferences for anesthesia and sedation.* Asking a few simple questions can help determine this aspect of the assessment. For example, does the patient really need to be sedated? Some patients are able to use relaxation techniques to calm themselves and may not need to be sedated to be able to tolerate brief discomfort. Mentally preparing a patient for anesthesia or sedation also plays an important role in decreasing anxiety and gaining the patient's cooperation.
- *Anxiety.* Anxiety can impair an individual's ability to focus, and it can influence clinical outcomes. For example, perioperative anxiety in young children may influence their recovery and lead to a higher incidence of sleep and other problems.[5] Providers should encourage patients to share their worries and fears, so that providers can acknowledge and address them prior to surgery.
- *Delirium.* This aspect is particularly important in older adults, who are more likely to have symptoms

Sidebar 4-2: Assessing Patients in the Ambulatory Setting

For ambulatory organizations offering surgery or other invasive procedures that require anesthesia, the U.S. Association of periOperative Registered Nurses (AORN) has specific standards and recommended practices that relate to the preadmission assessment. They require ambulatory surgery centers to have specific admission criteria and to ensure that all patients meet these criteria. The preadmission assessment should be done by a perioperative registered nurse and involve written guidelines for preadmission. The process can occur via telephone or face-to-face interview, but criteria should exist that indicate when each type of assessment method is warranted.

According to AORN, a comprehensive assessment should include but not be limited to the following:

- An appropriate baseline physical assessment
- Identification of allergies and sensitivities
- Signs of abuse or neglect
- A cultural, emotional, and socioeconomic assessment
- A comprehensive pain assessment
- Medication and anesthetic history
- Results of perioperative testing
- Preoperative patient education

Organization policy should dictate the content of the assessment, and the organizations should have a way of measuring whether the required information is obtained during the assessment process.

Source: Association of periOperative Registered Nurses (AORN): AORN Guidance Statement: Preoperative Patient Care in the Ambulatory Setting. In *Perioperative Standards and Recommended Practices*, 2010 ed. Denver: AORN, 2010, pp. 625–630.

of delirium. Delirium is one of the most serious and prevalent cognitive disorders among hospitalized elders.[6] Other risk factors for delirium[7] include prior cognitive impairment, presence of infection, severe illness, dehydration, psychotropic medication use, alcoholism, vision impairment, fractures, and family history of malignant hyperthermia. It is important to identify delirium in a preoperative assessment because it can influence sedation and anesthesia medication as well as increase the likelihood of postoperative complications. (*See* related Tip.)

- *Nutritional status.* Malnutrition has long been identified as a risk factor for surgical site infections.[8] It can also impact an individual's ability to recover quickly from a procedure. Serum albumin level is the marker most commonly used to classify nutritional status. Organizations should consider assessing patients for poor nutrition risk.[8]
- *Potential risk for deep vein thrombosis.* This potentially fatal condition can occur after surgery and originates in the calf or thigh due to a combination of venous stasis, vessel wall damage, and hypercoagulability.[9] Blood clots can then form and travel to the lungs, causing fatal pulmonary embolism. Some patients are at higher risk for this complication than others. Common risk factors include advanced age, obesity, history of smoking, family history of thrombosis, or the presence of another condition, such as cancer.[10] Certain preventive measures, such as the administration of anticoagulation medication prior to surgery, can help prevent this condition. More information on deep vein thrombosis and how to treat it can be found in Chapter 10.

TIP Use a Screening Tool for Assessing Delirium

One tool organizations can use to assess delirium in patients is the Confusion Assessment Method. This is a two-part assessment involving a screen for overall cognitive impairment and a specific assessment for four features that are found to have the greatest ability to distinguish delirium or reversible confusion from other types of cognitive impairment.[7]

A pain management plan developed with the patient's assistance should be a crucial part of the preprocedure assessment. Pain should be reassessed at regular intervals to determine the patient's pain intensity, discomfort, and response to treatment. As with all pain management, organizations should use tools appropriate to the patient for assessing pain and consider the patient's report of pain as

Sidebar 4-3: Using Allergy Bands

To help easily communicate a patient's allergies, some organizations choose to use allergy bands. These bands offer a clear warning that a patient has allergies. The bands also can serve as a reliable source of information for clinicians, even when the patient is medicated, sedated, or confused. To be effective, allergy bands must be readily available and used throughout an organization in a standardized manner. If the use of bands is inconsistent, health care providers will not be able to reliably differentiate when a patient does not have allergies versus when a staff person forgot to apply the allergy band. Policies regarding allergy bands should clearly identify who assesses allergies, when the allergy band is applied, and how the allergy band is updated and verified. In addition, the information on the band should be readily visible, pertinent, and readable.

Source: Beyea S., Hicks R.: Oops—The patient is allergic to that medication—Patient safety first. *AORN J* Mar. 2003. http://www.findarticles.com/p/articles/mi_m0FSL/is_3_77/ai_99237614/print (accessed Jul. 20, 2010).

the gold standard. For patients who are unable to verbally communicate their level of pain, alternative methods should be used to perform the assessment, including the use of visual assessment of patient response or facial gestures and by speaking with the patient's family or caregiver.

Verifying the Correct Site, Side, Patient, and Procedure

Significant medical errors involving the wrong procedure site, procedure, and patient can and do occur in health care organizations around the world. Despite efforts to reduce the number and frequency of these events, the number is in fact increasing.[11] To help organizations avoid these medical disasters, The Joint Commission created the Universal Protocol for Preventing Wrong Site, Wrong Procedure, Wrong Person Surgery.™ This is a systematic preprocedure verification process that requires surgical teams to collect, verify, and cross-reference information about the patient's surgery, site, and side of surgery, and any other information necessary to ensure the correct procedure, patient, and operative site.

The Joint Commission requires U.S. health care organizations to use the Universal Protocol to help prevent wrong surgery. Joint Commission International (JCI) requires organizations outside the United States to develop an approach to ensuring correct site, procedure, and patient surgery. JCI standards emphasize the use of evidence-based practices, such as those described in the Universal Protocol and other tools, including the World Health Organization (WHO) Surgical Safety Checklist.

The preprocedure assessment process is an opportune time to discuss the procedure with the patient and collect information to confirm the correct site, side, and procedure. During the assessment process, surgical team members should involve the patient in the verification process as much as possible, confirm the details of the procedure, and ensure that those details match previous information documented in the medical record. Some information to confirm includes the patient's identity, the surgical site, the procedure to be performed, and patient consent. Any missing information or discrepancies should be addressed promptly.

More information about preventing wrong-site, wrong-procedure, wrong-person surgery and using the Universal Protocol and/or the WHO Surgical Safety Checklist can be found in Chapter 6.

Systematizing the Assessment Process

Like other aspects of surgical care, a systematic approach to the presurgical assessment is warranted to ensure that all relevant information and risks are captured, evaluated, and addressed. To help systematize the process, organizations may wish to use a checklist designed specifically for assessing issues related to surgery. As mentioned in Chapter 1, checklists can help providers remember to consider various risks and parts of a process and can also foster communication around particular topics. Such a checklist may include verification opportunities for specific risks (such as weight, nicotine use, or alcohol use) as well as prompts for particular information (such as the site of the operation, the procedure, and other details used to prevent wrong-site, wrong-procedure, wrong-person surgery).

After the presurgical assessment is completed, nurses and physicians should review it in depth before surgery to identify questionable or confusing information. In addition, a designated staff person, typically a nurse, should ensure that all needed assessments, including the history and physical, are available and complete prior to surgery. He or she can also compare information available in the assessments, laboratory reports, and various forms to ensure consistency.

Managing Medications

According to the United States Pharmacopeia, surgical patients are three times more likely to experience a harmful medication error than other patients in the health care system.[12] Not only is this statistic worrisome, but the fact that medication errors in surgery are more likely to cause patient harm than any other type of medical error is particularly troubling.[12]

The prevalence of medication errors in the operating room or procedure area is due, in part, because surgery and other invasive procedures take place in a fast-paced environment in which complex care is provided using high-tech equipment and high-alert drugs. These factors come together to set the stage for medication errors. Medication errors in surgery and other invasive procedures often involve the wrong medication or the wrong dose of medication. Although most medication errors occur within the operating room or procedure area or within the postprocedure setting, proactive efforts to prevent these errors begin in the preprocedural setting.

Part of preparing the patient for surgery or other invasive procedure involves determining and ordering the medications needed for the procedure, reconciling a patient's current medications with those he or she will receive during the procedure, and preparing the medications for the procedure. When these activities are done well, they can help prevent medication errors down the line. The following sections take a closer look at these activities. Further discussion of the medication management process can be found in subsequent chapters.

Determining and Ordering Appropriate Medications

Based on the preoperative assessment process, any risks identified within this process, and the nature of the procedure, the surgeon and the anesthesiologist will determine which medications are necessary for use in the operating room or procedure area. These medications may be anesthesia and sedation medications, antibiotics to prevent infection at the surgical site, pain medications, or others. A patient's allergies, preexisting medical conditions, and other potential risk factors will influence which medications are selected.

An important aspect of determining a proper medication is identifying the correct dose and concentration of that medication for the patient. Delivering the wrong dose of medication is one of the more frequent types of medication error in the surgical setting. One study at a major children's teaching hospital showed that the overwhelming majority of medication errors that occurred in the surgical area involved ordering the wrong dose of medication.[13]

Health care providers must be particularly careful when dosing medication for pediatric versus adult patients. Many drugs used in surgery, including those used in anesthesia, are not packaged in dilutions or doses that are appropriate for children. Conversions must be made to ensure that the dose is appropriate for the age and weight of the patient.[14] Standardized doses, including those for pediatric and adult patients, may help avoid the need to convert doses in the surgical setting. According to the U.S. Association of periOperative Registered Nurses (AORN), medications that are ordered using weight-based doses—for both pediatric patients and adults—should be independently calculated and verified by two licensed individuals.[15]

To help ensure proper dosing of medications, organizations may want to dedicate a pharmacist to oversee the medication management process in perioperative units. According to U.S. AORN, any written orders for medications in this setting should be reviewed by a pharmacist before dispensing. By reviewing orders, the pharmacist can address concerns and issues related to medication, dose, frequency, route of administration, therapeutic duplication, allergies, potential interaction, and contraindication.[15]

As with other aspects of surgery and other invasive procedures, technology can help improve efficiency and reduce error in the medication management process. For example, to standardize medication ordering, some organizations are implementing a computerized provider order entry (CPOE) system. Although shown to be beneficial in inpatient settings, such a system can also improve efficiency in the surgical setting.[16] This technology can reduce, if not eliminate, handwriting errors, it can link to medical records systems to improve communication, and it can provide alerts to signal potential dosing, duplication, or drug interaction errors.

Despite its benefits, CPOE has some limitations. Because of its use in many organizations, staff members may perceive that a CPOE system will address all possible medication risks, which can lead to a sense of overconfidence and reduce the effectiveness of clinicians' diligence with orders. In addition, the alarm feature included in many CPOE systems—designed to help alert providers to issues—can cause potential problems. If alarms are too frequent, providers may start to ignore the alarms and miss a critical issue.

In addition to CPOE, some organizations use automated dispensing machines in the surgical setting to help improve medication availability, increase the efficiency of drug dispensing and billing, and reduce errors. Such systems store medications and then dispense them in a controlled fashion. They are typically stocked by centralized or decentralized pharmacies and, depending on the system, can be accessed via a user identification number or biometric verification.[17] In some cases, the automated dispensing system includes a list of the patients scheduled for surgery and thus can match the appropriate medication with the patient.

Avoiding Dangerous Abbreviations

Within the health care environment, critical and sometimes lifesaving information must be communicated quickly and clearly. Unfortunately, when health care providers use some abbreviations, the communication can be quick but many times far from clear. There are countless stories of medication mistakes that resulted from the use of an abbreviation, such as the use of "U" for *unit.* Sometimes these mistakes can have tragic consequences, such as patient injury or even death. For example, when a prescriber uses the letter "U" instead of writing out the word *unit,* staff reading the prescription can mistake the "U" for a "0" or "4," thus resulting in an overdose. Depending on the medication and the patient, the overdose could be fatal.

The issue of dangerous abbreviations is by no means new: the Institute for Safe Medication Practices (ISMP) has been discussing this topic for more than 20 years, and The Joint Commission and JCI have been addressing it as well (*see* Sidebar 4-4 below). There are many ways to address dangerous abbreviations, including developing a "do-not use" list based on research and organizational experience. When developing policies related to dangerous abbreviations, organizations should involve physicians, nurses, and other providers who would use the abbreviations on a daily basis.

Reconciling Medications

In conjunction with determining and ordering medications for a surgical procedure, perioperative teams must reconcile those medications against ones the patient is currently taking to ensure that any new medications will not conflict with any existing medications or allergies. The process of reconciling medications before

Sidebar 4-4: Prohibited Abbreviations

The Joint Commission requires that organizations follow their own list of prohibited abbreviations, acronyms, symbols, and dose designations, which includes the following:

- U, u
- IU
- Q.D., QD, q.d., qd
- Q.O.D., QOD, q.o.d., qod
- Trailing zero (X.0 mg)
- Lack of leading zero (.X mg)
- MS
- MSO_4
- $MgSO_4$

Joint Commission International also requires organizations outside the United States to follow their own list of prohibited abbreviations. The abbreviations to be included on the list will vary depending on local and national standards.

surgery is critical to safe care. When perioperative teams did not effectively reconcile medications, there have been severe consequences. Inadequate medication reconciliation accounts for nearly 50% of all medication errors and up to 20% of adverse drug events among hospitalized patients.[18]

Health care providers in the operating room or procedure area should not prescribe medication before reviewing the medications that the patient is currently taking. Effective reconciliation involves multiple sources often spread across organizations and communities, including but not limited to the patient, caregiver or family member, primary care physician, medical specialists, outpatient medical records, previous hospital discharge summaries, and community pharmacies.[19] Information coming from these sources can vary widely, resulting in duplication of information in some areas and insufficient information in others. Because of its many moving parts, the process of medication reconciliation is often haphazard and disjointed. If there is not a standardized approach for collecting, documenting, and reconciling information, there is the potential to collect incomplete patient medication information, which results in the opportunity for error.[20]

Some patients are more at risk for inadequate medication reconciliation than others. For example, older patients are increasingly receiving care from multiple specialists and other health care providers, each of whom may be prescribing medication. This can lead to the potential for conflicting prescriptions and adverse drug reactions. In addition, older adults are more likely to take multiple medications, which can increase the chance of negative drug interactions if providers are not aware of all the medications the patient is taking. Patients taking multiple medications prescribed from different providers may also be more likely to fill their prescriptions at multiple pharmacies, thus creating even more confusion.

In addition to older adults, people with chronic conditions who are taking multiple medications can be prone to medication error associated with inadequate medication reconciliation, particularly as more and more drugs are being introduced into the market and many of them have complex or look-alike/sound-alike names that can be easily confused with one another.

Studies have shown that limited health literacy is associated with a greater number of unreconciled medications.[21] Individuals with literacy issues can be prone to medication reconciliation–related errors because these individuals may not understand what medications they are taking and for what reasons. Medication reconciliation can be particularly challenging for patients with low literacy if they see one or more specialists in addition to their primary care physician and/or if they purchase their medications through several different venues (mail-order versus pharmacy with insurance versus discount pharmacy) to get the best prices.

Patients who have trouble remembering what medications they are taking—whether this poor recall is because of dementia, confusion, lack of understanding, stress, or a lack of commitment to the reconciliation process—also put themselves at risk. In addition, if a patient has an attitude that runs contrary to the reconciliation process, the chances that the provider will be able to adequately reconcile the patient's medications is slim. For example, if a patient believes that his or her medications are "nobody else's business," then he or she will be less or not involved in the reconciliation process, thus putting himself or herself at risk for poor reconciliation.

As with other aspects of surgical care, a systematic approach to medication reconciliation can ensure the efficiency, accuracy, and effectiveness of the process. Developing a team to tackle the reconciliation process across an organization, and specifically within the surgical setting, can be beneficial. As discussed in Chapter 2, using a systematic improvement methodology, such as Lean Six Sigma, may be helpful in redesigning the process.

One aspect to focus on when designing or redesigning reconciliation processes is the method by which information is collected in the surgical setting. A structured interview process can help providers obtain important information about a patient's medications and allergies and how frequently he or she takes those medications. To elicit the most comprehensive information, this interview process should involve specific, open-ended questions about patient health and medications. (*See* Sidebar 4-5 on page 66.)

Sidebar 4-5: Questions That Can Help with Medication Reconciliation

When asking patients about their medications, health care providers should try to use open-ended questions. Following are some possible categories of questions with specific examples that could be helpful when interviewing a patient about his or her medication list.

Questions about medical conditions

- What do you take for your high blood pressure? Diabetes? Asthma?
- I read on your chart that you had an ear infection a few weeks ago. What medication did you take to treat that? Are you still taking that medication?
- Six months ago you had knee surgery, yes? Are you taking any pain medication to help in recovery?

Questions about medication route

- What medications do you swallow in pill form?
- What medications do you take that are liquid?
- Do you put any medications on your skin?
- Do you take any eyedrops? If so, which ones?

Tip: Patients often forget to mention creams, ointments, lotions, patches, eyedrops, eardrops, nebulizers, and inhalers when citing their current medications. Asking specific questions about these types of medications may help improve the accuracy of the medication list.

Questions about the patient's various physicians and other providers who could prescribe medication

- Does your "arthritis doctor" prescribe any medications for you?
- Does your therapist prescribe medications for you?
- Have you visited an urgent care center recently for any reason? Did they prescribe medication for you?

Questions about medication timing

- What time of day do you take your medications?
- Are there some medications you take only once a week? Once a month? As needed?

Questions about new medications

- Have any of your doctors recently started you on new medication?
- If so, what was the name of the medication? When do you take it? How long have you taken it?

Questions about discontinuing medication

- Have any of your doctors told you to stop taking one or more of your medications?
- If so, which medications? How long ago did you stop taking these medications?

Questions about over-the-counter (nonprescription) medications, including herbal supplements and vitamins

- Are you taking any over-the-counter medications? Any herbal or dietary supplements? Or vitamins?
- What do you take when you get a headache?
- What do you take for allergies?
- Do you take anything to help you fall asleep?
- What do you take when you get a cold?
- Do you take anything for heartburn?

In addition to these questions, asking patients to describe their medication by color, size, shape, and other distinguishing characteristics may help determine dosage strength and formulation for particular medications.

To help capture information about patient medications, many organizations create a form that staff and/or the patient can fill out to document the patient's current prescription medications, over-the-counter (nonprescription) medications, herbal supplements, and dietary supplements as well as doses, providers, and other pertinent information. Such a form also allows documentation of whether medication information came from a patient-provided list, patient or family recall, a pharmacy, the primary care physician, information existing in the patient's medication record, or the medication administration record of another facility or institution.

This type of tool can be particularly helpful when reconciling medications across various providers. To help ensure consistent use, the form should be placed in a highly visibly location within the patient chart so it is easily accessible by all clinicians writing orders. Use of the form should also be clearly outlined within organization policy. The form may be electronic in organizations that use electronic health record systems.

Technology can be used to automate reconciliation forms. By integrating medication reconciliation with the organization's CPOE system and electronic medical record, for example, an organization can ensure an up-to-date list that can be easily accessed at critical points in the care continuum and can also be shared with other providers.

There are several benefits to electronic medication reconciliation, including the following:

- Medication lists are easily accessible, and health care providers will not need to keep track of paper lists.
- Patients, families, and the organization can all have printed copies of the current medication list at any time, particularly upon discharge or transfer.
- Medication lists have the potential for being more accurate.
- Multiple prescribers and staff members can easily access the medication list at the same time.
- Providers within various sites of an organization—for example, the surgery department, ambulatory care clinic, or home care program—can communicate better about patient medications.

Medication reconciliation technology can be particularly helpful in large integrated health systems where the organization can maintain a common medication profile for both outpatient and inpatient visits. Even in these cases, however, providers must rely on the patient to report prescriptions and over-the-counter medications obtained from outside the system. Patient portal products seem to have great potential to facilitate this partnership by allowing both provider and patient to view and modify select drug history content.[22]

Data about medication reconciliation in the surgical setting should be collected and analyzed to be certain that current reconciliation processes are effective. Such data collection can also reveal potential areas of improvement. Organizations can collect data on medication reconciliation in a variety of ways, including by monitoring the number of medication errors occurring in the surgical setting, asking patients about the medication reconciliation process, and observing the medication reconciliation process and documenting how it is performed. This may include a validation of the entire process by physically following the patient/list/orders through the entire system.

Although all of the previous performance measurement methods can be helpful in determining the effectiveness of a medication reconciliation program, a combination of these approaches may be most helpful in determining the success of the program.

Preparing Medications for Surgery

In the perioperative setting, the medication preparation process is different than in other settings. Medications are often removed from manufacturers' identifying containers and placed in cups, syringes, or other delivery devices. Often the individual administering the medication is not the person who prepares it. Depending on the situation, as many as three individuals can be involved before the patient receives the medication: the circulating nurse, the scrub nurse, and the physician.[23] Even though all these providers are members of the perioperative team, they often work in different locations and stages of the surgical continuum and thus may not communicate with one another. For example, to prepare a local injection, a circulating nurse may draw up the medication from the manufacturer's vial before a procedure. When he or she moves it to the sterile field, he or she then goes on to other tasks and responsibilities. At some point, the scrub nurse will prepare the delivery device so that it is available when the surgeon is ready to administer it. The surgeon is the individual who actually administers the medication. With each individual involved in the preparation and delivery process, the risk for medication error goes up.[23]

One critical effort to avoid medication errors involved in the preparation process is effective labeling. This includes labeling the container the medication or solution is in and the device used to deliver the solution. Errors have resulted from medications and other solutions being removed from their original containers and placed into unlabeled containers.

Despite its importance, medication labeling in the surgical setting does not take place as often as it should. A survey by the ISMP showed that 41% of individuals surveyed always label containers on the sterile field, 18% do not label at all, and 42% label inconsistently.[24] The Joint Commission National Patient Safety Goal requiring medication labeling often has been among the requirements that surveyors identify most frequently as "not compliant." In 2009, for example, 20% of organizations in the ambulatory care program and 19% of organizations in the office-based surgery program were found not compliant with the goal.[25] Hospitals also have found the goal challenging.

The Joint Commission, JCI, the World Health Organization (WHO), the ISMP, AORN, and other safety-focused organizations around the world have specific requirements or recommendations related to labeling medications. According to these organizations, providers should label all containers and syringes both on and off the sterile field except when an individual removes a medication from its original container and immediately administers it. If an unlabeled container or device is found, it should be discarded immediately because the content of the container cannot be verified.[24] JCI also requires that medications, and chemicals used to prepare medications, be accurately labeled with contents, expiration dates, and warnings.

Labels are the primary "drug/user" interface.[23] All labels should include the following information about the medication:

- Name
- Strength
- Amount
- Expiration date or time, depending on when the medication will expire
- Diluent and volume (if not apparent from the container)
- Preparation date

One recent study from Switzerland showed that standardizing information on drug labels substantially improved human performance when selecting medication. Specifically, standardized labels for injectable medication that mentioned concentration, amount, and volume produced the lowest rate of selection errors and the most rapid selection of the correct product.[26]

To help standardize labeling, organizations may want to consider premade labels for frequently used medications. They can be part of a drug labeling kit that contains both premade labels for frequently used medication and some blank labels to be filled in for infrequently used medications. Waterproof marking pens can also be included in these kits, which can be kept in the operative and preoperative areas.[23] One organization that tested a labeling kit found that scrub personnel were more likely to label medications and medication-delivery devices when preprinted labels were provided.[23]

When labeling syringes, organizations should consider different kinds of labels for various types of syringes. For example, sterile medication labels may adhere best to aseptos syringes because there is more flat surface on the cylinder of the syringe on which to apply the label. Labels may not adhere well to bulb syringes because the surface of such syringes is round, flexible, and often has ridges. Labels that do not adhere adequately to a bulb syringe could increase the risks of leaving foreign bodies in the surgical wound (*see* Chapter 8). Consequently, using a sterile indelible marker to write directly on the bulb may be a more suitable strategy for labeling bulb syringes.[27]

It is important to note that perioperative staff should not label more than one medication at a time but should completely label one medication and deliver it to the surgical field before preparing and labeling another medication. Doing so prevents inadvertent medication mix-ups and confusion.

TIP Consult the Manufacturer

Medication manufacturers can play an important role in medication safety in the operating room or procedure area. For example, organizations should work with manufacturers to use distinctive labels for medications and solutions. In addition, manufacturers should be encouraged to provide medications and solutions in ready-to-use or ready-to-administer containers that will allow for sterile delivery of medications to the sterile field.[28]

Determining, Ordering, and Preparing Antibiotics

One important type of medication, which is used in almost all surgical procedures, is antibiotics. Delivery of appropriate, intravenous antibiotics within one hour before surgical incision (some may be given at different intervals in accordance with manufacturer's guidelines) is the most effective method to reduce the risk of surgical site infection. It is estimated that 40% to 60% of all surgical infections could be prevented by appropriate antibiotic prophylaxis and other measures. Antimicrobial agents for prophylaxis for a particular procedure should be administered according to methods cited in scientific literature or endorsed by professional organizations.

The goal of antimicrobial prophylaxis is to reduce the risk of site contamination to a level that the patient's immune system can handle. Optimal administration requires appropriate antibiotics, initiation within 30 to 60 minutes of incision, and discontinuation within 24 hours after surgery. (Discontinuation within 48 hours is allowable for cardiothoracic procedures for adult patients.[30])Depending on the nature of the wound, the duration of antibiotics will vary. For example, dirty or contaminated wounds may require a longer course of antibiotics than clean ones. (*See* Chapter 10 for a discussion of different types of wounds.) If a procedure is delayed by more than one hour, antibiotics should be readministered.

TIP Standardize Timing of Antibiotics

To help ensure proper timing of antibiotics, organizations should consider standardizing the process as much as possible. This might include storing antibiotics in ready-to-administer doses in the operating room or procedure area.[29]

To ensure the appropriate timing of antibiotic administration, health care organizations should designate responsibility for administration. This responsibility could go to anesthesiologists, circulating nurses, or preoperative nurses. Electronic reminders in a medical record, anesthesia management system, or CPOE system can help trigger the designated provider to administer the antibiotics.

Someone should also be designated to document the dose and incision time. Verification of administration can be part of a preoperative checklist or another type of standardized documentation form. By assigning responsibility for both administration and documentation, the health care organization can review their timing and see whether improvements need to be made. Involving providers in designing the process of administering and documenting the use of antibiotics can help ensure that the process works well within existing work flow and practice.[30]

When organizations select the appropriate antibiotic for antibiotic prophylaxis, the selection will vary depending on the pathogens most commonly associated with the procedure being performed.[31] Published guidelines recommend that antibiotic selection should take into account the expected flora, the ability of the antibiotic agent to reach the target tissues at appropriate concentrations, bacterial resistance patterns, and drug pharmocokinetics.[32]

To ensure consistent and appropriate antibiotic selection, organizations may want to develop a protocol and standardized order form. The American Society of Health-System Pharmacists and the U.S. Centers for Disease Control and Prevention (U.S. CDC) have developed guidelines for appropriate antibiotic selection. When developing a prophylactic antibiotic protocol and order form, organizations should review and consider these guidelines. In addition, health care organizations should consider physician input and their formulary. By standardizing the process, organizations can decrease the need to write unique antibiotic orders for each patient, which can prevent prescription errors or omission. A preprinted or automated order form will specify antibiotic, timing, dose, and discontinuation time.[33] A good protocol will contain clear guidance for health care providers as to appropriate substitutions in case of allergies or when a physician should be contacted for a different order.[29]

TIP Pay Attention to the Blood Pressure Cuff

If the patient requires a blood pressure cuff during surgery, and the cuff is to be applied near the surgical site, the dose should be fully infused prior to cuff inflation, otherwise the cuff may prevent the full dose from reaching the site.[29]

Preparing the Surgical Site

A final step in getting the patient ready for surgery or another invasive procedure is preparing the surgical site. The surgical site must be prepared so as to limit the spread of bacteria and other contaminants into the incision area. Appropriately preparing the surgical site is essential to reducing the likelihood of surgical site infections (SSIs).

Surgical site infections are a problem for health care organizations worldwide. In the United States alone, SSIs occur in 2% to 5% of patients undergoing surgery, with approximately 500,000 SSIs occurring annually. In developing countries around the world, surgical site infections are the most frequent type of infection, occurring at a rate of 1% to almost 25% per 100 surgical procedures. SSI rates are 2% to 3% per 100 surgical procedures in developed countries.[34] Studies show that patients who develop surgical site infections are at least twice as likely to die, are more likely to require an intensive care unit admission, remain in the hospital between 7 and 10 days longer, and cost an organization in the United States between $3,000 and $29,000 more than surgery patients who do not develop an SSI.[35] Patients can experience significant pain with an SSI as well as a longer period of recuperation and an extended inability to return to activities of daily living.[36]

Surgical site preparation is a three-tiered process. The first tier involves having the patient perform a preoperative shower or bath using an antiseptic agent, preferably one containing chlorhexidine gluconate—this substance is preferred because of its persistence. Hair should also be washed with antiseptic solution.[37] For this first tier of the process to be most effective, the patient should bathe or shower the night before and the morning of the surgical procedure. If the patient is hospitalized, health care providers should make sure that the chlorhexidine bath is administered.

TIP Consider When Hair Removal Is Not an Option

In some cultures, removing facial hair is problematic, and patients may refuse to allow their hair to be clipped or trimmed. One study showed that the use of a synthetic leather mask on patients with facial hair resulted in no displacement of the endotracheal tube, no pressure on the neck veins, and no skin reaction. This mask is made in several sizes and can be reused. It is suitable for laryngoscopy, suctioning, and inserting the oral airway.[38]

The second consideration is hair removal. Hair removal at the site should be avoided unless it is absolutely necessary to do so to effectively carry out the procedure. When hair removal is necessary, use a method that is cited in scientific literature or endorsed by professional organizations. During this second phase of preparation, an organization's policy may dictate that the surgical site be marked to prevent wrong-site, wrong-procedure, and wrong-person surgery. This marking should be done with a marker or pen that ensures the site marking is clear and visible after the patient has been prepped and draped. There has been some concern about the infection risks associated with site marking. Various studies have shown this infection risk to be negligible. For example, a study conducted by a group of researchers at the University of Alberta in Edmonton found that Sharpie pens are safe to use as surgical markers.[39] (More information about marking the surgical site can be found in Chapter 6.)

The final phase of surgical skin preparation involves the use of antiseptics applied immediately prior to the surgical procedure. Such application helps remove soil and transient microorganisms from the skin, reduce the microbial count in a short period of time with minimal tissue irritation, and inhibit rapid rebound growth of microorganisms.[40]

There are several types of antiseptic agents appropriate for use in the operating room or procedure area, including isopropyl alcohol, povidone-iodine, chlorhexidine combined with isopropyl alcohol, and chlorhexidine alone.[41] Although effective as a rapid-acting skin antiseptic, the use of alcohol in surgical preparation is often limited because of potential flammability issues. (More about this topic can be found in Chapter 8.)

Chlorhexidine acts to disrupt bacteria at the cellular level and is known for its long-lasting activity against gram positive and gram negative bacteria.[42] In addition, chlorhexidine gluconate is not inactivated in the presence of blood and so can remain effective at preventing infection even during surgery.[43]

An antiseptic made up of a combination of two antiseptics with different mechanisms of action can be even better at fighting bacteria. For example, the use of chlorhexidine plus 70% isopropyl alcohol has demonstrated a positive effect against a wide range of bacteria, including antibiotic-resistant bacteria.[44] Although povidone-iodine is used in almost 75% of all surgeries to prepare patient skin, a chlorhexadine-alcohol solution may be more effective at preventing SSIs. In a recent clinical trial, the use of such a solution yielded a 41% reduction is SSIs.[45] Since 2002, the U.S. CDC has recommended the use of a chlorhexidine-alcohol solution for skin cleansing of the insertion site for vascular catheters; however, a similar recommendation does not currently exist for surgical site preparation.[45]

When choosing which antiseptic to use across the surgical setting, health care organizations should consider a number of factors, including the efficacy of the antiseptic, the type of procedures for which it will be used, the safety issues surrounding the product, and the effects it will have on the staff using it. Health care organizations should conduct careful research and determine a consistent antiseptic to use.

When preparing the patient's skin, health care providers should keep the antiseptic on the skin for one to two minutes or until it dries naturally on its own. Areas of higher microbial counts, such as the umbilicus or open wounds, should be prepared last. Any open, contaminated areas should be covered with an antiseptic-soaked sponge until it is time to prep the area. This area should be prepped last. When preparing the skin of burn patients, health care providers should use normal saline.[46,47]

After proper asepsis of the surgical or procedural site, a sterile drape should be used to cover the patient during surgery to further protect him or her from harm.[48] It is important to note that individuals preparing the site should not allow the antiseptic agent to pool beneath patients or other equipment placed on the patient—such as electrodes—to reduce the risk of chemical burns.[47]

One recent approach to reducing the potential for SSI is a microbial surgical sealant. This is a film-forming liquid that is applied to the site after the typical skin preparation. It coats the skin with the intent of isolating and immobilizing any surviving skin flora, including those that remain in hair follicles. In theory, this reduces the risk of surgical wound contamination by skin flora during the procedure. One study showed that patients treated with a sealant were more likely to have no bacterial cells found in the surgical wounds. None of the patients receiving the sealant developed an SSI.[49] Other studies have shown that a microbial sealant improves the effectiveness of povidone iodine by sealing it on the skin.[50] In general, sealants are thought to be easy to apply and use with a variety of skin preparation solutions and wound closure techniques.[50] More information on avoiding surgical site infections can be found in Chapter 8.

References

1. Fry D., et al.: Patient characteristics and the occurrence of never events. *Arch Surg* 145:148–151, Feb. 2010.
2. Halliday A.: Shades of sedation: Learning about moderate sedation and analgesia. *Nursing* 36:36–41, Apr. 2006.
3. Gawande A.: *The Checklist Manifesto: How to Get Things Right.* New York: Metropolitan Books, 2009.
4. Blaney-Koen L., Dickey N.: Safe surgery: A patient's guide. *J Patient Saf* 3:56, Mar. 2007.
5. Kain Z., et al.: Preoperative anxiety, postoperative pain, and behavioral recovery in young children undergoing surgery. *Pediatrics* 118:651–658, Aug. 2006.
6. McCurren C., Cronin S.: Delirium: Elders tell their stories and guide nursing practice. *Medsurg Nurs* 12:318–323, Oct. 2003.
7. Waszynski C.: Confusion Assessment Method (CAM). *Try This: Best Practices in Nursing Care to Older Adults* 13, Hartford Institute for Geriatric Nursing, Nov. 2001. http://consultgerirn.org/uploads/File/Confusion%20 Assessment%20Method%20(CAM).pdf (accessed Jul. 24, 2010).
8. Pear S.: Patient risk factors and best practices for surgical site infection prevention. *Managing Infection Control,* pp. 56–64, Mar. 2007.
9. Lieberman J., Hsu W.: Prevention of venous thromboembolic disease after total hip and knee arthroplasty. *J Bone Joint Surg AM* 87:2097–2112, Sep. 2005.
10. American Academy of Orthopaedic Surgeons (AAOS): *Clinical Guideline on Prevention of Pulmonary Embolism in Patients Undergoing Total Hip or Knee Arthoplasty.* Rosemont, IL: AAOS, 2007.
11. World Health Organization Collaborating Centre for Patient Safety Solutions: Performance of correct procedure at correct body site. *Patient Safety Solutions* 1, May 2007.
12. ABCNews.com: *Study Finds Widespread Medication Errors During Surgery: When Do Mistakes Most Often Occur and What Should Patients Do?* Mar. 6, 2007. http://abcnews.go.com/GMA/OnCall/story?id=2927047&page=1 (accessed Jul. 24, 2010).
13. Engum S., Breckler F.: An evaluation of medication errors—The pediatric surgical service experience. *J Pediatr Surg* 43:348–352, Feb. 2008.

14. Thompson C.: Surgical units have high potential for harmful medication errors, USP says. *Am J Health Syst Pharm* 64:917, 920, May 2007.
15. AORN guidance statement: Safe medication practices in perioperative settings across the life span. *AORN J* 84:276–283, Aug. 2006.
16. Stone W., et al.: Impact of a computerized physician order-entry system. *J Am Coll Surg* 208:960–967, May 2009.
17. Murray M.: Automated medication dispensing devices. In Shojania K., et al. (eds.): *Making Health Care Safer: A Critical Analysis of Patient Safety Practices.* Agency for Healthcare Research and Quality, Jul. 20, 2001. http://archive.ahrq.gov/clinic/ptsafety/chap11.htm (accessed Jul. 24, 2010).
18. Varkey P., Cunningham J., Bisping D.: Improving medication reconciliation in the outpatient setting. *Jt Comm J Qual Patient Saf* 33:286–292, May 2007.
19. Poon E., et al.: Design and implementation of an application and associated services to support interdisciplinary medication reconciliation efforts at an integrated healthcare delivery network. *J Am Med Inform Assoc* 13:581–592, Nov.–Dec. 2006.
20. Health Forum: Medication reconciliation: Medication safety issue brief. *Hospitals & Health Networks* 79, Sep. 2005.
21. Persell S., et al.: Limited health literacy is a barrier to medication reconciliation in ambulatory care. *J Gen Intern Med* 22:1523–1526, Nov. 2007.
22. Pinakiewicz D. (moderator), O'Donnell S., Scheckelhoff K., Chochinov J.: High-Tech Medication Management [podcast]. Future Healthcare. Q1:66–74, 2008.
23. Jennings J., Foster J.: Medication Safety: Just a label away. *AORN J* 86:618–625, Oct. 2007.
24. Institute for Safe Medication Practices (ISMP): Loud wake-up call: Unlabeled containers lead to patient's death. *ISMP Medication Safety Alert! Acute Care,* Dec. 2, 2004. http://www.ismp.org/newsletters/acutecare/articles/20041202.asp (accessed Jul. 24, 2010).
25. Top 10 standards compliance issues in 2009. *Jt Comm Perspect* 30:5–10, May 2010.
26. Garnerin P., et al.: Drug selection errors in relation to medication labels: A simulation study. *Anaesthesia* 62:1090–1094, Nov. 2007.
27. Connor R.: Clinical issues: Medication labeling. *AORN J* 82:869–879, Nov. 2005.
28. AORN guidance statement—Safe medication practices in perioperative practice settings. *AORN J* 79:674–676, Mar. 2004.
29. Griffin F.: Best-practice protocols: Preventing surgical site infection. *Nurs Manage* 36:20–26, Nov. 2005.
30. O'Reilly M., et al.: An anesthesia information system designed to provide physician-specific feedback improves timely administration of prophylactic antibiotics. *Anesth Analg* 103:908–912, Oct. 2006.
31. Owens C., Stoessel K.: Surgical site infections: Epidemiology, microbiology, and prevention. *J Hosp Infect* 70(suppl. 2):3–10, Nov. 2008.
32. Dohmen P.: Antibiotic resistance in common pathogens reinforces the need to minmise surgical site infections. *J Hosp Infect* 70(suppl. 2):15–20, Nov. 2008.
33. Institute for Healthcare Improvement (IHI): *Getting Started Kit: Preventing Surgical Site Infections How-to Guide.* Boston: IHI, 2008.
34. World Health Organization: *The Burden of Health Care–Associated Infection Worldwide.* http://www.who.int/gpsc/country_work/burden_hcai/en/index.html (accessed Jul. 24, 2010).
35. Anderson D., et al.: Strategies to prevent surgical site infections in acute care hospitals. *Infect Control Hosp Epidemiol* 29(suppl. 1):S51–S61, Oct. 2008.
36. Murkin C.: Pre-operative antiseptic skin preparation. *Br J Nurs* 18:665–668, Jun. 2009.
37. Tanner J., Khan D.: Surgical site infection, preoperative body washing and hair removal. *J Perioper Pract* 18:232, 237–243, Jun. 2008.
38. Kamalipour H., Kardan K.: New method for the fixation of the endotracheal tube in patients with facial hair. *East Mediterr Health J* 9, Jan. 2003. http://www.emro.who.int/publications/emhj/0901_2/newMethods.htm (accessed Jul. 24, 2010).
39. Smith M.: ICAAC-IDSA: Re-using Sharpie pens as surgical marker in OR gets clean bill. *Medpage Today,* Oct. 23, 2008. http://www.medpagetoday.com/MeetingCoverage/ICAAC-IDSA/11440 (accessed Jul. 24, 2010).
40. Association of periOperative Registered Nurses (AORN): *Recommended Practices for Safe Preoperative Skin Antisepsis.* Denver: AORN, 2008.
41. Hibbard J.: Analyses comparing the antimicrobial activity and safety of current antiseptic agents: A review. *J Infusion Nurs* 28:194–207, May–Jun. 2005.
42. Fletcher N., et al.: Prevention of perioperative infection. *J Bone Joint Surg Am* 89:1605–1618, Jul. 2007.
43. Florman S., Nichols L.: Current approaches for the prevention of surgical site infections. *Am J Infect Dis* 3:51–61, Jan. 2007.
44. Paulson D.: Efficacy of preoperative antimicrobial skin preparation solutions on biofilm bacteria. *AORN J* 81:492–501, Mar. 2005.
45. Game changer: Clinical trial sets new standard of care for preventing surgical-site infections. *Hospital Infection Control & Prevention* 37:13–24, Feb. 2010.
46. Blanchard J., Chobin N.: The operating room. In Jarvis W. (ed.): *Bennett & Brachman's Hospital Infections,* 5th ed. Philadelphia: Lippincott Williams & Wilkins, 2007, pp. 449–460.
47. Association of periOperative Registered Nurses (AORN): Recommended practices for skin preparation of patients. In *Standards, Recommended Practices, and Guidelines.* Denver: AORN, 2007, pp. 654–655.
48. Roy M.: Operating room. In Wenzel R., Brewer T., Butzler J. (eds.): *A Guide to Infection Control in the Hospital.* Boston: International Society for Infectious Diseases, 2002, pp. 68–71.
49. Towfigh S., et al.: Significant reduction in incidence of wound contamination by skin flora through use of microbial sealant. *Arch Surg* 143:885–891, Sep. 2008.
50. Wilson S.: Microbial sealing: A new approach to reducing contamination. *J Hosp Infect* 70(suppl. 2):11–14. Nov. 2008.

Chapter 5

Preparing the Surgical Team

A team is group of people who work together to achieve a common purpose. In sports, teams around the world work together to execute plays, interact fairly, and win games or matches. Before every sporting event, a team comes together to prepare for the event. This preparation process involves donning appropriate uniforms and conferring just prior to the event to exchange information, identify issues, and plan strategy.

A surgical team is like a sports team whose common purpose is to safely and effectively perform a procedure that improves a patient's quality of life. Before every procedure, the surgical team should come together and prepare. This preparation involves donning proper attire and briefly meeting to set the stage for the procedure and the events to come. This chapter takes a brief look at the surgical team's preparation process and provides some tips and strategies on how to enhance that process.

Surgical Attire

To prevent the spread of infection to and from the patient, health care providers involved in surgery and other invasive procedures must wear specific surgical attire—for example, gowns, shoes, and caps—that contains any bacterial shedding from the provider and promotes environmental control.[1,2] In addition, health care providers must wear other personal protective equipment that serves as barrier precautions to protect mucous membranes, airways, skin, and clothing from contact with infectious agents.[3] Such personal protective equipment includes masks, protective eyewear (if a splatter is anticipated), a face shield (if a splash is anticipated), and fluid-resistant attire during activities that generate splashes, splatters, sprays, or aerosols.[4] In addition, health care providers must wear gloves.

In 2010 the U.S. Association for periOperative Registered Nurses (AORN) released a comprehensive list of recommended practices for surgical attire. Following is a summary of several of the recommended practices[5]:

- Surgical attire selected for use in the perioperative setting should be made of low-linting material; minimize bacterial shedding; and provide comfort, safety, and a professional appearance. Surgical fabrics should be breathable and lightweight while promoting stain resistance, minimal linting, and durability. Surgical attire should not be made of cotton because the pores in cotton may allow microorganisms to pass through the material. Cotton is also flammable and is not as effective at reducing bacterial load as noncotton materials.[1,6–8]
- Protective shoes must be worn in the perioperative environment. Shoes should have closed toes, low heels, and nonskid soles. Closed toes will help protect staff from falling or rolling objects, sharps injuries, spilled liquids, or other items that are inadvertently dropped or kicked in the surgical setting. In addition, low heels and nonskid soles reduce the risks of slips and falls. Shoes should be cleaned regularly and have no visible soiling.
- Facility-approved, clean, and freshly laundered surgical attire should be donned in a designated dressing area of the perioperative suite before entry or reentry into semirestricted and restricted areas of the suite.[9] (*See* Chapter 3 for definitions of these areas.) Doing so ensures privacy, prevents cross-contamination, and helps traffic control, as well as provides an area for secure storage of personal and facility-owned attire. Any surgical attire worn from outside of the health care facility should be changed before entering the semirestricted or restricted areas.

- Before donning surgical attire, all persons entering the perioperative suite should clean their hands with soap and water, antiseptic and water, or an antiseptic hand rub if visible soil is not present upon arrival.[10] As discussed in Chapter 2, hand washing removes soil, organic material, and microorganisms, thus helping prevent the spread of infection in the surgical area.
- Surgical attire should be changed daily and also when it becomes visibly soiled, contaminated, or wet.[9,11] When wearing a two-piece scrub suit, the top of the scrub suit should be secured at the waist, tucked into the pants, or fit close to the body. Loose scrub tops may contaminate the sterile field and allow shedded skin cells to disperse into the environment.
- All personnel should cover head and facial hair, including sideburns and nape of the neck, when in the semirestricted and restricted areas of the surgical suite. A clean, low-lint surgical head cover or hood that confines all hair and covers scalp skin should be worn. The head cover or hood should be designed to minimize microbial dispersal. It is important to note that skullcaps may fail to contain the side hair above and in front of the ears and hair at the nape of the neck. Consequently, these types of head coverings should be avoided if they do not cover all head and facial hair.
- Persons entering the semirestricted or restricted areas for a brief time for a specific purpose—such as law enforcement officers, administrators, parents, or biomedical engineers—should cover all head and facial hair and may don either freshly laundered surgical attire or a single-use jumpsuit (sometimes known as a coverall or bunny suit) designed to totally cover outside apparel.
- Personal protective equipment must be made available and worn to reduce the risk of exposure to potentially infectious material.[3,11] Specifically, protective equipment, including liquid-resistant eyewear, masks, respirators, gowns, gloves, aprons, and shoe covers, must be worn when exposure to blood or other potentially infectious materials is anticipated, such as during trauma procedures.[3]
- All individuals entering the restricted areas of the perioperative suite should wear a mask when open sterile supplies and equipment are present.[9] All individuals should don a mask before setting up a sterile procedure. A surgical mask protects both the surgical team and the patient from transfer of microorganisms.[9] The mask should cover the mouth and nose and be secured in a manner to prevent venting.
- Surgical attire should be laundered in a health care–approved or accredited laundry facility. This is one of the more controversial topics addressed in the AORN guidelines. Currently some organizations require their health care providers to launder used surgical attire at home in order to save on organization costs. However, the use of health care–approved and accredited laundry facilities is preferred because they follow industry standards in the United States. The Healthcare Laundry Accreditation Council offers voluntary accreditation for those laundry facilities that process reusable textiles and which incorporate U.S. Occupational Safety and Health Administration (OSHA) and U.S. Centers for Disease Control and Prevention (U.S. CDC) guidelines and professional association recommended practices. Using a laundry facility that is accredited ensures that the laundry facility has met stringent guidelines for cleaning, drying, and ironing. Home laundries may not meet the specified measures necessary to achieve a decrease in microbial levels in soiled surgical attire and thus can present a risk to providers and their families for the spread of infection.
- Health care personnel should receive education, guidance, and competency validation on appropriate surgical attire. Competency assessment should verify that health care personnel have an understanding of the articles and purpose of surgical attire. This knowledge is essential in reducing the risk of health care–associated infections.[12]

For a complete listing, see AORN's *Perioperative Standards and Recommended Practices,* 2010 edition.

When considering policies and procedures for surgical attire and other personal protective equipment, organizations should consider reviewing the AORN guidelines in full as well as standards and requirements from the U.S. CDC, U.S. OSHA, and the international Association for Professionals in Infection Control and Epidemiology. Providers should be well trained on the policies and procedures of the organization, and a monitoring process should be in place to ensure that appropriate apparel is being worn and cleaned according to organization policy.

Ensuring the Proper Use of Gloves

Although all surgical attire plays a critical role in the surgical setting, gloves are probably the most important personal protective equipment worn during surgery because they protect health care providers from pathogen exposure. Regarding infection, gloves reduce hand contamination by 70% to 80%, prevent cross-contamination, and protect patients and health care personnel from infection.[13]

In addition to its surgical attire recommendations, AORN also recommends the following gloving strategies to help prevent and control infections. Many of these apply to the surgical setting[4]:

- Gloves should provide an effective barrier against infectious materials, including blood and body fluids.
- PVC gloves should be used only during short, low-risk exposures.
- The manufacturer's guidelines should be consulted for glove use with chemicals. Some chemicals may cause breakdown of the gloves.
- Nonsterile gloves should be changed after each patient contact, when a visible defect or perforation is noticed or suspected, and according to organization policy.
- Sterile gloves should be changed after each patient contact, when a visible defect is noticed, when suspected or actual contamination occurs, when perforation is suspected, immediately following contact with uncured methyl methacrylate, when unintentional electrical shock is received to the hands, and according to organization policy.
- Gloves should not be washed and reused.
- During invasive procedures, health care providers should wear two pairs of gloves, one on top of the other.

Throughout a procedure, gloves can become contaminated and should be changed frequently. When changing contaminated gloves in the operating room or procedure area, health care providers should work with a partner, if possible. It is preferred that one member of the sterile team glove another. If this is not possible, then the individual should advance his or her scrubbed hands through the sleeves and cuffs of the surgical gown before placing them into the gloves.[14]

There are many varieties of surgical gloves, including latex, polyisoprene, nitrile, neoprene, and others. Despite the variety, many health care providers in the surgical department prefer powder-free latex gloves because of their fit, feel, comfort, and level of protection.[14] In fact, alcohol-based hand rubs can interact with powder in gloves and produce a gritty feeling on the hands.[15]

When choosing gloves, health care organizations should seek the opinion of health care providers who work in the surgery department or procedure area to ensure that the gloves available in the organization will be worn. Working with manufacturers to host a testing session of different types of gloves can provide personnel who actually will wear the gloves with an opportunity to try different options and provide feedback before the organization decides which kind to choose. Seeking input in this manner can increase user support and compliance with gloving policies.

It is important to note that gloves do not reduce hand contamination completely. Although wearing gloves can help reduce the transmission of infectious agents, they should be used in conjunction with effective hand hygiene, not as a substitute for it. As discussed in Chapter 2, hand hygiene must take place before putting on gloves and after gloves are removed even if a health care provider is going to put on another pair of gloves. Some studies have shown that aloe vera–impregnated medical exam gloves can help preserve skin condition and thus promote better hand hygiene.[16] After cleaning their hands, providers must allow the hands to thoroughly dry before gloving.[17]

Although gloves can serve as a barrier between the provider and the patient, that barrier can be compromised. Perforation rates as high as 61% for thoracic surgeons and 40% for scrub nurses have been reported.[18] The practice of double gloving involves wearing two pairs of surgical gloves to prevent and mitigate the effects of barrier failure—the ripping, tearing, or puncturing of a glove.[19] On average, an outer operative glove is perforated within 40 minutes of being used. Yet, although the puncture of the outer glove is common, corresponding punctures of both the inner and outer gloves are rare. In those cases in which a double puncture does occur, the volume of blood is significantly reduced, thus reducing the likelihood of infection.[20]

Although double gloving has been shown to be effective, many practitioners have objections to the practice, including poor fit, loss of tactile sensitivity, and increased costs. Following are some suggestions on how organizations can overcome those objections:

- Work with glove manufacturers to offer a "glove-fitting" station where practitioners can try on many glove options and find a fit that works for them. This will allow practitioners to evaluate performance characteristics of two gloves worn together before entering the operating room or procedure area. This process can be conducted at no cost to the organization.
- Educate practitioners on the value of double gloving to justify the time and effort involved in implementation.
- Enlist the support of individuals who are already double gloving, such as surgeons or scrub nurses who can testify to the effectiveness of the procedure and allay any concerns.

Although some organizations may view double gloving as an unnecessary increase in cost, the reduction of bloodborne pathogen exposure and the decrease in infections for both patients and providers offer significant savings for health care organizations.

In addition to double gloving, providers should change gloves at regular intervals during surgery because fresh gloves may be less likely to perforate than ones that have been in use for a period of time. Regular glove changing also can reduce the amount of time that a perforated glove remains in use. In one study, participants changed gloves approximately every 16 minutes, and this interval was associated with a significant reduction in the incidence of glove perforations for surgeons and nurses.[21] More information on avoiding glove perforations and other sharps injuries can be found in Chapter 8.

Setting the Tone for Collaboration

The operating room or procedure area is ready. The patient is prepped. All surgical team members have scrubbed and donned appropriate attire and personal protective equipment. There are a few minutes before the procedure starts, and these may be the most critical minutes in the entire preparation process. For in these minutes, the team members must come together, introduce themselves if they do not know one another, briefly discuss the procedure, and set the tone for teamwork, communication, and problem solving.

As discussed in Chapter 1, communication among surgical team members is paramount to successful outcomes and avoiding errors in the surgical setting. If providers skip this critical preparation step, the entire procedure can be compromised.

The surgical team leader—typically the surgeon—consciously or unconsciously sets the tone for interactions in the operating room or procedure area through his or her verbal communication, body language, facial expressions, and attitudes. In a recent observational study of 300 surgical cases, researchers noticed that surgeons were vital to setting the tone for team interaction. As they prepared for the next surgical case, operating room team members—nurses, technicians, and anesthesia providers—participated in active dialogue about the case, social issues, how their day was going, and other conversation before the surgeon entered the room. Within 10 seconds of entering the room, the surgeon's behavior had shown a profound effect on the communication pattern in the room. If the surgeon engaged the team, set a positive tone, and shared the plan, the previous level of communication continued. However, if the surgeon set a negative tone, virtually all team communication stopped.[22]

Consider this example, based on a true story. A surgeon strides into the operating room as the team is setting up for a hernia repair. He loudly announces with a distinct edge in his voice, "I have a plane to catch in four hours and we have a bunch of cases to do. Get on with it!" As the first procedure begins, the surgeon is so fixated on getting the cases done and pushing the pace that he makes the incision on the wrong side as the nurses helplessly watch, not knowing how to tell him he is making an error and not willing to challenge him or speak up.[23]

Although not every surgical team leader will be as terse as the one in the previous example, many surgeons will squelch communication and interactions inadvertently by skipping preprocedure checklists, not introducing themselves, or simply appearing uninterested in hearing anyone else's thoughts on the case. Even when providers set a positive tone, it is often done informally or by default. A far better idea is to actively set the stage by greeting everyone by name; introducing those team members who are new to the team; making eye contact with team members as appropriate; sharing the plan for the case; encouraging feedback from all members of the team, including nurses and residents; and continuously inviting team members into conversation for their expertise, knowledge, and concerns.[24]

TIP Write Down Team Member Names

To help with introductions in the operating room or procedure area, team leaders should consider writing all team members' names on a wall-mounted whiteboard for reference.

The action of creating an environment conducive to two-way communication is sometimes referred to as "establishing psychological safety."[23] Within psychologically safe environments, everyone is comfortable speaking up, every individual and what he or she has to say is treated with respect at all times, and disrespectful behavior is not tolerated.

Consider this example, in which a provider set a positive tone for the surgical experience and established psychological safety. Like the previous example, this one is also based on a true story. A vascular surgeon was doing a new procedure on a very high-risk patient. The procedure was complicated and was to be performed in an unfamiliar setting requiring the coordinated efforts of several individuals, many of whom did not know one another. The surgeon walked into the room and announced, "I have no pride invested in this procedure; I just want us to get it right. If you see anything that is helpful or see me getting off in the weeds, please speak up." He then went around the room and introduced himself to everyone by his first name. This simple action created a collaborative, open environment in which people could participate and speak up easily and hierarchy was eliminated.[24] The surgical procedure continued without complications, and the patient had a successful outcome.

The previous two examples illustrate the two extremes of team behavior. The usual interactions among members of surgical teams are somewhere between these two extremes, with the typical team including a relatively close group of people who know one another. They may not always like one another, but in general they know how the team is going to work. Most surgical teams can improve their level of teamwork and communication by striving to be more like the team in the second example and taking care to avoid the behavior of the team members in the first.

Psychological safety is essential for surgical teams because people act tentatively and defensively when they do not feel safe, thereby inhibiting their willingness to participate and speak up.[25] When team members think they or their suggestions are being criticized, an unhealthy dynamic occurs, eroding team cohesion.[23] Surgical team leaders must establish psychological safety before proceeding with a case in order to maintain open lines of communication during the procedure.

After a team leader has set the tone for collaboration, the team should use structured communication techniques, such as the ones discussed in Chapter 1—preprocedure briefing, callouts, and read-backs—to outline what will happen in the procedure, ensure that all preparation efforts are complete, and continue effective communication and information exchange during the procedure. These techniques can thrive in a positive, interactive environment and can help teams successfully navigate the complex surgical process. More information about using a specific preprocedure briefing—the time-out portion of the Universal Protocol for Preventing Wrong Site, Wrong Procedure, Wrong Person Surgery™—can be found in Chapter 6. To guide, supplement, or enhance its use of the Universal Protocol, an organization may want to use a checklist, such as the World Health Organization Surgical Safety Checklist, also discussed in Chapter 6.

As mentioned in Chapter 1, teamwork and communication, including establishing the tone for team interactions and fostering psychological safety, do not necessarily come easily to health care providers. Many, if not most, providers have not been trained in these skills. Therefore, comprehensive, interactive training involving role playing is critical to ensure that team leaders can effectively set a positive tone in which other providers feel comfortable speaking up about issues, offering opinions, and giving feedback.

References

1. Andersen B., Solheim N.: Occlusive scrub suits in operating theaters during cataract surgery: Effect on airborne contamination. *Infect Control Hosp Epidemiol* 23:218–220, Apr. 2002.
2. Tammelin A., et al.: Dispersal of methicillin-resistant *Staphylococcus epidermidis* by staff in an operating suite for thoracic and cardiovascular surgery: Relation to skin carriage and clothing. *J Hosp Infect* 44:119–126, Feb. 2000.
3. Siegel J., et al.: *2007 Guideline for Isolation Precautions: Preventing Transmission of Infectious Agents in Healthcare Settings.* Healthcare Infection Control Practices Advisory Committee, 2007. http://www.cdc.gov/hicpac/2007IP/2007isolationPrecautions.html (accessed Jul. 24, 2010).
4. Association of periOperative Registered Nurses (AORN): Recommended practices for prevention of transmissible infections in the perioperative practice setting. In *Perioperative Standards and Recommended Practices.* Denver: AORN, 2008.
5. Association of periOperative Registered Nurses (AORN): Recommended practices for surgical attire. In *Perioperative Standards and Recommended Practices,* 2010 ed. Denver: AORN, 2010, pp. 67–73.
6. Whyte W., et al.: An investigation of occlusive polyester surgical clothing. *J Hosp Infect* 15:363–374, May 1990.
7. Barrie D.: How hospital linen and laundry services are provided. *J Hosp Infect* 27:219–235, Jul. 1994.
8. Wu X., Yang C.: Flame retardant finishing of cotton fleece fabric: Part III—The combination of maleic acid and sodium hypophosphite. *Journal of Fire Sciences* 26:351–368, Jul. 2008.
9. Mangram A., et al.: Guideline for prevention of surgical site infection, 1999. Hospital Infection Control Practices Advisory Committee. *Infect Control Hosp Epidemiol* 20:250–278, Apr. 1999.
10. Conner R., Blanchard J., Reno D. (eds): *Perioperative Standards and Recommended Practices.* Denver: AORN, 2009.
11. Occupational exposure to bloodborne pathogens—OSHA. Final rule. *Fed Regist* 56:64004-64182, Dec. 1991.
12. Gerba C.: Application of quantitative risk assessment for formulating hygiene policy in the domestic setting. *J Infect* 43:92–98, Jul. 2001.
13. Boyce J., Pittet D.: Guideline for hand hygiene in health-care settings. *MMWR Recomm Rep* 51(RR16), 2002. http://www.cdc.gov/mmwr/preview/mmwrhtml/rr5116a1.htm (accessed Jul. 24, 2010).
14. Church N., Bjerke N.: Surgical services. In *APIC Text of Infection Control and Epidemiology,* 3rd ed. Washington, DC: Association for Professionals in Infection Control and Epidemiology, 2009, pp. 45-1–45-14.
15. Trampuz A., Widemer A.: Hand hygiene: A frequently missed lifesaving opportunity during patient care. *Mayo Clin Proc* 79:109–116, Jan. 2004.
16. Korniewicz D., Masri M.: Effect of aloe-vera impregnated gloves on hand hygiene attitudes of health care workers. *Medsurg Nurs* 16:247–252, Aug. 2007.
17. World Health Organization: *WHO Guidelines on Hand Hygiene in Health Care (Advanced Draft): A Summary: Clean Hands Are Safer Hands.* 2005. http://www.who.int/patientsafety/events/05/HH_en.pdf (accessed Jul. 24, 2010).
18. Tokars J., et al.: Percutaneous injuries during surgical procedures. *JAMA* 267:2899–2904, Jun. 3, 1992.
19. Twomey C.: Double gloving: A risk reduction strategy. *Jt Comm J Qual Saf* 29:369–378, Jul. 2003.
20. Berguer R., Heller, P.: Preventing sharps injuries in the operating room. *J Am Coll Surg* 199:462–467, Sep. 2004.
21. Al-Maiya M., et al.: Glove perforation and contamination in primary total hip arthroplasty. *J Bone Joint Surg BR* 87:556–559, Apr. 2005.
22. Mazzocco K., et al.: Surgical team behaviors and patient outcomes. *Am J Surg* 197:678–685, May 2009.
23. Leonard M., Frankel A., Simmonds T.: Effective teamwork and communication. In Frankel A., et al. (eds.): *The Essential Guide for Patient Safety Officers.* Oak Brook, IL: Joint Commission Resources, 2009, pp. 49–60.
24. Leonard M., Frankel A., Simmonds T.: *Achieving Safe and Reliable Healthcare: Strategies and Solutions.* Chicago: Health Administration Press, 2004.
25. Edmondson A.: Managing the risk of learning: Psychological safety in work teams. In West M., Tjosvold D., Smith K. (eds.): *International Handbook of Organizational Teamwork and Cooperative Working.* London: Blackwell, 2003, pp. 255–275.

Chapter 6

Completing the Universal Protocol for Preventing Wrong Site, Wrong Procedure, Wrong Person Surgery™

Each year, an estimated 234 million people around the world undergo a major operation.[1] Although most of these procedures are completed successfully, it is estimated that major complications occur in 3% to 16% of inpatient surgical procedures in industrialized countries.[1] One specific type of complication that occurs more often than it should is wrong-site, wrong-procedure, wrong-person surgery.

What Is Wrong-Site Surgery?

Wrong-site, wrong-procedure, wrong-person surgery—sometimes referred to simply as wrong-site surgery or wrong surgery—happens when a medical procedure is executed on the wrong body part, the wrong side of the patient's body, or the wrong patient.[2] According to the U.S. Centers for Medicare & Medicaid Services, wrong surgery occurs when a surgical or other invasive procedure is not consistent with the correctly documented informed consent.[3] Wrong surgery procedures are considered "never events," which means they are, in theory, completely preventable and thus should never happen.[4]

Despite the fact that they are preventable, wrong surgery errors continue to plague the surgical setting. Although the frequency of these types of errors is difficult to quantify because of possible underreporting issues, the statistics that are available are quite alarming. For example, since 1995, when The Joint Commission began reviewing sentinel events and their root causes, wrong-site surgery has become the most frequently reported category of sentinel events.[5] Although this increase may be due to increased awareness and reporting of the issue, the fact is that surgical errors of this type are continuing to occur.[6]

One study conducted in the United States suggests wrong-site surgery happens in 1 out of 112,994 cases.[7] These numbers represent actual cases; however, the number of near misses (also called close calls) is much higher.[8] The Patient Safety Authority of Pennsylvania—which collects data on wrong-site surgery, both actual and prevented—indicates receiving reports of an average of one wrong-site surgery event (either actual or near miss) every six days since mandatory state reporting began in the early 2000s.[9] Although many of these near misses and surgical confusions cause little or no permanent injury, the risks are present for a serious, irreversible event that can permanently scar a patient, family, and provider.[10]

According to a recent study from the *Journal of the American Medical Association*, surgery on the wrong side is the most frequent type of surgical adverse event, followed by surgery involving the wrong patient, and then wrong implant.[11] Many wrong surgery cases occurred in outpatient settings, where the number of surgeries performed and the time pressures involved continue to increase.[12]

Wrong-site surgery is not just a problem for the United States. This type of medical error is occurring all around the world, and several safety-focused organizations are working with health care facilities to implement systematic processes to reduce wrong surgery errors. For example, in March 2005 the National Patient Safety Agency in the United Kingdom developed a national safety alert for all National Health Service hospital trusts in England and Wales, which offered recommendations on how to prevent surgical errors.[13] In Australia, the Australian Commission for Safety and Quality in Health Care requires reporting for eight sentinel events, including procedures involving the incorrect patient or body part. In the most recent yearly figures, 53 such wrong surgery procedures were reported.[14]

Many health care providers believe that because they happen infrequently, wrong surgeries could never happen under their supervision. However, every physician, surgical nurse, other surgical team member, and organization leader needs to recognize that failures involving wrong-site, wrong-procedure, and wrong-person surgery *can* happen anywhere. The American Academy of Orthopaedic Surgeons reports that during a 35-year career, an orthopedic surgeon has a 1 in 4 chance of performing a wrong-site surgery.[15] No one who works in the surgical arena is immune to the problem, and, therefore, everyone needs to maintain a high degree of awareness of the possibility of this type of event.

What Causes Wrong-Site Surgery?

As with other types of medical errors, the causes of wrong-site surgery are, in essence, systemic and thus complex in nature.[16] With that said, these types of events are largely the result of miscommunication and or unavailable or incorrect information. A lack of standardized processes to collect, interpret, and talk about information creates opportunities for error.[5] In addition, a lack of safety culture and teamwork among surgical teams can create a negative environment conducive to error. Within these teams, providers do not value systematic processes to proactively reduce the possibility of error and can sometimes feel uncomfortable speaking up about issues when they do occur. A lack of education and understanding of the problem of wrong-site surgery and the risks associated with it can also lead providers to dismiss the importance of systematic improvement in this area, including the use of structured preprocedure briefings.

Wrong surgery errors can stem from human error, mistakes, omissions, and miscommunications in various aspects of the surgical preparation process. For example, an error in documenting the correct site in the medical record, if not corrected, can continue throughout the preprocedure process and cause a problem during surgery. Likewise, an error in site marking or a lack of correct paperwork—if not caught before the start of a procedure—can lead to tragedy.

Certain surgical situations present a greater likelihood for wrong surgery. Some high-risk situations include the following:

- More than one surgeon is involved in the case, either because multiple procedures are contemplated or because the care of the patient is transferred to another surgeon.
- Multiple procedures are conducted on the same patient during a single trip to the operating room, particularly when the procedures are on different sides of the patient's body.
- Unusual time pressures exist related to an unusual start time or pressure to speed up the preoperative procedure, such as during an emergency situation.
- The patient has unusual characteristics, such as a physical deformity or massive obesity that might alter the usual process for equipment setup or positioning of the patient.
- The patient has a similar site, procedure, or name as another patient being operated on at the same time.

Although wrong-site surgeries have been reported in all surgical specialties, some have inherently greater risk of exposure than others. For example, in orthopedic surgery the potential for right/left confusion is almost an occupational hazard.[17] In addition, there is a high prevalence of wrong-level surgery among spine surgeons, with 50% of spine surgeons performing a wrong-level surgery at some point during their career.[18]

Like any complex problem, solving the issue of wrong-site surgery cannot be accomplished with a single remedy or action. Organizations cannot merely ask providers to "be more careful" or "try harder." Reducing the likelihood of wrong surgery requires a systematic approach, not only by the surgeon or a nurse but also by the entire team of health care professionals working together with a supportive health system for the benefit of the patient.[1]

The balance of this chapter discusses some systematic approaches to reducing the likelihood of wrong-site surgery, including the Universal Protocol for Preventing Wrong Site, Wrong Procedure, Wrong Person Surgery™ and the World Health Organization Surgical Safety Checklist.

Understanding the Universal Protocol for Preventing Wrong Site, Wrong Procedure, Wrong Person Surgery

In 2004, to address the issue of wrong-site surgery, The Joint Commission released its Universal Protocol for Preventing Wrong Site, Wrong Procedure, Wrong Person Surgery. Joint Commission International (JCI) recommends the evidence-based practices described in the Universal Protocol as part of its International Patient Safety Goal to ensure correct-site, correct-procedure, correct-patient surgery. The International Patient Safety Goal also requires organizations to create a policy, which includes a definition of *surgery* that incorporates at least those procedures that investigate and/or treat diseases and disorders of the human body through cutting, removing, altering, or insertion of diagnostic or therapeutic scopes. The policy applies to any location in the organization where these procedures are performed.

Fundamentally, the Universal Protocol describes a series of organizational systems. These systems are designed to prevent human error from reaching and affecting the patient.[17] The Universal Protocol applies to all operative and other invasive procedures that expose patients to more than minimal risk, including procedures done in settings other than the operating room, such as a special procedures unit, endoscopy unit, or interventional radiology suites. Certain routine, "minor" procedures such as venipuncture, peripheral intravenous line placement insertion of a nasogastric tube, and Foley catheter insertion are not within the scope of the Universal Protocol.

The Universal Protocol is made up of the following three components:

1. A preprocedure verification process
2. Marking of the procedure site
3. A time-out that is performed before the procedure

Ideally, the preprocedure verification process starts when surgery or another invasive procedure is scheduled and continues throughout the patient preparation process up until the time the patient enters the procedural area. The surgical site is marked in the preoperative holding area, and the time-out occurs just before the start of surgery in the operating room or other procedural area. The following sections take a closer look at these three components.

The Preprocedure Verification Process

A preprocedure verification process should ensure that any procedure is what the patient needs and is performed on the correct person. As mentioned in Chapter 4, this process is designed to be an ongoing effort of information gathering and confirmation that makes sure all relevant documents and related information are available prior to the start of the procedure; are correctly identified, labeled, and matched to the patient's identity; and are reviewed and consistent with the patient expectations and with the team's understanding of the intended patient, procedure, and site. Any missing information or discrepancies must be addressed as soon as they are discovered.

It is helpful to look at the preprocedure verification process as a series of progressive steps taken to reduce the risk of error associated with operative and invasive procedures. The first step requires a process—defined by the organization—to verify the correct procedure, for the correct patient, at the correct site. It is up to the organization to determine when this information is collected, such as at the time of scheduling or preadmission testing, and by which team member. Whenever possible, consideration should be given to involving the patient in this process.

The next step requires a standardized preprocedure verification list of items that, at a minimum, are or may be required at the time of the operative or invasive procedure.

Activities to address such items may start days—or perhaps weeks—prior to the actual procedure. Such activities may include ordering medical devices, implants, or special equipment; ordering blood products; and/or obtaining copies of reports or radiographic images to ensure their availability at the time of the procedure. Working from a standard verification list reduces variability and thus the potential for error.

The final step in the process involves comparing information about the patient and procedure with the items identified in the preprocedure verification list that are required to proceed with the procedure. This step occurs before the patient leaves the preprocedure area or enters the procedure room. Missing information, supplies, or discrepancies are addressed before starting the procedure.

To help ensure a thorough preprocedure verification process, organizations should consider creating a checklist that can be used to make sure the patient's identity is verified using at least two patient identifiers—such as the patient's name and birth date—and also confirm the availability and review of any relevant documentation, images, implants, or special equipment. Documentation that may be helpful in verifying the correct site, procedure, and patient can include the patient's history and physical examination findings, preoperative assessment, and informed consent. Although a checklist is not required by The Joint Commission or JCI, it is a common approach to ensuring a comprehensive, consistent, and effective preoperative verification process.

TIP Ensure a Current History and Physical

When the history and physical is used in the preoperative verification process, organizations should make sure that it is current and the intended procedure, site, side, level, implants, and planned donor sites are accurately and comprehensively described on it.

Marking the Procedure Site

Organizations must mark the procedure site to unambiguously identify the intended site of incision or insertions. The mark should be visible after the patient has been prepped and draped. To effectively mark the site, the person performing the procedure should make the mark at or near the incision site. When making the mark, health care providers should use a marker that is sufficiently permanent to remain visible after completion of the skin preparation. Adhesive site markers should not be used as the sole means of marking the site.

In addition to being sufficiently permanent, the mark also must be distinct and unambiguous. For example, organizations may want to use the surgeon's initials or the word "YES" to mark the site. It is important to note that an "X" could be considered ambiguous and should be avoided. Regardless of the method chosen for marking, the method and type of mark should be consistent throughout the organization.

It is required that organizations *not* mark any nonoperative site unless necessary for some other aspect of care. Although some surgeons do not wish to have ink on the surgical site, marking the nonoperative site can be risky. Consider the following example:

> A surgeon was going to repair a man's ruptured right Achilles tendon. The patient was anesthetized while he was lying on his back, and the left leg was marked "No." While the surgeon scrubbed, the scrub nurse and anesthesiologist turned the patient on his stomach. After scrubbing, the surgeon returned to the same side of the table, not realizing the patient had been flipped over, causing the leg to change positions. The surgeon made an incision on the wrong side before realizing his mistake.[19]

What sites should be marked. Although The Joint Commission and JCI recommend marking all surgical sites, health care organizations are required, at a minimum, to mark all cases involving laterality, multiple structures (for example, fingers, toes, lesions), or multiple levels (for example, the spine). If a patient requires multiple surgeries while in a health care organization, the site mark should be removed at the end of the procedure unless the next surgical procedure will continue on the same site.

Site marking is not required (nor is it prohibited) for some procedures such as midline sternotomy, Cesarean section, laparotomy, and laparoscopy. Most procedures that involve puncture or incision of the skin or insertion of an instrument or foreign material into the body are within the scope of the Universal Protocol and JCI requirements; however, these procedures do not necessarily require site marking. Procedures that do *not* require site marking include, but are not limited to, the following:

- Single organ cases (for example, Cesarean section, cardiac surgery)
- Interventional cases for which the catheter/instrument insertion site is not predetermined (for example, cardiac catheterization)
- Dental procedures involving the teeth. Although the Universal Protocol does not require marking on the teeth, organizations must indicate operative tooth name(s) on documentation *or* mark the operative tooth or teeth on the dental radiographs or dental diagram. (*See* Sidebar 6-1 below.)
- Procedures involving premature infants, for whom the mark may cause a permanent tattoo

Each organization will need to identify which procedures being performed at the organization would expose the patient to more than minimal risk and require site marking for those procedures. Surveyors will use the organization's definition in evaluating compliance with the Universal Protocol and JCI standards.

The surgeon's role in site marking. The Universal Protocol for Preventing Wrong Site, Wrong Procedure, Wrong Person Surgery states that the individual performing surgery or an invasive procedure should be the one who marks the surgical site. Often, this individual is a surgeon. By marking the site, the surgeon can have contact with the patient before surgery, make sure that the proper site is marked, and prevent any confusion in the procedural area.

In cases where the person performing the procedure does not mark the surgical site, another member of the surgical or patient care team who is fully informed about the patient and the intended procedure must do the marking. Any delegation of responsibility for marking the surgical site must be consistent with applicable law and regulation.

In circumstances where it is not feasible for the person performing the procedure to mark the site, the reason that the person performing the procedure cannot mark the site must be explained. These exceptions to the policy should be handled on a case-by-case basis and not as a routine activity for the organization. The organization must ensure that whenever the responsibility for site marking is delegated to someone other than the person who will be performing the procedure, the safety of the patient will not be compromised.

Regardless of whether the surgeon marks the site or another designated qualified individual does, the surgeon must look for the mark before beginning surgery and

Sidebar 6-1: Identifying Teeth for Surgery

When the Universal Protocol for Preventing Wrong Site, Wrong Procedure, Wrong Person Surgery was created, the American Dental Association (ADA) acknowledged, and The Joint Commission supported, that no reliable method exists to directly mark teeth intended for extraction. In lieu of directly marking the teeth, the ADA recommends the following:

- Review the dental record, including the medical history, laboratory findings, appropriate charts, and dental x-rays. Indicate the tooth number(s) or mark the tooth site or surgical site on the diagram or x-ray to be included as part of the patient's records.
- Ensure that x-rays are properly oriented and visually confirm that the correct teeth or tissues have been charted.
- Conduct a time-out to verify the correct patient, correct tooth/teeth, and correct procedure with the surgical assistant present at the time of the extraction.

Source: Joint Commission: Wrong site surgery summit: Working toward solutions. *Joint Commission Perspectives on Patient Safety* 3:7–8, Aug. 2003.

reconfirm that it is in the right location during the time-out process.

Involving the patient in site marking. When possible, the marking process should involve the patient. For this to be done in a meaningful way, it should happen before the patient is significantly sedated. Participation may be precluded by a disease state or heavy sedation; however, sedation by itself does not necessarily prevent the patient from participating in the site-marking process. The patient's capacity to participate must be based on an individual assessment. In cases of nonspeaking, comatose, or incompetent patients, or children, the "patient involvement" in the site-marking process should be handled in the same way as the informed consent process. Whoever has authority to provide informed consent for the patient to undergo the procedure would, as appropriate, participate in the site-marking process.

Although it rarely occurs, the patient always has the right to refuse site marking. This situation should be handled the same way as for any other refusal by a patient offered care, treatment, or services. The organization's responsibility is to provide the patient with information to understand why site marking is appropriate and desirable as well as the implications of refusing the site marking. If a patient continues to refuse site marking, the organization should have a procedure in place to appropriately identify the site. This alternative method may involve a bedside consult with the surgical team so that everyone understands the location of the site and the patient's refusal to be marked.[20]

Ensuring proper marking instruments. Both the Joint Commission and JCI require organizations to have clear site marking. To help with effective surgical site marking, organizations should ensure the availability and use of appropriate surgical marking pens. Several manufacturers offer special surgical marking pens and other direct skin-marking methods that will not be washed off when the surgical site is prepped but which can be removed following the procedure. For patients with dark skin, a marker in a color other than black or dark blue may be used to ensure that the site marking is clearly visible. Some organizations have found red markers useful in this regard.[20] Other organizations opt to use a special-purpose wristband in addition to a mark with a surgical pen to communicate the appropriate site on a dark-skinned patient.[21]

As mentioned in Chapter 4, there has been some concern that marking the surgical site could introduce bacteria to the surgical site, thus affecting its sterility. Several studies from around the world—including ones from China and Australia—have shown that surgical site marking with a nonsterile surgical marking pen did not contaminate the surgical site.[14,22]

TIP Consider a Two-Stage Marking Process

When marking the site for spinal surgery, organizations may want to consider using a two-stage marking process.

1. Mark the general level of the procedure (cervical, thoracic, or lumbar) preoperatively.
2. Mark the exact interspace to be operated on interoperatively, using the standard intraoperative radiographic marking technique.

Wrong-site surgery of the spine can also be eliminated by using markers that do not move and by double-checking the level of the spine with an intraoperative x-ray.[15]

The Time-Out

The purpose of the time-out, or "huddle," is to bring the surgical team together to conduct a final assessment of the correct patient, procedure, site, patient position, and, as applicable, availability of implants and special equipment. Some providers believe that a time-out should occur before anesthesia to involve the patient. Although organizations may choose to perform the time-out this way, they can also conduct two time-outs: one before the start of anesthesia and one just prior to incision. Organizations also should consider conducting a time-out after a change in position, after redraping (*see* Sidebar 6-2 on page 85), or after an intraoperative x-ray or fluoroscopy.[23]

Although the task of conducting a final confirmation before proceeding with surgery may seem straightforward, some health care organizations are not conducting time-outs when they should or are not doing them at all. During the first six months of 2009, The Joint

Sidebar 6-2: Changing Direction During Surgery

When a clinician is facing a patient, the patient's right side is the clinician's left. However, if the direction of the patient is changed during the procedure—for example from supine to prone or the entire table is rotated 180 degrees—it is easy to forget that the patient's position relative to the clinician may have changed. If a patient is rotated onto one side and his or her arms or legs are flexed, then, from some viewing angles, it may require significant mental effort to determine which is the patient's right or left side in relation to the clinician's right or left side. It is not surprising that this type of process is subject to errors, especially in a distraction-rich environment like the operating room. Frequent and regular communication during surgery can help avoid errors, even when the patient is being moved throughout surgery. Team members may want to take a brief time-out to verbally state and reconfirm the correct surgical site every time a patient is moved during surgery.

Source: Seiden S., et al.: Wrong-side/wrong-site, wrong-procedure, and wrong-patient adverse events: Are they preventable? *Arch Surg* 141:931–939, Sep. 2006.

Commission surveyed accredited organizations in the United States about their compliance with the time-out process. The results of the survey indicated that 24% of ambulatory care organizations, 34% of hospitals, and 13% of office-based surgery practices surveyed were not fully compliant with the time-out function. These lapses in compliance took many forms, including not conducting a time-out for each procedure when the same physician performed multiple procedures, not suspending activity to conduct the time-out, and not appropriately documenting the time-out.

The most effective and safest method of performing a time-out includes the following processes:

- A designated member of the surgical team should be in charge of initiating the time-out. This person could be a circulating nurse, the anesthesiologist, or the surgeon; however, it must be someone who is considered an immediate member of the procedure team or someone who will be participating in the procedure from the beginning. Although it does not always need to be the same person, the individual doing the time-out should know the elements to be reviewed during the time-out for the particular surgery or procedure. Whoever holds the responsibility must have the respect and attention of the entire surgical team. Organization leaders must reinforce this respect to ensure that the time-out occurs as it should. (*See* Sidebar 6-3 on page 86.)
- Active communication between team members must take place in a *fail-safe mode*—that is, communication is interactive, and the procedure is not started until any and all questions or concerns are resolved. Remember, the purpose of the time-out is to reach an agreement between team members. If there is no agreement, then something is wrong!
- All activities should be suspended to the extent possible so team members can focus on active confirmation of the patient, site, and procedure. Doing so can be difficult for some organizations and may be a source of compliance failure.
- The entire surgical team should be involved. At a minimum, this includes active participation by the surgeon, anesthesia provider, and circulating nurse. Participation by the other members of the team, as appropriate to their involvement in the procedure, is also encouraged. In particular, there should be no barrier to anyone speaking up if there is concern about a possible error. To include some members of the team but not others sends the wrong message. It could imply that the input and opinions of some of the staff members are not valued.
- If multiple procedures are conducted by the same physician, a time-out must take place for each procedure.
- If a situation arises in which there is a discrepancy in staff response, an organization should have processes and systems in place for reconciling these differences. The procedure should not be started until all questions or concerns are resolved.
- The time-out must, at a minimum, include a verification of the following:

— Correct patient identity
— The correct site
— The procedure to be done

- The time-out must be documented. There are many ways to document the time-out procedure, and each organization will need to determine the method appropriate for it. Although organizations can document each aspect of the time-out, a simple statement that confirms that all the components of the time-out were completed is sufficient.

Even if a nurse is put in charge of calling the time-out, surgeons and anesthesiologists must actively participate in the process, verifying information and responding to concerns. If an inconsistency is identified in the time-out process, surgeons must be willing to stop the procedure until the inconsistency is identified and reconciled. As mentioned in Chapter 5, the surgeon is often the leader of the surgical team. As a leader, he or she must create an environment in which the time-out is part of the surgery preparation and is a valuable communication tool. If physicians do not establish this precedent, they can make the time-out a useless exercise that does not identify or prevent error. Actively participating in a time-out takes no more time than actively working to avoid the time-out, and the consequences of active participation can have positive effects on patient safety, team morale, and quality of care.

TIP Develop a Time-Out Process for Bedside Procedures

Time-outs must occur not only for surgical procedures in the operating room but before any procedures that put the patient at more than minimal risk. Some organizations have found that developing a time-out process for bedside procedures is challenging. Often there is only one individual—typically the physician—performing the procedure, and thus following the same process as a surgical time-out is not appropriate. To address this difference, organizations may consider examining the bedside procedures performed in the organization that require a time-out process and developing a targeted policy for these procedures.

Sidebar 6-3: Remember Anesthesia Blocks

To ensure the complete and consistent verification of the correct site, organizations should consider conducting a time-out any time there is a question of site or laterality. This includes not only before a surgical incision but also before the administration of a regional anesthesia block, which is itself an invasive procedure and is a frequently reported type of wrong-site procedure. Consider this example:

An elderly woman was scheduled for a hip replacement on her left side. The patient's evaluation before surgery was conducted in the preoperative holding area, and anesthesia consent was obtained for a spinal epidural and a regional block for postoperative analgesia. The surgical site alone was marked with the surgeon's initials per the hospital's protocol.

A scheduling change in the operating room occurred. An operating room had been prepared for a patient who was scheduled to receive a right hip replacement, but that procedure was canceled. The current patient was brought into this operating room, and monitors were applied. The patient was given the spinal epidural and was not responsive to verbal stimulation. The regional block was administered. After administration of the anesthetic, the surgical team began final positioning of the patient and discovered—during the time-out before incision—that the patient was positioned on the incorrect side and the block had been performed on the wrong side. After she was positioned correctly, the surgical procedure proceeded uneventfully. A block on the left side was given after the procedure was completed to ensure postoperative analgesia.

Although in this example the time-out before the surgical incision prevented the wrong-site surgery, it did not prevent the regional block being administered on the wrong site. By conducting an additional time-out before the administration of the regional block, this error could have been prevented. To address this issue, the organization could have required a preanesthetic site verification at the time patient consent was obtained and a preanesthesia time-out to confirm the appropriate site.

Source: Adapted from Edmonds C., Ligouri G., Stanton M.: Two cases of a wrong-site peripheral nerve block and a process to prevent this complication. *Reg Anesth Pain Med* 30:99–103, Jan.–Feb. 2005.

Verification, site-marking, and time-out procedures should be as consistent as possible throughout an organization, including in the operating room and other locations where invasive procedures are performed. This consistency helps the process be the most effective, as all individuals involved in performing invasive procedures in an organization know what will happen when, and how discrepancies will be resolved.

Taking a Systematic Approach to Implementing the Universal Protocol for Preventing Wrong Site, Wrong Procedure, Wrong Person Surgery

Although the Universal Protocol has specific elements that must be present to ensure safety in the operating room, how an organization incorporates the Universal Protocol into its daily processes will depend on the organization. As with other aspects of improving safety in surgery, a systematic approach to implementing the components of the Universal Protocol is warranted. To help with implementation, organizations may want to pull together a multidisciplinary team to assess the current process, identify areas of improvement, and design initiatives to address those areas. (*See* Figure 6-1 on pages 88–92 for a self-assessment checklist that organizations can adapt to identify potential flaws in their processes to prevent wrong-site surgery. *See* Sidebar 6-4 below for a standardized patient safety protocol developed specifically to test the feasibility and effectiveness of standardization in reducing the risk of wrong-patient, wrong-procedure, or wrong-site surgery.)

As with the discussion in Chapter 2 about improving hand hygiene, improving compliance with the Universal Protocol can benefit from the use of systematic improvement

Sidebar 6-4: The High 5s Standard Operating Protocol (SOP) for Correct Site Surgery

The High 5s Standard Operating Protocol (SOP) for Correct Site Surgery is one of several standardized patient safety protocols developed specifically to test the feasibility and effectiveness of standardization in reducing the risk of certain types of adverse events. The High 5s Project is a collaboration among a group of countries, the World Health Organization (WHO), and the WHO Collaborating Centre for Patient Safety (designated as The Joint Commission and Joint Commission International) in support of WHO Patient Safety Programme's efforts to improve patient safety worldwide.

The High 5s SOP for Correct Site Surgery focuses on reducing the risk of wrong-patient, wrong-procedure, or wrong-site surgery. To achieve the goals of the High 5s Project, participating hospitals are required to adhere to the SOP as written and to measure their performance both in implementing the protocol and in achieving success in reducing or eliminating wrong-patient, wrong-procedure, and wrong-site surgery. Testing takes place in a modest number of volunteer hospitals in four countries and includes a robust measurement and evaluation component that provides for the use of standardized performance measures, data collection procedures, event analysis protocols, and other evaluation tools and techniques.

Like both the Universal Protocol and the WHO Surgical Safety Checklist, the High 5s SOP for Correct Site Surgery requires certain preoperative checks, surgical site marking, and a "time out" before surgery. Despite their similarities, there are some differences, including the range of perioperative activities included in each. The High 5s SOP for Correct Site Surgery has a more fully developed preoperative verification process that begins when the surgical procedure is first scheduled and continues throughout the preoperative process. All of these approaches to surgical safety have value and, indeed, should be considered by all organizations that provide surgical services.

Note: *The Standard Operating Protocol for Correct Site Surgery has been developed solely for use within the context of the High 5s Project, an internationally coordinated, limited-participation activity for testing the feasibility of implementing standardized patient safety protocols and determining the impact of the implementation on certain specified patient safety outcomes. Because the efficacy of this and other High-5 SOPs has not yet been demonstrated, the SOP is not available to the public at this time. Results of this initiative, when completed, will be published and the refined SOPs, as appropriate, will be made available for general implementation.*

For more information on the High 5s Standard Operating Protocol for Correct Site Surgery, go online to https://www.high5s.org.

Figure 6-1: Self-Assessment Checklist

Self-Assessment Checklist for Program Elements Associated with Preventing Wrong-Site Surgery

	Yes	No	NA
Scheduling			
1. Does your facility have a policy or procedure for verifying the exact description of the procedure, including side or site as applicable, when a request is made to schedule an operation?	☐	☐	
2. Does your facility require the use of a standardized form when scheduling a case?	☐	☐	
If yes, does the standardized form include verifying the exact description of the procedure and side or site, as applicable?	☐	☐	☐
Consent			
3. Does your facility's policy or procedure require that the surgeon obtain consent for surgery from the patient or legal representative prior to or at the time the procedure is scheduled?	☐	☐	
4. Does your policy or procedure require that the consent for surgery include the following:			
a) correct patient name?	☐	☐	
b) exact description of the procedure?	☐	☐	
c) site or side, as applicable?	☐	☐	
Preoperative Verification			
5. Does your facility's policy or procedure require that patients are informed, as part of their preoperative preparation, that all healthcare providers will be verifying the following information:			
a) name?	☐	☐	
b) procedure?	☐	☐	
c) site or side, as applicable?	☐	☐	
6. Does your facility's policy or procedure require that verification and reconciliation of the schedule, consent, and history and physical examination be performed at the following times:			
a) at the time the surgical procedure is scheduled?	☐	☐	
b) at the time of pre-admission testing and assessment?	☐	☐	
c) prior to the patient arriving in the preoperative area?	☐	☐	☐
d) prior to the operating room (OR) being set up for the procedure?	☐	☐	
e) prior to the patient leaving the preoperative area or entering the OR?	☐	☐	
7. Does your facility's policy or procedure require the use of a standardized checklist prior to the day of surgery for documentation of the preoperative verification and reconciliation?	☐	☐	
If yes, does the standardized checklist include verification using the following items:			
a) schedule?	☐	☐	☐
b) consent?	☐	☐	☐
c) history and physical examination?	☐	☐	☐

(continued on page 89)

Figure 6-1: Self-Assessment Checklist *(continued)*

	Yes	No	NA
8. Does your facility's policy or procedure require that the verification and reconciliation on the day of surgery include the following:			
a) schedule?	☐	☐	
b) consent?	☐	☐	
c) history and physical examination?	☐	☐	
d) pathology reports, radiology reports, and/or radiographs, as applicable?	☐	☐	
e) patient or his or her legal representative's verbalized understanding of the procedure?	☐	☐	
9. Does your facility's policy or procedure require that the verification and reconciliation be performed independently on the day of surgery by at least two healthcare providers?	☐	☐	
10. Does your facility's policy or procedure designate which healthcare providers are required to perform the verification and reconciliation?	☐	☐	
11. Does your facility's policy or procedure designate which of the following providers are required to perform the verification and reconciliation:			
a) preoperative nurse?	☐	☐	☐
b) anesthesia provider?	☐	☐	☐
c) operating surgeon?	☐	☐	☐
d) circulating nurse?	☐	☐	☐
12. Does your facility's policy or procedure require that if any discrepancies are identified in the preoperative documents, a review of documents occur before the patient enters the OR?	☐	☐	
If yes, does the review include the following documents;			
a) Schedule?	☐	☐	
b) Consent?	☐	☐	
c) History and physical examination?	☐	☐	
d) Pathology reports, radiology reports, and/or radiographs, as applicable?	☐	☐	
e) Office records?	☐	☐	
13. Does your facility's policy or procedure designate that the operating surgeon is responsible for the resolution of any discrepancies in the preoperative document review verification process?	☐	☐	

Site Marking

	Yes	No
14. Does your facility's policy or procedure require the following;		
a) the operative site is marked after reconciliation of ALL relevant documents?	☐	☐
b) the operative site is marked after an alert patient's or legal representative's verbalization of understanding of the procedure?	☐	☐
c) the operative site is marked by the operating surgeon?	☐	☐
d) the operative site is marked by a preoperative nurse?	☐	☐

PA PSRS

(continued on page 90)

Figure 6-1: Self-Assessment Checklist *(continued)*

	Yes	No	NA
15. If your facility's policy or procedure requires that the operating surgeon verify the accuracy of the mark, is the surgeon required to verify the accuracy of the mark with the following:			
a) an alert patient's or surrogate's verbal understanding of the procedure?	□	□	□
b) consent?	□	□	□
c) schedule?	□	□	□
d) history and physical examination?	□	□	□
e) pathology reports, radiology reports, and/or radiographs, as applicable?	□	□	□
16. Does your facility's policy or procedure require that the operative site is marked prior to the administration of regional or local anesthesia?	□	□	
17. Does your facility's policy or procedure require that a provider who is responsible for marking the operative site has received instruction about how to mark the site?	□	□	
If yes, does the policy or procedure require that the instruction include the following:			
a) mark only the site?	□	□	□
b) mark the site unambiguously?	□	□	□
c) mark the site using a marker that is sufficiently permanent?	□	□	□
d) mark the site to be visible at all times, including:			
1) after positioning the patient on the operating table?	□	□	□
2) after prepping the operative site?	□	□	□
3) after draping the patient?	□	□	□
4) during the final time out?	□	□	□
18. Does your facility have a policy or procedure in place regarding patients who refuse site marking?	□	□	

Time Out

	Yes	No	NA
19. Does your facility's policy or procedure require that the anesthesiologist participate in a formal time out, with either the preoperative or circulating nurse, before administering a regional or local anesthetic block to the patient?	□	□	
If yes, does the policy or procedure require that the anesthesiologist reference the site marking as part of the formal time out verification?	□	□	
20. Does your facility's policy or procedure require that the operating surgeon conduct a preoperative briefing before care is given to the patient in the OR?	□	□	
If yes, does the policy or procedure require that the preoperative briefing include identification of the following items:			
a) the procedure?	□	□	□
b) the site?	□	□	□
c) the side?	□	□	□
d) implants, devices or special equipment?	□	□	□

(continued on page 91)

Figure 6-1: Self-Assessment Checklist *(continued)*

	Yes	No	NA
21. Does your facility's policy or procedure require that a final time out verification be done, involving all members of the surgical team, after prepping and draping and prior to starting the procedure?	☐	☐	
If yes, does the policy or procedure require that the surgeon state that other members of the operating team speak up if their understanding of the situation is different than the one stated in the time out?	☐	☐	☐
If yes, does the policy or procedure require that the final time out verification include secondary procedures and sites, such as vein harvest sites, when more than one procedure is being done at a site or a procedure involves operating at more than one site?	☐	☐	☐
22. Does your facility's policy or procedure designate who is responsible for conducting the final time out verification?	☐	☐	
If yes, who is designated:			
a) circulating nurse?	☐	☐	☐
b) anesthesia provider?	☐	☐	☐
c) operating surgeon?	☐	☐	☐
d) other? ______________________________(specify)	☐	☐	☐
23. If the designated person is other than the operating surgeon, does your policy or procedure require the following during the final time out verification:			
a) the operating surgeon has access to the consent?	☐	☐	☐
b) the operating surgeon states the correct patient's name, procedure, site and side as appropriate?	☐	☐	☐
c) the accuracy of the surgeon's statements is verified with an independent read-back confirmation by the designated person using information from the schedule, consent, history and physical examination, AND the site marking?	☐	☐	☐
24. Does your facility's policy or procedure require that during the time out, all other activities stop, except support of the patient's ventilation?	☐	☐	
25. Does your facility's policy or procedure require that if the patient is repositioned in the OR, the location of the operative site is confirmed at once by each member of the operative team?	☐	☐	
26. Does your facility have a policy or procedure addressing when a patient has more than one distinct procedure performed?	☐	☐	☐
If yes, does the policy or procedure require the following:			
a) separate verifications are done for the separate procedures?	☐	☐	☐
b) separate site markings are done for the separate procedures?	☐	☐	☐
c) separate time outs are done for the separate procedures?	☐	☐	☐
27. When an operation is done at the level of a particular vertebra or rib, does your facility's policy or procedure require the following;			
a) the target vertebra or rib is marked with a firmly affixed radiopaque marker by the operating surgeon?	☐	☐	

(continued on page 92)

Figure 6-1: Self-Assessment Checklist *(continued)*

	Yes	No	NA
b) the identity of the vertebra or rib is verified by fluoroscopy or radiograph (x-ray)?	☐	☐	
c) the identity of the vertebra or rib is verified in writing by a radiologist before the target structure is disturbed?	☐	☐	
Specimen Collection			
28. Does your facility's policy or procedure require that the identification of the specimen be verified?	☐	☐	
If yes, does the policy or procedure require that the verification include:			
a) the surgeon?	☐	☐	☐
b) the surgical technician?	☐	☐	☐
c) the surgical nurse?	☐	☐	☐
If yes, does the policy or procedure require that the verification include:			
d) the patient's name?	☐	☐	☐
e) the type of tissue?	☐	☐	☐
f) the specific location or site of the specimen, including side as applicable?	☐	☐	☐
Upon Completion of the Procedure			
29. Does your facility's policy or procedure require the removal of all patient information from the room after the patient leaves the OR and before the next patient arrives?	☐	☐	

For more information visit: http://www.psa.state.pa.us

This checklist, revised as of March 2008, accompanies the following:
Insight into preventing wrong-site surgery.
PA PSRS Patient Saf Advis
2007 Dec;4(4):109,112-123.

Created by the Pennsylvania Patient Safety Authority, this checklist allows organizations to gauge the quality of their verification, site marking, and time-out processes.

Source: Pennsylvania Patient Safety Authority.

methodologies, such as Lean Six Sigma, that use failure mode and effects analysis (FMEA)—which is a proactive risk reduction strategy that involves identifying potential areas where a process may fail and correcting them before they cause problems—and formal change management strategies. Preliminary results from the Joint Commission Center for Transforming Healthcare show that Robust Process Improvement™ (RPI) methods can be used to successfully reduce variation in the perioperative process. The learnings from the Center's wrong-site surgery project are currently being tested in other hospital and ambulatory care operating rooms.

TIP Review Center for Transforming Healthcare Initiative

The Joint Commission Center for Transforming Healthcare in mid-2009 began work on a project to prevent wrong-site, wrong-person, and wrong-procedure surgery. The project is being led by an obstetric and gynecologic surgeon, a Master Change Agent, and a Master Black Belt, all trained in Robust Process Improvement™ management processes, at Lifespan system hospitals and three ambulatory surgery centers. The project includes hospital leadership, surgeons, operating room directors, and staff. The team is examining all activities that take place in an operating room from the time the procedure is scheduled through confirmation that the intended procedure was performed. Solutions are expected to be available in late 2010. For more information, check the center's Web site, http://www.centerfortransforminghealthcare.org.

Health care organizations can comply with the Universal Protocol by using a variety of strategies and processes. Checklists, site-marking protocols, and documentation tools that verify completion of the time-out process can all be used to comply with the Universal Protocol. It is important to note, however, that merely putting protocols and processes in place will not guarantee compliance with the Universal Protocol. Organizations must work with the staff, including physicians, to develop and sustain a culture that values patient safety and ensures that compliance with the Universal Protocol is a matter of course.

Some further points to consider when designing processes and procedures related to the Universal Protocol include the following:

- *Structure the time-out process.* In addition to fostering a culture of safety within the team, organizations may want to structure team interactions to ensure that no critical information is missed. Although an organization may be conducting time-outs, if the time-outs are not specific enough, they may not catch an error before it occurs. Consequently, it is important to have a well-defined process for conducting the time-out. This process can involve a script or checklist for the time-out that declares the elements of the time-out, who needs to articulate them, and when they need to be articulated. The script also can encourage documentation in the medical record.[24] To be effective, a script or checklist should require active response from as many surgical team members as possible.
- *Educate team members on the importance of the Universal Protocol.* Some surgical teams skip or race through the presurgical verification and time-out processes because they do not understand the importance of them. Sharing data, including real-life incidents, that show how a focused, collaborative verification and time-out process can reduce the chance of wrong-site surgery can be helpful. One study conducted at National Taiwan University Hospital noted that an education program that used case-based materials, information feedback, and clinical guidelines reduced the incident of wrong-site tooth extraction.[25]
- *Involve the patient.* Patients are an important ally in preventing wrong surgery. By systematically including the patient in site verification and time-out, organizations can tap into this critical resource. Organizations that strive to achieve a patient-focused approach to care will naturally include the patient in these processes.
- *Target champions for change.* Few things are more frustrating for a health care provider than a required process or protocol, designed by an administrator, that does not fit well with daily work, does not result in improved patient care, and adds time. To avoid this situation with regard to the Universal

Protocol, organizations should involve surgeons, nurses, and physicians who are actively involved in surgical procedures in the development process. These individuals can not only contribute valuable opinions and thoughts to the process but also ensure that the elements of the Universal Protocol work in the surgical environment. These individuals can serve as champions for change and help drive the improvement process.

- *Consider technology.* Technology, such as electronic whiteboards, automated medical records, and radiofrequency identification (RFID), have the potential to reduce wrong-site operations. Electronic whiteboards can help improve communication among team members and provide a visual cue to the time-out process. RFID involves a tag, which is placed close to the surgical site, that can hold medical history, prescribed medications, allergies, and other pertinent information. Data are read remotely using a scanner.[26] This technology also can help ensure that all documentation is present at the beginning of a procedure and can help with correct patient identification.

  As with other technology, however, installation of state-of-the-art systems will not solve issues with wrong-site surgery if the organization culture is not committed to addressing the issue. Simply throwing technology at a problem does not fix it. Organizations must make sure their processes are safe and effective, and they should consider technology to help improve efficiency and reliability. (*See* Case Study 6-1 below.)

Case Study 6-1: Vanderbilt University Hospital

About the Organization: Vanderbilt University Hospital is an 832-bed tertiary care hospital in Nashville, Tennessee. With nearly 35,000 patients admitted annually, the hospital is a principal referral center for physicians and patients throughout the region.

Purpose of the Project: To enhance the organizationwide use of the Universal Protocol, including its use in both operative and nonoperative procedural settings.

Preventing wrong-site, wrong-procedure, wrong-patient surgery is part of the overall culture of safety at Vanderbilt University Hospital. The organization has based its culture on the principles of teamwork and communication, stressing that everyone who works in the organization has the right and responsibility to speak up if they see potential problems or inaccuracies or if they have questions or concerns.

For several years, Vanderbilt has been using the Universal Protocol for Preventing Wrong Site, Wrong Procedure, Wrong Person Surgery™ to improve patient safety in the surgical setting. Recently, the hospital has strengthened its application of the Universal Protocol process by enhancing its use of technology and measuring not only the performance of the Universal Protocol but also the quality of the effort.

Enhancing Technology

Within each of Vanderbilt's 54 operating rooms, there is an electronic whiteboard (*see* Figure 6-2 on page 95), which displays the preoperative checklist for all surgical team members to see. Information for the whiteboard is fed from the Vanderbilt computer system, so handwriting errors are eliminated. The whiteboard lists any important facts about the case as well as the patient's name, surgeon's name, anesthesiologist's name, and any other staff person present in the operating room.

Recently a group of medical students, key surgeon leaders, anesthesiologist leaders, and nurses redesigned the whiteboard to make it more interactive and ensure that the whiteboard fits well into current work processes. Now, at the beginning of a procedure, the presurgical checklist appears all in red on the whiteboard. Once the time-out is announced, the entire room watches as the circulating nurse begins the time-out process. As the nurse works down the checklist, asking a scripted series of questions and receiving confirmation from members of the surgical team that the checklist item is complete, the nurse clicks the answer to each question, and a green "check" appears for that portion of the checklist. The team cannot proceed to the next question until the previous question is answered and checked. At the point that all the elements of the time-out have been reviewed and agreed on by the surgical team, the entire checklist and the banner across the top of the whiteboard turn green and remain

(continued on page 95)

Case Study 6-1: Vanderbilt University Hospital (continued)

Figure 6-2: Whiteboard

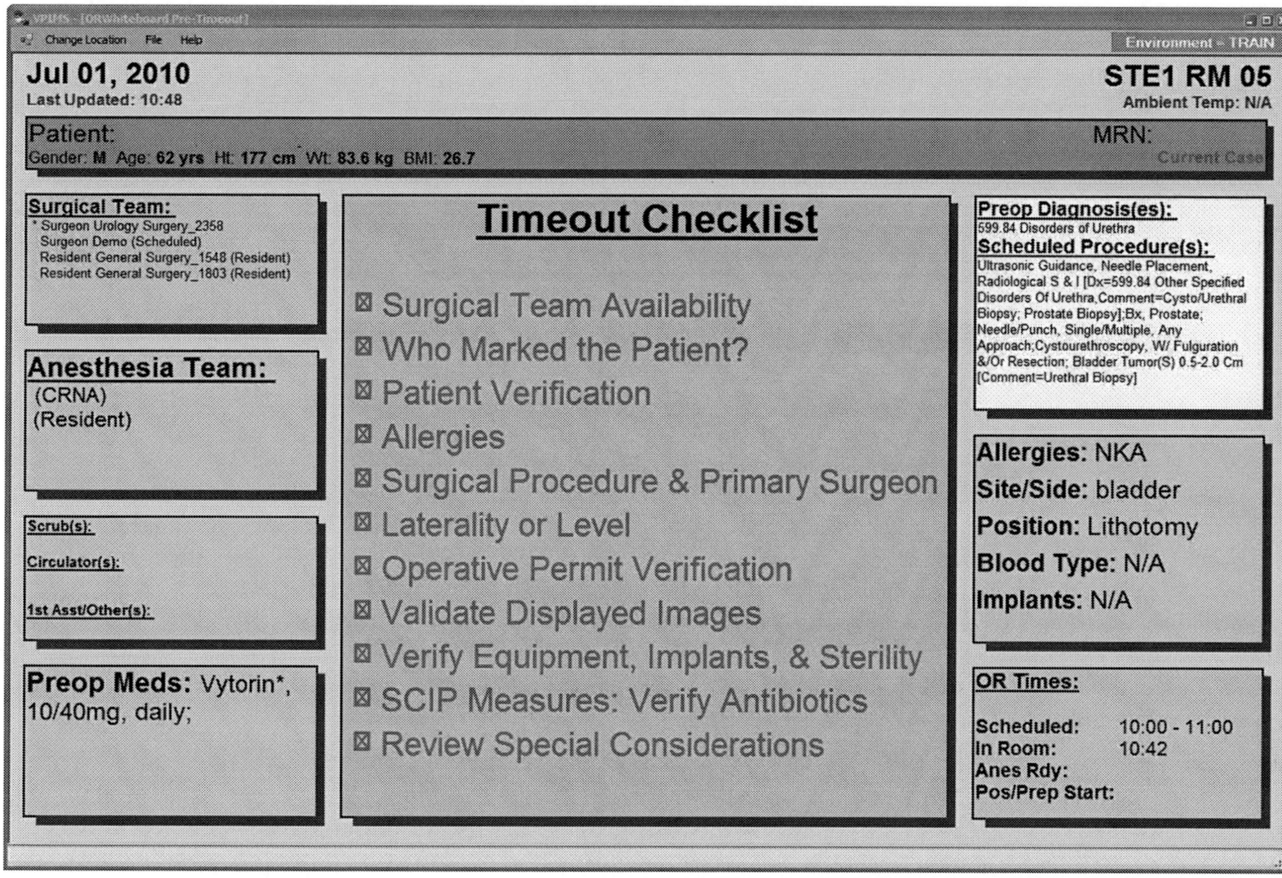

Vanderbilt University Hospital uses this electronic whiteboard to display the preoperative checklist in the operating room. As shown here, the central checklist screen and the banner across the top are red. The elements of the checklist will be confirmed one by one during the time-out, and the "X" in each box will change to a check mark (√). After the last element is confirmed, the screen and banner will change from red to green.

Source:

green throughout the surgical case. The term *Complete* also appears on the electronic whiteboard screen. This process step identifies, to any member of the surgical team entering the operating room, that a time-out was completed and all the critical elements have been met. Because the electronic whiteboard is more interactive and visual, it allows team members to quickly see if the time-out process occurred. The scripting of the key elements for the circulating nurse to read aloud ensures a standardized, sustainable performance process. If there is any disagreement among team members,

(continued on page 96)

Case Study 6-1: Vanderbilt University Hospital (continued)

they are charged to "stop the line" and reconcile the difference before proceeding.

Although the circulating nurse is assigned responsibility for initiating the time-out, all members of the surgical team are aware of the role they play in verifying the correct site, procedure, and patient. Each individual acknowledges the nurse's request and confirms readiness to proceed. After the time-out is completed, the nurse documents the process in the organization's electronic nursing documentation tool. Once the documentation is complete, it is reflected in the organization's electronic medical record, allowing compliance with the time-out to be monitored in real time.

Although an electronic whiteboard is not present in other settings throughout the organization that perform invasive procedures, such as the intensive care unit, interventional radiology, nursing units, and physician-owned clinics, the same principles of using interactivity and forcing functions apply. The organization uses a scripted series of questions to frame the time-out process in other procedural areas. For those areas with a computer at the bedside—such as the intensive care unit—the nurse or individual in charge of completing the time-out uses the script on the computer as a framework for conducting the time-out. As each step in the time-out is completed, the user checks off the step on the script. For those areas without a bedside computer, a paper template is provided that allows the user to enter the time-out information into the medical documentation system at a later time.

Vanderbilt uses a partnered approach to the Universal Protocol in procedure settings outside the operating room. Any time an individual is performing an invasive procedure that requires a time-out, he or she must conduct that time-out with a partner before starting the procedure. This provision ensures that there are two sets of eyes on the patient, confirming the necessary details for correct procedures.

Measuring Quality, Not Just Completion

Although the operating room setting at Vanderbilt has long been able to measure whether a time-out occurred, the new, interactive electronic whiteboards allow the organization to capture more information on the quality of the time-out. The scripted time-out process used in nonoperative settings also is conducive to measuring quality instead of just completion. Thus, it allows the organization the opportunity to truly measure performance, identify deficiencies, and work with providers to enhance their performance of the Universal Protocol. A strong educational program helps target areas of improvement and enhances the organization's performance even further.

To continuously improve and enhance the organization's Universal Protocol performance, a strong educational program has been established. A strong educational program targets areas of improvement and enhances the organization's performance even further. This is accomplished through various modalities of education and training such as interactive learning management software and the traditional classroom instruction. The entire multidisciplinary surgical team comprised of surgeons, anesthesiologist, CRNA [certified registered nurse anesthetist], residents, surgical technologist, and circulating nurse receive the Universal Protocol education and training to provide a shared approach to the time-out process.

The measure of successful training is demonstrated utilizing a series of questions asking the learner to evaluate his or her perception of safety when using the Universal Protocol Time Out checklist. To further evaluate the effectiveness of the training at various intervals after implementation of the Universal Protocol Time Out, the medical students will return to the operating room to observe the time-out process to ensure a hardwired work flow.

As with any process or procedure, the only way to know if it is being followed is to monitor compliance. Ambulatory surgery centers can benchmark their organization's use of the Universal Protocol with others throughout the United States by participating in the ASC Association's Outcomes Monitoring Project.[27]

There are a variety of ways to monitor compliance with systems and processes in place to meet the requirements of the Universal Protocol, such as through regular observation or surgical staff surveys. (*See* Figure 6-3 on page 97 for an example of a monitoring tool.) Another successful approach to measuring compliance is conducting daily, weekly, or monthly audits of the medical record to check for the completion of the preoperative verification, site-marking, and time-out processes. Regardless of how data are collected, information to capture could include the following[28]:

Figure 6-3: Wrong-Site Surgery Prevention Observational Monitoring Tool

Wrong-Site Surgery Prevention Observational Monitoring Tool

Perform 10 unannounced observations of operating room (OR) cases, preferrably orthopedic with laterality, spinal, eye, and other procedures on extremities. Exclude cardiac and upper abdominal surgeries.
For each blank box, indicate: *Yes* if element/action was completed as described, *No* if element/action was not completed as described, or *N/A* if not applicable.
Document time in minutes where indicated.

Scheduling/Consent (a standardized form is suggested)	**Case #1**	**Case #2**	**Case #3**	**Case #4**	**Case #5**	**Case #6**	**Case #7**	**Case #8**	**Case #9**	**Case #10**
Exact description of procedure was on OR schedule (including site, level, side, digit)										
Exact description of procedure was on consent (including site, level, side, digit)										
Consent was completed (including exact procedure, all required signatures, and dates)										
Preoperative Verification (a standardized checklist is suggested)	**#1**	**#2**	**#3**	**#4**	**#5**	**#6**	**#7**	**#8**	**#9**	**#10**
Verification and documentation were done independently by at least two providers										
Verification included OR schedule										
Verification included consent										
Verification included history and physical (H&P)										
Verification included the patient's understanding of the procedure										
Site Marking	**#1**	**#2**	**#3**	**#4**	**#5**	**#6**	**#7**	**#8**	**#9**	**#10**
Duration for the surgeon to complete the verification process and marking process	min	min	min	min	min	min	min	min	min	min
OR staff member marking the site used his or her initials										
Site marking occurred after reconciliation of all documents (schedule, consent, H&P)										
Site marking occurred before administration of sedation and/or anesthesia										
Site marking included discussion with patient										
Site marking was visible after patient was positioned, prepped, and draped										
Site marking was confirmed by intraoperative radiography for vertebrae and/or ribs										
Time Out (a standardized tool is suggested)	**#1**	**#2**	**#3**	**#4**	**#5**	**#6**	**#7**	**#8**	**#9**	**#10**
Duration to complete the time out	min	min	min	min	min	min	min	min	min	min
Time out was conducted prior to regional or local anesthesia, if applicable										
Final time out was conducted after patient was positioned, prepped, and draped										
All documents (schedule, consent, H&P) were verified during time out										
Diagnostic, radiology, and pathology results were verified during time out										
Surgeon was engaged—all work stopped and verbal acknowledgement occurred										
Anesthesia provider was engaged—all work except ventilation stopped and verbal acknowledgement occurred										
Nurses were engaged—all work stopped and verbal acknowledgement occurred										
Surgeon encouraged surgical team to speak up if there were any concerns										
OR Turnover	**#1**	**#2**	**#3**	**#4**	**#5**	**#6**	**#7**	**#8**	**#9**	**#10**
All patient information and specimens were removed from the room before the next patient arrived										

Adapted with permission from the Health Care Improvement Foundation.
2008 Pennsylvania Patient Safety Authority

Developed by the Pennsylvania Patient Safety Authority, this tool can help document observations of cases occurring in either the operating room or another area where invasive procedures take place.

Source: Pennsylvania Patient Safety Authority.

- Number or percentage of preoperative checklists completed
- Number or percentage of sites marked by patient
- Number or percentage of sites that were unmarked
- Number or percentage of time-outs completed before incision
- Number or percentage of time-outs completed before administration of regional anesthesia
- Percentage of films taken without sides marked with lead markers
- Percentage of times the side and site are noted correctly on the consent form
- Percentage of times "left" and "right" are spelled out in the medical record throughout the perioperative process and whether all side designations are in agreement

Simply collecting data is not sufficient. Organizations should regularly review compliance data and determine whether health care providers are complying with the systems and processes, and if they are not, why not. Feedback is critical to discuss with providers why they are not complying and how compliance can be improved. One study conducted in Switzerland showed that audits and feedback helped change practice and increase compliance with patient identity and site-of-surgery checks.[29]

TIP A Helpful Site for Resources

The U.S. Association of periOperative Registered Nurses (AORN) sponsors a National Time Out Day to call attention to the importance of the time-out process and other efforts involved in preventing wrong surgery. To support this effort, AORN has assembled several tools and resources in one convenient location. To access this helpful compendium, go to http://www.aorn.org/AboutAORN/PartnersInHealth/NationalTimeOutDay/.

Understanding the World Health Organization (WHO) Surgical Safety Checklist

As discussed earlier in this chapter and in other chapters, an organization may want use a checklist to guide, supplement, or enhance its use of the Universal Protocol. One specific checklist that is gaining popularity around the world is the World Health Organization (WHO) Surgical Safety Checklist. Although use of this particular checklist is not a requirement of The Joint Commission or JCI, it can serve as a useful tool in an organization's collection of strategies for reducing and eliminating wrong surgery and other avoidable errors in the surgical setting.

The WHO Surgical Safety Checklist was created to assist surgical teams and those performing other invasive procedures in reducing patient harm and enhancing safety.[1] At its core, the WHO checklist focuses on enhancing teamwork and communication while catching omissions before they result in errors. Like checklists used in aviation, the WHO checklist helps the surgical team coordinate discussions about safety during various phases of the surgical continuum.

The development of the checklist was guided by three overarching principles: simplicity, wide applicability, and measurability. Simplicity was important because if the checklist became too detailed, it might sacrifice ease of use and therefore negatively impact adoption among health care providers. Wide applicability was important because this principle allowed the checklist to reach all environments and settings and not be narrowly focused on specific procedures or specific settings. Measurability was important to allow users to clearly see if implementing the checklist results in improvement. By using meaningful metrics, organizations can get a sense of how the checklist is working and what alterations need to be made.[1]

The checklist was designed to help health care organizations in nations around the world evaluate their own processes of care and improve safety. Evidence, expert consensus, and input from anesthesiologists, operating room nurses, surgeons, patients, and other professionals helped shape the content of the checklist to ensure that tangible, lifesaving improvements could be achieved through its use.[1] These individuals considered a number of standards that could be used to improve surgical care and evaluated evidence for each before deciding what should be included in the checklist. They also estimated the potential effectiveness of each of the components of the checklist and developed measures to assess this potential.[1] (A copy of the checklist can be found in Figure 6-4 on page 99.)

Taking only a few minutes to complete, the checklist addresses 19 activities that occur at three specific points in the surgical process: before the patient is anesthetized, before skin incision, and before the patient is taken from the operating room.[30] Activities before the patient is anesthetized focus on obtaining consent, verifying identity, marking the surgical site, checking equipment, reviewing risks—including allergies and airway problems—and making sure appropriate equipment, blood, fluids, and other supplies are available if needed.

Activities before incision focus on confirming the correct patient and procedure, verifying that appropriate antibiotics were given if necessary, and checking that any radiology images are displayed. Within this step, teams brief about the case, with surgeons, anesthesiologists, and nurses each providing details and offering any concerns.

Activities at the end of the operation focus on documenting the completed procedure; labeling any tissue specimens; performing needle, sponge, and equipment counts; and identifying any equipment problems that need to be addressed before the next procedure.[31]

Figure 6-4: WHO Surgical Safety Checklist

Surgical Safety Checklist

World Health Organization | Patient Safety
A World Alliance for Safer Health Care

Before induction of anaesthesia → **Before skin incision** → **Before patient leaves operating room**

Before induction of anaesthesia

(with at least nurse and anaesthetist)

Has the patient confirmed his/her identity, site, procedure, and consent?
- ☐ Yes

Is the site marked?
- ☐ Yes
- ☐ Not applicable

Is the anaesthesia machine and medication check complete?
- ☐ Yes

Is the pulse oximeter on the patient and functioning?
- ☐ Yes

Does the patient have a:

Known allergy?
- ☐ No
- ☐ Yes

Difficult airway or aspiration risk?
- ☐ No
- ☐ Yes, and equipment/assistance available

Risk of >500ml blood loss (7ml/kg in children)?
- ☐ No
- ☐ Yes, and two IVs/central access and fluids planned

Before skin incision

(with nurse, anaesthetist and surgeon)

- ☐ **Confirm all team members have introduced themselves by name and role.**
- ☐ **Confirm the patient's name, procedure, and where the incision will be made.**

Has antibiotic prophylaxis been given within the last 60 minutes?
- ☐ Yes
- ☐ Not applicable

Anticipated Critical Events

To Surgeon:
- ☐ What are the critical or non-routine steps?
- ☐ How long will the case take?
- ☐ What is the anticipated blood loss?

To Anaesthetist:
- ☐ Are there any patient-specific concerns?

To Nursing Team:
- ☐ Has sterility (including indicator results) been confirmed?
- ☐ Are there equipment issues or any concerns?

Is essential imaging displayed?
- ☐ Yes
- ☐ Not applicable

Before patient leaves operating room

(with nurse, anaesthetist and surgeon)

Nurse Verbally Confirms:
- ☐ The name of the procedure
- ☐ Completion of instrument, sponge and needle counts
- ☐ Specimen labelling (read specimen labels aloud, including patient name)
- ☐ Whether there are any equipment problems to be addressed

To Surgeon, Anaesthetist and Nurse:
- ☐ What are the key concerns for recovery and management of this patient?

This checklist is not intended to be comprehensive. Additions and modifications to fit local practice are encouraged.

Revised 1 / 2009

This checklist was developed by the World Health Organization to help improve the safety of the surgical process. The checklist is also available in Chinese, Arabic, French, Russian, and Spanish and can be downloaded at http://whqlibdoc.who.int/publications/2009/9789241598590_eng_Checklist.pdf.

Source: © World Health Organization 2010. http://whqlibdoc.who.int/publications/2009/9789241598590_eng_Checklist.pdf. Used with permission.

Before releasing the checklist to the world in 2009, the WHO implemented the checklist in eight hospital sites around the world. The results of this implementation were striking. The final results showed that the rate of major complications fell by 36% and deaths fell by 47% across all hospitals.[31] (*See* Case Study 6-2 below for the story of one hospital's journey in implementing the checklist.)

It is important to note that the aim of the WHO checklist is not to prescribe a single approach to improving surgical safety but to ensure that key safety elements are incorpo-

Case Study 6-2: University Hospital of Monastir, Tunisia

About the Organization: The University Hospital of Monastir is an 800-bed public and general hospital located in Monastir, Tunisia.
Purpose of the Project: To test the use of the World Health Organization (WHO) Surgical Safety Checklist. The checklist was first tested in the pediatric surgery operating room and now is being implemented in the digestive surgery department.

To implement the World Health Organization (WHO) Surgical Safety Checklist, the University Hospital of Monastir followed three distinct steps:

1. Getting leadership support
2. Testing the checklist within the pediatric surgery department
3. Sustaining improvement and transitioning the use of the checklist to other areas of the organization

Getting Leadership Support
"Gaining the support of hospital leadership was an important requirement in this process," says Mondher Letaief, M.D., M.P.H., professor of preventive medicine for University Hospital of Monastir. "After soliciting the support of the head of the pediatric surgery department as well as the hospital manager, who were motivated to implement the checklist, we organized a multidisciplinary meeting, where we presented the objective and the required process for introducing the checklist in the operating room. The surgical team was invited to contribute to the process of translating the checklist into French and adapting it to the hospital's environment."

Testing the Checklist
Beginning in April 2009, the organization introduced the use of the checklist into its pediatric surgery operating room. A nurse was fully assigned for checklist administration for each surgical intervention. This individual also gave leadership regular feedback (either positive or negative) about the use of the checklist. Between June 2009 and December 2009, the organization used the checklist on more than 600 consecutively enrolled patients who underwent surgery. During this time, the organization assessed adherence to the checklist. "The reported stories from the nurse revealed that checking for the patient identification avoided at least one possible error," says Dr. Letaief. "Moreover, asking about potential blood loss was very important as it reinvited the team to guarantee the availability of blood before starting the operation."

In reviewing data from the pilot study, the organization found that checklist implementation also improved the compliance with prophylactic antibiotic administration within 60 minutes before incision, as it rose from 32.5% to 43.2%. The use of the checklist also enhanced interpersonal communication and teamwork in the operating room.

Sustaining Improvement
To sustain the use of the checklist and widen its utilization by additional teams at the local level as well as at the national level, the hospital conducted a meeting with all surgical team members to discuss and review the feasibility of the checklist. "Indeed, some notifications were added to complete the checklist and adapt it to our own context," says Dr. Letaief. "At this time, other teams showed their willingness to use the checklist." In this phase the organization also held a meeting with representatives from surgery-related scientific societies across the country, aiming at involving them in the implementation initiative on a national level.

"Fundamentally, we found that the WHO safe surgery checklist represented a driving opportunity to test the feasibility of implementing risk prevention strategies in the field practice," says Dr. Letaief. "It has also improved communication among surgical teams and consistency of care, as well as provided a way to assess safety indicators in order to reduce adverse events in surgery. We recommend that surgical departments practice with the checklist and examine how to sensibly integrate these essential safety steps into normal operative work flow."

rated into the operating room routine.[1] The checklist is not regulatory in nature or a component of official policy but a guide for developing processes to improve safety in the surgical setting. Although the content of the checklist was considered thoroughly before being finalized, the checklist is not meant to be all-inclusive. Organizations are encouraged to add to, edit, and modify the checklist to meet the needs of their local practice. The checklist comes with an implementation manual and guidelines to help organizations use it in a constructive manner.

Complying with the Universal Protocol and the WHO Surgical Safety Checklist do not have to be mutually exclusive. For example, the Surgical Safety Checklist can be used as part of an organization's approach to using the Universal Protocol because the checklist covers many of the components found in the preprocedure verification, site-marking, and time-out processes. Because both tools address many of the risks involved in surgery and other invasive procedures, using them in conjunction with each other can be beneficial, as one tool can inform the other, resulting in a comprehensive approach to reducing the risk for wrong surgery. Continued use of the checklist or a revised version of the checklist that reflects the characteristics of the organization should result in long-term improvement, particularly if such a checklist is used in conjunction with an organized approach to the Universal Protocol.

References

1. World Alliance for Patient Safety: *The Second Global Patient Safety Challenge: Safe Surgery Saves Lives.* Geneva: World Health Organization, 2008.
2. Senders J., Kanzki R.: The egocentric surgeon or the roots of wrong side surgery. *Qual Saf Health Care* 17:396–400, Dec. 2008.
3. Centers for Medicare & Medicaid Services: National Coverage Determination. Manual Section Number 140.6, 140.7, 140.8. http://www.cms.hhs.gov/center/coverage.asp (accessed Mar. 24, 2010).
4. Stahel P., et al.: The 5th anniversary of the "Universal Protocol": Pitfalls and pearls revisited. *Patient Saf Surg* 3, Jul. 1, 2009. http://www.ncbi.nlm.nih.gov/pmc/articles/PMC2712460/ (accessed Jul. 24, 2010).
5. Joint Commission International: Performance of correct procedure at correct body site. *Patient Safety Solutions* 1, May 2007.
6. Wrong-site surgery is no. 1 among sentinel events—Are you at risk? *Same Day Surgery* 31:113–124, Oct. 2007.
7. Kwaan M., et al.: Incidence, patterns, and prevention of wrong site surgery. *Arch Surg* 141:353–357, Apr. 2006.
8. Edwards P.: Ensuring correct site surgery. *J Perioper Pract* 18:168–171, Apr. 2008.
9. Blanco M., Clarke J., Martindell D.: Wrong site surgery near misses and actual occurrences. *AORN J* 90:215–218, 221–222, Aug. 2009.
10. Simon J., Ngo Y., Khan S.: Surgical confusions in ophthalmology. *Arch Ophthalmol* 125:1515–1522, Nov. 2007.
11. By the numbers. *Mod Healthc* 39:9, Nov. 23, 2009.
12. The Joint Commission: A follow-up review of wrong site surgery. *Sentinel Event Alert* 24, December 5, 2001. http://www.jointcommission.org/SentinelEvents/SentinelEventAlert/sea_24.htm (accessed Jul. 24, 2010).
13. Rhodes P., et al.: Assessment of the implementation of a national patient safety alert to reduce wrong site surgery. *Qual Saf Health Care* 17:409–415, Dec. 2008.
14. Rooney J., et al.: Surgical site marking does not affect sterility. *ANZ J Surg* 78:688–689, Aug. 2008.
15. American Academy of Orthopaedic Surgeons: *Wrong Site Surgery.* http://www5.aaos.org/wrong/viewscrp.cfm (accessed Jul. 24, 2010).
16. Chassin M., Becher E.: The wrong patient. *Ann Intern Med* 136:826–833, Jun. 2002.
17. O'Leary D.: The Universal Protocol. *American Medical Association Policy Forum,* Jun. 10, 2005.
18. Mody M., et al.: The prevalence of wrong level surgery among spine surgeons. *Spine* 33:194–198, Jan. 2008.
19. Adapted from: Wrong-site protocol is more than one year old, but problems mount. *Same Day Surgery* 29:121–132, Nov. 2005.
20. American Health Consultants: Effective strategies to comply with Joint Commission's Universal Protocol. *Hosp Peer Rev* 28:149–151, Nov. 2003.
21. National Center for Patient Safety: *Ensuring Correct Surgery Directive FAQ.* http://www.va.gov/NCPS/faq.html#Pen (accessed Jul. 24, 2010).
22. Zhao X., et al.: Surgical site marking will not affect sterility of the sterile field. *Med Hypotheses* 73:319–320, Sep. 2009.
23. Morley J.: New York State Procedural and Surgical Site Verification Panel. Presented at the Wrong Site Surgery Summit II, Chicago, Feb. 23, 2007.
24. Avoiding wrong-site surgery for 5 years isn't long enough. *Same Day Surgery* 33:84, Aug. 2009.

25. Chang H., et al.: Effectiveness of an educational program in reducing the incidence of wrong-site tooth extraction. *Oral Surg Oral Med Oral Pathol Oral Radiol Endod* 98:288–294, Sep. 2004.
26. Michaels R., et al.: Achieving the National Quality Forum's "Never Events": Prevention of wrong site, wrong procedure, and wrong patient operations. *Ann Surg* 245:526–532, Apr. 2007.
27. Martin S.: Best practices for preventing wrong site surgery. *Focus*, Jan.–Feb. 2009. http://www.ascassociation.org/csarticle/ASCAssociationWrongSiteSurgeryArticle.pdf (accessed Aug. 4, 2010).
28. Effective strategies to comply with Joint Commission's Universal Protocol. *Hosp Peer Rev* 28:149–160, Nov. 2003.
29. Garnerin P., et al.: Verifying patient identity and site of surgery: Improving compliance with protocol by audit and feedback. *Qual Saf Health Care* 17:454–458, Dec. 2008.
30. Anderson L.: Safe surgery to save lives. *Nurs N Z* 15:21–22, Jul. 2009.
31. Gawande A.: *The Checklist Manifesto: How to Get Things Right.* New York: Metropolitan Books, 2009.

PART 2

During the Procedure

This part of the book examines important considerations while the surgery or other invasive procedure is under way. Chapter 7 discusses aspects of the patient's condition that must be carefully monitored throughout the procedure. Chapter 8 looks at problems that can occur during the procedure and discusses ways to avoid them.

Chapter 7

Monitoring the Patient

Even with a comprehensive patient assessment and preparation process and a skilled surgical team, it is not always possible for health care providers to predict how a patient will respond to surgery or other invasive procedures, and a certain degree of ambiguity will still be present during the procedure. Professional skill and knowledge of a patient are not sufficient to determine outcomes of procedures because there are many interdependent variables in the surgical setting, some of which are not necessarily under one's control.[1] Due to this unpredictability, surgical team members must understand how to effectively manage patients undergoing procedures. Such management involves a variety of efforts, including monitoring anesthesia and sedation, administering medications safely, and monitoring glucose level, body temperature, and blood use. The following sections take a closer look at these various efforts.

Monitoring Anesthesia and Sedation

A particularly complex part of the surgical process involves anesthesia and sedation. Historically, this part of the surgical experience was one of the riskiest. In the 1970s, a patient receiving general anesthesia as part of a surgical procedure had an estimated 1 in 5,000 chance of death. With improvements in knowledge and basic standards of care, this risk has dropped to 1 in 200,000 in the developed world.[2] Although the administrating and monitoring efforts of organizations in developed countries have made the use of anesthesia and sedation safer, there are still risks. For example, a patient can experience any one of the following complications as a result of anesthesia and sedation[3]:

- Aspiration of gastric contents
- Failed intubation
- Esophageal intubation
- Inadequate ventilation
- Airway obstruction
- Respiratory failure
- Cardiac arrest
- Local anesthetic toxicity
- Drug reaction
- Anaphylaxis
- Medication overdose
- Prolonged hypotension or hypertension
- Malignant hyperthermia
- Anesthesia awareness

The degree of complexity involved in administering and monitoring anesthesia and sedation cannot be overstated. Within this process, anesthesiologists or other highly skilled health care providers competent to administer anesthesia and sedation must insert equipment, monitor and adjust equipment, administer medication, monitor the patient, and communicate with colleagues.[4] Different aspects of care must be attended to simultaneously, and the chances of error during this time are significant. Inadequate patient monitoring and lack of knowledge of the pharmacology of the medications being administered—such as benzodiazepines, opioids, etomidate, propofol, ketamine, sodium thiopental, and neuromuscular blocking agents, to name a few—can lead to disaster. In addition, distractions, conflicting priorities, mistakes in judgment, and poor communication among providers can further exacerbate risks.

According to The Joint Commission and Joint Commission International (JCI), there are several levels of anesthesia and sedation with which a health care provider must be familiar:

- *Minimal sedation (anxiolysis).* This is a drug-induced state during which patients respond normally to verbal commands. Although cognitive function and coordination may be impaired, ventilatory and cardiovascular functions are unaffected.

- *Moderate sedation/analgesia.* This is a drug-induced depression of consciousness during which patients respond purposefully to verbal commands, either alone or accompanied by light tactile stimulation. Reflex withdrawal from a painful stimulus is not considered a purposeful response. No interventions are required to maintain a patent airway, and spontaneous ventilation is adequate. Cardiovascular function is usually maintained.
- *Deep sedation/analgesia.* This is a drug-induced depression of consciousness during which patients cannot be easily aroused but respond purposefully following repeated or painful stimulation. The ability to independently maintain ventilatory function may be impaired. Patients may require assistance in maintaining a patent airway, and spontaneous ventilation may be inadequate. Cardiovascular function is usually maintained.
- *Anesthesia.* This category consists of general anesthesia and spinal or major regional anesthesia. It does not include local anesthesia. General anesthesia is a drug-induced loss of consciousness during which patients are not arousable, even by painful stimulation. The ability to independently maintain ventilatory function is often impaired. Patients often require assistance in maintaining a patent airway, and positive pressure ventilation may be required because of depressed spontaneous ventilation or drug-induced depression of neuromuscular function. Cardiovascular function may be impaired.

Anyone designated to administer anesthesia should be familiar with and competent to handle all these levels.

Because of its complexity and propensity for error, the anesthesia and sedation function should involve a systematic approach that includes competent professionals, effective medications, careful execution, structured processes, and good communication. Without such an approach, the intricate function of anesthesia and sedation becomes more susceptible to error and harm.

When creating a systematic approach to anesthesia and sedation, surgical teams should consider the following strategies:

- *Communicate about risks before the start of a procedure.* As discussed in Chapter 4, the risk assessment is a critical factor in determining the success of anesthesia and sedation administration. If providers are aware of patient risks before the start of a procedure, they can plan accordingly. All team members should be aware of any concerns or potential risks and initiate appropriate patient monitoring based on the level of sedation and the patient's identified needs. To foster communication about risks before the start of the surgery or other invasive procedure, organizations may want to include this discussion in a structured preprocedure briefing process or preprocedure checklist.
- *Ensure competency.* When anesthesia and sedation are used in a surgical procedure, they must be administered by qualified individuals who have credentials and privileges and/or proven competencies to (1) administer medications to predictably achieve the desired level of sedation, (2) monitor patients to maintain them at the desired level of sedation, and (3) reverse anesthesia or sedation agents and rescue patients if they go "too deep."

    Generally, anesthesiologists are in charge of administering anesthesia/sedation agents, but sometimes these medications also may be administered by a nurse anesthetist.

    It is important to note that the person administering the anesthesia and sedation must be the first responder to any anesthesia/sedation emergencies. Although another anesthesiologist or code team can serve as an additional backup, the individual administering the medication should be competent to perform any necessary reversals. Ways that clinicians can demonstrate competency might include advanced cardiac life support certification, passing a written test, and/or demonstrating competence in the presence of an anesthesiologist or other qualified individual. Organizations can also conduct mock exercises to demonstrate ongoing competency. These might be done at predetermined intervals to demonstrate continued competency for recredentialing.

For providers who administer sedation or anesthesia but who are not licensed independent practitioners—for example, nurses—organizations should include the ability to administer moderate sedation in their job descriptions and as a designated competency. The criteria for demonstrating competency might be developed and observed by the anesthesiologist, who should then deem the professional competent. Competency demonstration might include passing a written examination, demonstrating processes in the presence of an anesthesiologist, responding to drills, and orally responding to questions posed by the anesthesiologist.

Joint Commission and Joint Commission International standards call for sufficient numbers of staff to administer and monitor anesthesia and sedation safely. Some organizations have difficulty determining the number of staff members or specific equipment needed to administer sedation or anesthesia, monitor the patient, perform the procedure, and respond with possible airway maintenance, oxygenation, and ventilation. According to Jane Schetter, R.N., M.S.N., C.N.S., senior consultant for Joint Commission Resources, "It is the level of sedation and the patient-specific history and physical rather than the medications given that determine the monitoring requirements and equipment that needs to be available."

- *Have reversal medications ready.* To be prepared for the unexpected, surgical teams should ensure that reversal agents that are appropriate to the medication and the patient are readily available in the operating room or procedure area. Processes should exist to verify that a reversal agent is the correct dose, is the appropriate agent for the anesthesia medicine in use, and has not expired. As mentioned in Chapter 3, a checklist can be helpful. Using such a tool to help prepare the operating room or procedure area and ensure the availability of reversal agents may be beneficial.
- *Address medication risks.* Several studies have suggested that medication error is a leading cause of adverse events in anesthesia.[5] Medication-related events, including syringe swaps, medication ampoule swaps, overdoses, and incorrect medication choices, can all occur. In fact, the risk of serious medication errors in anesthesia may be higher than in other specialties.[6] In part this is due to the sheer volume of medications an anesthesiologist administers each year. It is estimated that a typical anesthesiologist administers at least a quarter of a million medications during a practice lifetime.[7]

In addition to the high volume of medications administered by an anesthesiologist, there are many other reasons for medication error in patients undergoing anesthesia, including the use of potent drugs that carry a risk of serious injury or death when administered in excessive doses or without adequate patient support. In addition, the complex and ever-changing environment of the operating room or procedure area and the time pressures that require providers to administer several high-risk medications over a short period can add to the risk of error. Finally, the fact that one person—the anesthesiologist—is typically responsible for prescribing, dispensing, and administering the anesthetic and monitoring the patient, and therefore has no one ensuring that the correct dose and medication are being used, can further exacerbate risk.[5]

Taking a close look at the anesthesia medication management process may be beneficial in reducing errors associated with anesthesia medication. Using structured improvement techniques that reduce the number of steps in the process; include forcing functions; standardize elements of the process; and improve communication can all be helpful.

Developing specific protocols for anesthesia and sedation administration and monitoring can also be useful. Such tools can reduce the likelihood of adverse events by reducing the variability of the anesthesia and sedation process and ensuring consistency. Studies have shown that the use of anesthesia and sedation protocols or algorithms can yield great benefits, including decreased ventilation time, shortened hospital intensive care unit stays, fewer tracheotomies, and lower costs.[8,9] Such protocols direct that the dosage of an anesthesia or sedation agent be adjusted to an end point defined at the start of therapy using a standardized assessment scale and reevaluated regularly.[10] When developing protocols and algorithms, organizations should consult anesthesiologists and nurse anesthetists because these individuals know how the anesthesia administration process currently functions and where improvement opportunities lie. In addition, reviewing evidence-based practices, such as clinical pathways and clinical practice guidelines, can be helpful.

- *Monitor vital signs.* After anesthesia administration begins, health care providers should regularly monitor vital signs, including the following:
  — Blood pressure
  — Heart rate and rhythm
  — Respiratory rate
  — Oxygen saturation
  — Adequacy of intravenous access
  — Pain
  Such monitoring can help call attention to problems with anesthetics and cue staff to respond quickly to issues.
- *Consider technology.* For the administration of anesthesia and sedation, including regional blocks, the use of technology is becoming more common. For example, ultrasound-guided regional blocks allow real-time viewing of anatomical structures and can allow the anesthesiologist to watch the progression of the needle and the spread of the local anesthetic, which is thought to increase the safety of regional blocks and possibly reduce the risk of intraneural or intravascular injection of anesthetics.[11] However, the technology does not entirely remove these risks and, like other technology, should be used with well-designed processes that ensure safety.

  To help with documentation, organizations can also consider using a form of technology called an *anesthesia information management system*. This system records anesthesia information in a database, allowing for high-quality documentation.[12] An anesthesia information management system allows providers to document their care in near real time, and it automatically records vital signs from patient monitors.[13] Not only does the system help improve safety during the procedure, but information generated from the system can be used in performance improvement efforts targeted at improving anesthesia administration.
- *Use mnemonics to improve crisis response.* Because of the complexity of anesthesia and sedation, anesthesiologists and other providers administering anesthesia and sedation medication must be able to manage complex, rapidly evolving, life-threatening crises with little or no warning. In some cases, events may unfold at a rate that exceeds an individual's ability to keep up. A person's ability to manage a crisis is not necessarily dependent on experience. Several studies have shown that even experienced anesthesiologists may have trouble managing a crisis.[14] Effective crisis management is more dependent on the ability to identify problems quickly and respond consistently to unfolding events. Crisis response is best if providers can carry out predetermined sequences of actions that have been shown to be safe in responding to dangerous problems.[14] For that reason, it can be helpful for providers to use a mnemonic device that reminds them to cycle systematically through a basic series of thoughts and actions, the intensity of which will depend on the circumstances.[14]

  For example, the COVER ABCD – A SWIFT CHECK mnemonic is designed for use when any patient is undergoing general or regional anesthesia. It applies whether the patient is ventilated or spontaneously breathing. The elements of the mnemonic are as follows[14]:
  - **C** Circulation, Capnograph, and Color (saturation)
  - **O** Oxygen supply and Oxygen analyzer
  - **V** Ventilation (intubated patient) and Vaporizers
  - **E** Endotracheal tube
  - **R** Review monitors and Review equipment
  - **A** Airway (with face or laryngeal mask)
  - **B** Breathing (with spontaneous ventilation)
  - **C** Circulation (in more detail than above)
  - **D** Drugs (consider all given or not given)
  - **A** Awareness of Air and Allergy
  - **SWIFT CHECK** of patient, surgeon, process, and responses

The four levels of intensity for each of these components are represented by another, supplementary mnemonic:

SCARE, standing for SCAN, CHECK, ALERT/READY, EMERGENCY

Organizations should encourage surgical teams to follow the SCAN sequence on a regular basis, such as every 5 minutes, during any anesthetic procedure. By doing so, the sequence rapidly becomes second nature and can usually be completed in 40 to 60 seconds. Teams should consider using the CHECK sequence whenever all is not going according to plan. Providers can escalate to the ALERT/READY and EMERGENCY levels when warranted.

It is important to note that the sequence becomes AB COVER CD – A SWIFT CHECK when the patient is breathing spontaneously via any mask (including a laryngeal mask), and some components become redundant in certain circumstances.[14]

One important issue to keep in mind when monitoring anesthesia is *anesthesia awareness.* Also called *unintended intraoperative awareness,* anesthesia awareness occurs under general anesthesia when a patient becomes aware of some or all events during surgery or a procedure and has direct or indirect recall of those events. Although it does not happen frequently, the consequences of anesthesia awareness can be devastating to a patient.

A patient's experience with anesthesia awareness can take many forms. For example, a patient may hear events during surgery, such as alarms, doctors speaking to one another, or loud music. In addition, he or she could have pain, sensations of weakness or paralysis, and feelings of helplessness, anxiety, panic, and impending death.[15] The patient may be able to mentally comprehend what is happening but most times is physically unable to let anyone know. Sometimes the patient may not remember what happened but will start experiencing painful, often inexplicable, psychological difficulties, including sleep disturbances, dreams, flashbacks, and anxiety. Long-term effects of the experience can include emotional problems, nightmares, anxiety, and even posttraumatic stress disorder.[16] Anesthesia awareness can also adversely affect a patient's ability to recover from an operation.

To help consistently and appropriately address anesthesia awareness, organizations should consider developing and implementing an anesthesia awareness policy (*see* Sidebar 7-1 on page 110). Actions the policy could address include the following:

- *Identifying patients at risk.* Certain types of patients are at higher risk for anesthesia awareness than others. For example, very young patients, female patients, and chronic drug and alcohol users may be more likely to experience this problem.[17] Identifying these patients before surgery and discussing with them their risk for awareness can help avoid some of the fear associated with the issue. To help identify high-risk patients, providers should be educated on the characteristics of high-risk patients and how to identify them. During assessment, nurses should screen patients for a previous history of anesthesia awareness and listen carefully for cues of any risks.
- *Maintaining equipment.* Equipment failure is one of the causes of anesthesia awareness that can be virtually eliminated. Regularly scheduled maintenance and testing on anesthesia equipment can help prevent breakdowns that can lead to awareness. In addition, the anesthesia machine and its vaporizers should be meticulously checked before any administration of anesthesia.
- *Monitoring patients for anesthesia awareness.* Monitoring patients for anesthesia awareness can be challenging. Clinical monitoring, such as regularly checking blood pressure and heart rate, cannot reliably identify or prevent awareness episodes.[18] Another method of monitoring involves asking patients to respond to a question while they are sedated. Such a question might be, "If you can hear me, could you please squeeze my hand?" Although sometimes effective, there are obvious drawbacks to this method. For example, if a patient is unable to move because of the muscle relaxants or other similar medication, then he or she might hear the anesthesiologist but not be able to respond.

  A more recent monitoring method involves brain monitoring devices. These can be used to measure depth of consciousness. Studies have shown that these monitoring devices can help anesthesia providers further reduce the risk of awareness, although they alone are not guaranteed to prevent awareness.[16]

  When assessing for anesthesia awareness, providers may want to ask patients postoperatively whether they experienced any symptoms of anesthesia awareness. Although important to do, this will identify patients after the fact. In addition,

Sidebar 7-1: Joint Commission *Sentinel Event Alert* on Anesthesia Awareness

As part of a 2004 *Sentinel Event Alert* on preventing and managing the impact of anesthesia awareness, The Joint Commission recommended that organizations develop and implement an anesthesia awareness policy. The alert describes what to include in the policy and offers a detailed discussion of the issue of anesthesia awareness. The full text of the *Sentinel Event Alert* is available at http://www.jointcommission.org/SentinelEvents/SentinelEventAlert/sea_32.htm.

it may not capture all patients who have experienced this problem because an individual might have experienced it but not fully remembered it or not be sure enough to report it. Also, a patient may, in fact, remember something that did not occur or perhaps did not occur during surgery. Anesthesia awareness during surgery can be difficult to distinguish from awareness during awakening in the postanesthesia care unit.[19]

Sometimes, regardless of an organization's best intentions, a patient can experience anesthesia awareness. In these cases, health care practitioners must be prepared to acknowledge and manage the occurrence. Early identification of the problem is critical to adequately acknowledge the situation. Compassion, respect, and diligence are all important in interacting with a patient who has experienced this problem.

Administering Medications

During most surgical procedures, surgeons, anesthesiologists, and/or nurses must administer medication. The act of medication administration in the surgical setting is different than in other locations throughout a health care organization. As with anesthesia medications, many times, the clinician prescribing the medication is also the one dispensing and administering it, leaving little chance to detect an error before it reaches the patient. In other cases, even if one clinician prescribes a medication and another administers it, communication of the medication order is often verbal, which can present risks for medication error.[20]

Following are some activities in which surgical teams can engage that will help reduce the risks associated with administering medications in the surgical setting.

- *Identify the patient and confirm any medication allergies.* Before a medication is administered, the perioperative staff should verify the patient's identity to ensure the correct patient gets the correct medication. When conducting this verification process, it is important to use two identifiers. This can be done through the patient's identification band, if appropriate. If the band is not visible due to positioning or draping, the circulating nurse and anesthesia care provider may verify the patient's identity by using the patient's medical record.

  During patient verification, the circulating nurse should also verify the presence of any allergies. Providers should check the patient's chart for allergies and reconfirm any allergies with the patient before surgery. Verifying allergy information can be challenging in the operating room or procedure area because the pace of a procedure is quick and there often is not enough time to do an extensive review of the medical record to determine allergies. Organizations that incorporate allergy verification in a preoperative checklist or provide a specific location in the medical record for the documentation of allergy information can help ensure that such information is easily accessible during the procedure. Electronic medical records are particularly helpful in this process, as organizations can designate a particular field for allergy information.
- *Verify medications before administration.* Although Chapter 4 discussed properly preparing and labeling medications for use in the surgical setting as part of the patient preparation process, surgical team members must still verbally and visually verify medications before administering them. Within this verification process, each medication's name, strength, dosage, and expiration time, when applicable, should be verified. Verification must be

completed by two qualified individuals before the start of a procedure. If only a circulating nurse is present, he or she should be empowered to confirm the medication with another licensed professional (for example, the anesthesiologist or surgeon) performing the surgical procedure. Using structured techniques, such as repeat-back, can help with the verification process.

Shift changes can be particularly risk-prone for medication errors. When staff members are entering and exiting the operating room or procedure area, communication can break down. To prevent confusion at shift change or break relief, entering and exiting personnel should note and verify concurrently all medications on and off the sterile field and their labels. Communication about the amount of medication administered should take place at this time as well.[21]

- *Structure the use of verbal orders.* Verbal orders are often used in the surgical setting when surgeons and anesthesiologists need to order medications in the midst of a procedure. These types of orders present significant risks in the operating room or procedure area. When misheard or misinterpreted, such orders can result in the administration of incorrect medications or inappropriate dosages.

Verbal orders in the operating room or procedure area are subject to misinterpretation for a variety of reasons. For example, the multicultural backgrounds of the health care providers in the room, masks worn in the operating room or procedure area that muffle speech, and background noise—telephones ringing, alarms sounding, music playing—can all impede the clear receipt of a verbal order.[22] In addition, the person receiving a verbal order may be distracted, and if that individual is inexperienced, a lack of familiarity with the situation can further cause confusion.

In addition to the hectic, fast-paced environment of the operating room or procedure area, many of the medications used in the surgical setting have similar-sounding names, which can lead to confusion, particularly when the previously mentioned environmental factors are present. Some experts believe that 25% of medication errors involve similar medication names.[22,23]

To help prevent medication errors, all verbal orders in the operating room or procedure area should ideally be verified out loud and repeated back. For example, a surgeon could say "Give Mr. Sanchez ten thousand units of heparin," and the anesthesiologist should then repeat "ten thousand units of heparin." The surgeon should then confirm this is correct. Dry erase boards mounted in the operating room or procedure area can allow health care personnel, such as the circulating nurse, to write down the order and facilitate the surgeon or ordering clinician to visually and verbally confirm it.[22] For further verification, the individual administering the drug could announce the drug and dose just before administration.[24] Although this verbal verification may require extra effort on the part of the surgeon and surgical team, performing such verifications will likely improve not only communication between team members but also patient safety.

To further ensure that verbal orders are clear, organizations should encourage health care providers to spell words out, using such aids as "A as in Alfa," "B as in Bravo," "C as in Charlie," and so on. (*See* Sidebar 7-2 on page 112.) Providers should also use a digit-by-digit technique. This technique involves stating each digit of a number, such as saying "one-six" instead of "sixteen." Providers should also avoid abbreviations where possible. Organizations may choose to modify the list shown in Sidebar 7-2 or create their own list, but they should have one.

Although all the structured communication techniques presented here are helpful in improving clarity and reducing the likelihood of error, providers should still ask themselves whether an order makes sense in the context of the patient's procedure, condition, and indication for use. For example, a verbal order for Cerebyx during a craniotomy makes sense; however, a verbal order for Celebrex during the same procedure should raise a red flag. Practitioners should be empowered to question and reclarify that order.[22]

Sidebar 7-2: International Radiotelephony Spelling Alphabet

Developed in 1927, the following internationally recognized phonetic alphabet assigns code words to each letter of the alphabet so that critical combinations of letters (and numbers) can be pronounced and understood by those who transmit and receive verbal messages, regardless of their native language.

A - Alfa	J - Juliett	S - Sierra
B - Bravo	K - Kilo	T - Tango
C - Charlie	L - Lima	U - Uniform
D - Delta	M - Mike	V - Victor
E - Echo	N - November	W - Whiskey
F - Foxtrot	O - Oscar	X - X-ray
G - Golf	P - Papa	Y - Yankee
H - Hotel	Q - Quebec	Z - Zulu
I - India	R - Romeo	

Source: International Civil Aviation Organization: *The Postal History of ICAO.* http://www.icao.int/icao/en/hist/stamps/annex_10_aeronautical_telecommunications.htm (accessed Jul. 20, 2010).

Organizations should develop a verbal order policy for the operating room or procedure area, educate the health care providers on that policy, and monitor its consistent use.

- *Identify and address the use of high-alert medications.* High-alert medications are drugs that bear a heightened risk of causing significant patient harm when they are used in error. Although mistakes may or may not be more common with these drugs, the consequences of an error with them can be more devastating to patients.[25] Some examples of high-alert medications used in surgical settings include heparin, epinephrine (*see* Case Study 7-1 on page 113 and Sidebar 7-3 on page 114), and phenylephine. Many of the adverse events associated with these medications are related to incorrect dilutions, inappropriate concentrations, or medication mix-ups.[26] In addition, some events have resulted when medications are transferred to unlabeled vials or when indications and administration procedures are misinterpreted.

  To reduce the risks associated with high-alert medications, organizations can take a variety of actions. In addition to following the aforementioned safe medication practices, organizations should also consider the following:
  - Standardize preparation of all diluted solutions. These standardized solutions should be prepared before surgery so that they are in ready-to-use or ready-to-administer containers that will allow for sterile delivery of the container's contents.
  - Refrain from diluting medications on the surgical field. Although organizations should refrain from using nonstandardized dilutions, if a dilution is necessary, it should be done by a registered pharmacist. If a medication must be diluted in the operating room or procedure area, diluting instructions should be precalculated by a pharmacist and readily available for clinical use.
  - Use only premixed solutions, and limit the number of medication concentrations.
  - Clinicians in the operating room or procedure area should communicate all doses of all medications to be administered and clarify the maximum dose with the anesthesia care provider and surgeon.
  - Educate nurses and other personnel who work in the operating room or procedure area about the safe handling and administration of high-alert medications.
  - Assess and validate clinical competency with handling and administering these medications.

Monitoring Glucose Level

Inadequate control of glucose in surgical patients, particularly those patients with diabetes and those undergoing cardiac surgery, can increase the risk of surgical site infections. Maintaining tight control of blood glucose levels is reported to not only reduce the risk of surgical site infections but also reduce mortality in both diabetic and nondiabetic patients.[27,28]

Organizations can sometimes struggle with effective blood glucose monitoring. One way to facilitate blood glucose management is through the use of continuous glucose monitoring systems, which determine blood glucose levels on a continuous basis every few minutes. These systems use monitors that are placed under the

Case Study 7-1: Institute for Safe Medication Practices Canada

About the Organization: The Institute for Safe Medication Practices Canada (ISMP Canada) is an independent, not-for-profit agency committed to the advancement of medication safety in all health care settings within Canada. ISMP Canada works collaboratively with the health care community, regulatory agencies and policy makers, provincial, national, and international patient safety organizations, the pharmaceutical industry, and the public to promote safe medication practices.

Purpose of the Project: To identify areas of exposure and risk in the operating room environment and to inform the development of a medication safety self-assessment specific to the operating room.

In the early 2000s, an interdisciplinary team of consultants from the Institute for Safe Medication Practices Canada (ISMP Canada), along with representatives from the United States–based Institute for Safe Medication Practices (ISMP US), were invited to participate in a medication safety project for operating rooms in a large teaching hospital and in a community hospital in the province of Ontario, Canada. This interdisciplinary team conducted an assessment of the operating rooms within the organization based on the following 10 key elements of medication use from ISMP US:

1. Patient information
2. Drug information
3. Communication of drug information
4. Drug labeling, packaging, and nomenclature
5. Drug storage, stock, standardization, and distribution
6. Drug device acquisition, use, and monitoring
7. Environmental factors
8. Staff competency and education
9. Patient education
10. Quality processes and risk management

The review team directly observed same-day surgical wards and individual operating rooms. During the assessment, the team interviewed physicians—both surgeons and anesthesiologists—nurses, pharmacists, pharmacy technicians, educators, and representatives from surgical management. The team also toured the pharmacy and examined various supporting documents, including protocols, policies, and procedures and education materials.

Based on the results of this assessment, as well as on review of patient safety literature and medication incident analyses, ISMP Canada—in collaboration with the Canadian Anesthesiologists' Society, the Operating Room Nurses Association of Canada, and ISMP US, and with support from the Ontario Ministry of Health and Long-Term Care—developed a systematic checklist to help organizations assess, identify goals for, and determine opportunities within their operating room medication safety processes.

After creating an initial version of the checklist, ISMP Canada sent the document out to Ontario hospitals for review and comment. After revising the checklist based on feedback from this review, it was piloted by 18 Ontario hospitals, 4 of which had multiple sites. The hospitals provided direct, interactive feedback on the checklist and were also provided with the opportunity to participate in a follow-up survey about the checklist items. Within this interactive process, ISMP Canada tried to gauge the usefulness of the checklist as well as its clarity and effectiveness. Based on the feedback and survey findings, ISMP Canada made further changes and released Version One.

Shortly after the release of its checklist, ISMP Canada became aware of a fatal medication mix-up involving concentrated epinephrine 1 mg/mL intended for topical use and injectable local anesthetic containing dilute epinephrine. Based on the review of this incident and recommendations developed as a result of it, ISMP Canada changed its checklist to incorporate assessing for potentially dangerous mix-ups between drugs intended for topical use and those intended for injection. A second version of the checklist was released in 2009.

The checklist is intended for internal use by facilities to systematically review their operating room processes, especially with regard to medication safety. It is particularly useful as repeat assessments are performed to see where improvements have been achieved over time. To use the checklist, organizations must first establish a multidisciplinary team that includes representation from all providers involved with medication use in the surgical setting. Through the ISMP Canada Web site, organizations can examine their results over time and also compare them with the aggregate findings of other respondents on both a national and a regional basis.

Although the checklist may not directly apply to all organizations, it can provide a useful place to start when considering medication safety in the operating room. For more information about the ISMP Canada Operating Room Medication Safety Checklist, go online to https://www.ismp-canada.org/operatingroomchecklist/.

Additional Sources:

Institute for Safe Medication Practices: *Frequently Asked Questions (FAQ)*. http://www.ismp.org/faq.asp#Question_3 (accessed Jul. 24, 2010).

Institute for Safe Medication Practices Canada: *Operating Room Medication Safety Checklist (Version 2)*. https://www.ismp-canada.org/operatingroomchecklist/ (accessed Jul. 24, 2010).

Sidebar 7-3: Ephedrine vs. Epinephrine—A Risk for Confusion

One potential medication mix-up of which health care providers should be aware is the confusion between ephedrine and epinephrine. Not only do the names of these medications look and sound similar, they are often stored next to each other because they are both used as vasopressors and vasoconstrictors. Also, both drugs may be packaged in 1 mL ampoules or vials.

Following are several recommendations from The Institute of Safe Medication Practices (ISMP) for reducing the possibility of mix-ups between these two medications:

- Avoid storing epinephrine and ephedrine side by side.
- Use "tall man" letters on computer inventory listings, shelf labels, and other places where the medication names appear.
- Use screen alerts on automated dispensing cabinets.
- Where possible, use prefilled epinephrine syringes.
- Keep large vials of epinephrine out of clinical areas to reduce chances of preparing large amounts of the medication.
- To ensure an independent double check, have the pharmacy prepare infusions and bolus doses for these drugs, except in emergencies.
- When conveying orders verbally, use the "read-back" technique.

Epinephrine can also cause medical error if topical and injectable doses are used in the same procedure and are inadvertently mixed up. One such error occurred during an outpatient ear-nose-throat procedure in which the surgeon requested local anesthetic for injection and was handed a predrawn syringe. The surgeon injected the medication into the surgical site. Immediately afterward, the patient experienced a cardiac arrhythmia leading to cardiac arrest. The injection contained topical epinephrine at a significantly higher concentration than the injectable dose. Despite full resuscitation measures, the patient died.

To avoid these types of tragic errors, organizations should consider the following recommendations from the Institute of Safety Medication Practices Canada:

- Develop distinct processes for preparing and handling epinephrine for topical application. In particular, medications intended for topical application should not be placed into a parenteral syringe. Conversely, a medication intended for injection should not be placed into an open container.
- Supply epinephrine for topical use in a pour-bottle format.
- Use effective labeling strategies, such as the ones described in Chapter 4.
- Keep local anesthetics for injection in their original vials, and withdraw such medications into a syringe (and label the syringe) immediately before use. Doing so allows the surgeon to participate in a reliable verification process using the manufacturer's product and the syringe label.
- Inject the surgical site with local anesthetic before scrubbing and gowning for ear-nose-throat procedures. Subsequent injection is seldom needed, but if it is required, additional local anesthetic can be withdrawn directly from the vial.
- Do not stock the multidose vial of injectable epinephrine 1 mg/mL (a high-alert drug) in any operating room or procedure area.
- Ensure that the word TOPICAL appears on the label of any container used to hold a solution intended for topical application.
- Store and prepare medications intended for topical use in distinctly separate areas from those used for storing and preparing medications for injection.

Sources:

Guzmán F.: Drug name confusion: Ephedrine and epinephrine. *FDA Patient Safety News*, Dec. 10, 2008. http://pharmacologycorner.com/fda-video-on-ephedrine-and-epinephrine-how-to-prevent-mistakes-in-their-administration/ (accessed Jul. 22, 2010).

Institute for Safe Medication Practices: Worth repeating ... EPINEPHrine-ePHEDrine mix-ups. *ISMP Medication Safety Alert!* 13, Aug. 14, 2008. http://www.ismp.org/newsletters/acutecare/articles/20080814-1.asp (accessed Jul. 22, 2010).

Institute for Safe Medication Practices Canada: ALERT: Fatal outcome after inadvertent injection of epinephrine intended for topical use. *ISMP Canada Safety Bulletin*, Mar. 5, 2009. https://www.ismp-canada.org/download/safetyBulletins/ISMPCSB2009-2-InadvertentInjectionofEpinephrineIntendedforTopicaUse.pdf (accessed Jul. 22, 2010).

Institute for Safe Medication Practices Canada: Risk of tragic error continues in operating rooms. *ISMP Canada Safety Bulletin* 4, Dec. 2004. http://www.ismpcanada.org/download/ISMPCSB2004-12.pdf (accessed Jul. 22, 2010).

skin or intravenously.[28] One recent study by Yamashita et al. showed that a continuous glucose monitoring device may be useful for following blood glucose level changes continuously and reducing the frequency of intermittent measurement.[29]

Organizations can maintain a patient's glucose level by administering insulin during or after surgery. There are several protocols in existence that can help an organization determine a continuous insulin infusion strategy or a sliding scale for insulin administration. Organizations should carefully consider these protocols when developing their own process for insulin administration. Protocols should be easy to implement, be easy to follow, and allow for continuous patient monitoring.[30]

Monitoring Body Temperature

One of the most common complaints from people who are having surgery or other invasive procedures is being cold. Not only is being cold uncomfortable and unnecessary, it can also contribute to an increased risk of certain complications, including surgical site infections. In fact, hypothermia can triple the risk of surgical site infection in patients undergoing some surgeries.[31] In addition, monitoring and maintaining body temperature during the perioperative period has a significant impact on the risk of myocardial ischemia, cardiac morbidity, surgical bleeding, and patient discomfort.[32] Even a 1.5-degree drop in temperature may result in serious consequences.[33]

There are several risk factors for heat loss among patients. Some are directly related to the patient, including general ill health, female gender, and age—both pediatric and geriatric patients are more at risk. Also, long procedures and those that involve presurgery fasting can affect temperature. Cold rooms, prepping solutions, operating tables, and intravenous fluids also are factors.[33]

Anesthesia can also significantly impair an individual's ability to regulate his or her temperature and therefore can predispose patients to hypothermia. Without temperature monitoring, hypothermia during anesthesia may be missed and thus not prevented or treated. Even when conscious, patients receiving anesthesia are often asymptomatic from hypothermia because of impaired responses. Patients are thus unable to report the sensation of being cold.[32]

To help prevent hypothermia, health care organizations may use a combination of blankets, forced-air patient warming systems, warmed intravenous fluids, thermal pads, thermal lamps, and slightly elevated room temperatures. Organizations can also have patients wear a hat and booties perioperatively.[31] It is also important to have consistent equipment and methods for measuring and monitoring patient temperature.[34] Such equipment may include liquid crystal skin-surface monitoring or axillary temperature probes.

To ensure consistent temperature monitoring, organizations should document the effort in the medical record or other surgical notes. Such documentation will allow monitoring of the activities and identification of opportunities for improvement. It is important to note that perioperative temperature management has recently become one of the Surgical Care Improvement Project (SCIP) core measures. (*See* Sidebar 7-4 on page 116.)

Monitoring Blood Use

Another critical area of monitoring in the surgical setting is blood use. Although there are no widely accepted data on the optimal levels of blood use and when to perform blood transfusions during surgery, the concept of conserving blood is a valid one in the interest of both patient safety and financial stewardship.

Blood transfusions are associated with several postsurgical complications, including surgical site infections, pneumonia, slower wound healing, prolonged ventilator use, and increased length of stay. One study showed that the five-year mortality rate for transfused patients was more than double the five-year mortality rate for nontransfused patients.[35] In addition, blood is expensive, and organizations should try to use only as much as is necessary for safe patient care.

Sidebar 7-4: The Surgical Care Improvement Project (SCIP)

The Surgical Care Improvement Project (SCIP) is a national quality partnership of organizations in the United States that are interested in improving surgical care by significantly reducing surgical complications. Partners in SCIP believe that a meaningful reduction in surgical complications depends on health care providers from multiple disciplines—surgeons, anesthesiologists, perioperative nurses, pharmacists, infection control professionals, and hospital executives—working together to make surgical care improvement a priority. The SCIP goal is to reduce the incidence of surgical complications nationally by 25% by 2010. (The project was still under way at the time this book was published.)

SCIP Partners include the Steering Committee of the following 10 national organizations that have pledged their commitment and full support for SCIP:

- Agency for Healthcare Research and Quality
- American College of Surgeons
- American Hospital Association
- American Society of Anesthesiologists
- Association of periOperative Registered Nurses
- Centers for Disease Control and Prevention
- Centers for Medicare & Medicaid Services
- Institute for Healthcare Improvement
- The Joint Commission
- Veterans Health Administration

As part of the SCIP program, hospitals must collect core measure data with patient discharges regarding several surgical issues, including adverse cardiac events, surgical site infections, postoperative pneumonia, deep vein thrombosis, and end-stage renal disease. Each surgical issue has several associated core measures that drive data collection.

To ensure that SCIP measures are fully supported by evidence-based research, each of the SCIP target areas—related to the previously mentioned different surgical issues—is advised by a technical expert panel. These panels have provided hours of technical expertise and resources to the effort.

It is important to note that many of the SCIP measures are also ORYX CORE Measures and thus can be collected at the same time. For further details on the particular measures and their specifications, go online to https://www.qualitynet.org/dcs/ContentServer?c=MQParents&pagename=Medqic%2FContent%2FParentShellTemplate&cid=1228694349383&parentName=Category. (These measures apply to U.S. organizations only. Joint Commission International has its own International Library of Measures.)

The American College of Surgeons also has a program to improve the quality of surgical care. Called the American College of Surgeons National Surgical Quality Improvement Program (ACS NSQIP), it is a nationally validated, risk-adjusted, outcomes-based program that employs a prospective, peer-controlled, validated database to quantify 30-day risk-adjusted surgical outcomes, which allows valid comparison of outcomes among all hospitals in the program. The difference between SCIP and ACS NSQIP is that SCIP focuses on *process* improvement while ACS NSQIP focuses on *outcomes* improvement.

Source: QualityNet: *SCIP Project Information.* http://www.qualitynet.org/dcs/ContentServer?c=MQParents&pagename=Medqic%2FContent%2FParentShellTemplate&cid=1122904930422&parentName=Topic (accessed Jul. 22, 2010).

Historically, surgeons have transfused blood for a variety of reasons, including low hematocrit and/or hemoglobin levels; prophylaxis in case a patient bleeds too much during surgery; to prevent organ failure; or because of established practice. Surgeons often transfuse blood because that is how they were taught and it is what they have always done. In some cases, surgeons choose to transfuse just in case there are problems. This is not an effective use of transfusion. Although there are cases in which transfusions are necessary, proactively increasing hematocrit and lowering risk factors for bleeding can be more beneficial for the patient and more cost-effective for the organization.

Case Study 7-2 on pages 117–118 discusses the work of one organization in conserving blood use within cardiac surgery. This work resulted in increased safety for patients and significant cost reduction for the organization.

Case Study 7-2: Providence Regional Medical Center

Name of the Organization: Located in Everett, Washington, Providence Regional Medical Center is a 372-bed hospital that performs more than 12,000 surgeries annually.

Purpose of the Project: To enhance the safety of surgical patients by reducing the number of blood transfusions and the quantity of blood transfused.

In 1999 Dr. James Brevig, a cardiac surgeon at Providence Regional Medical Center, was performing multiple surgeries every week, many of which required blood transfusions. To ensure that he was performing these transfusions at the right time and as a result of warranting clinical circumstances, Dr. Brevig looked for evidence-based recommendations about blood use and blood transfusions during cardiac surgery. To his surprise, there was no consistent evidence relating to when to perform transfusions. Instead, he found incredible variation in transfusion rates across hospitals. Dr. Brevig was concerned that his organization did not have a consistent method of determining when transfusions were necessary and how much blood to transfuse.

Dr. Brevig approached organization leadership with his concerns and, as a result, the organization began a multipronged effort to improve the efficiency and safety of blood use throughout its cardiac surgery program. This effort included the following components:

- *Collecting data.* A first step in Providence's work was to collect data on its surgeons' performance of blood transfusions and the quantity of blood transfused. The organization collected data on transfusion rates across the hospital as well as complication rates. The data showed that transfused patients had higher rates of kidney failure, longer time on a ventilator, longer length of stay, and a greater chance of surgical site infection. These data ran contrary to many preconceived notions held within the organization about the safety of blood transfusions and their benefits to patients.
- *Sharing data with surgeons.* By sharing the data, surgeons were able to see their own transfusion and complication rates and understand the correlation between high transfusion rates and potential complications. Through this effort, Providence was able to convince cardiac surgeons that transfusing patients unnecessarily is not safe.
- *Hiring a blood management specialist.* To help with the organizationwide improvement effort, Providence hired a blood management specialist. This is a clinical specialist who consults with surgeons on how to avoid blood transfusions. This individual works closely with surgeons to treat anemia without transfusion, such as through the use of presurgical vitamins. This person also works to educate surgeons and other clinical staff to consider the risks associated with transfusions, manage data collection, and present results.
- *Developing an anemia treatment protocol.* A key part of Providence's work in this area was the development of a blood use protocol. Created by surgeons and the blood management specialist, this protocol requires surgeons to evaluate every cardiac surgery patient for transfusion risk before surgery and manage anemia without transfusion, when possible. To further ensure that any transfusions that do occur are absolutely necessary, the protocol requires that a surgeon be consulted prior to his or her patient receiving a blood transfusion. Something to note about this protocol is that there are no standard triggers for blood transfusion; each patient is assessed individually, and transfusion is used as a last resort. This represents a shift in thinking for the organization—one that tries to eliminate the use of transfusions unless absolutely necessary.
- *Encouraging surgeons to slow down.* One simple way the organization reduced the number of transfusions involved encouraging surgeons to slow down and proceed carefully during surgery. Providence educated surgeons about the importance of taking their time and using meticulous surgical techniques. This approach to surgery limits the possibility of blood loss and can prevent the need for a transfusion. It can also help avoid bringing a patient back to the operating room to stop his or her bleeding. By avoiding repeat visits to the operating room, surgeons can reduce the possibility of complications and also make processes more efficient and less costly.

Outcomes of the Initiative

As a result of the previously mentioned interventions, Providence transfused nearly 500 fewer cardiac patients over a six-year period and saved 1,800 units of blood. In 1999 the organization transfused 36% of all coronary artery bypass patients. By 2009 Providence transfused only 6.5% of coronary artery bypass surgery patients. Taking into consideration both the cost of the blood itself and the staff time and effort to transfuse the blood, this reduction in blood use translated into an estimated cost savings for the organization of $4.5 million.

(continued on page 118)

Case Study 7-2: Providence Regional Medical Center (continued)

Providence's work on conserving blood not only increased the safety of patients receiving cardiac surgery but also saved the organization money. Although the transfusion rate declined significantly within the organization, the level of complications among surgical patients remained relatively stable and in some cases decreased.

After the blood conservation effort showed positive results within cardiac surgery, Providence applied its improvement strategies to other types of surgeries. For example, orthopedic surgeons also began to conserve blood and minimize transfusions within total joint replacement surgeries, and the success of the program spread quickly throughout the organization.

Today Providence has an organizationwide focus on blood conservation. From organization leadership to surgeons to frontline staff, Providence has a commitment to proactively address risks for transfusion and to transfuse only when necessary.

References

1. Healey A., Primus C., Koutantji M.: Quantifying distraction and interruption in urological surgery. *Qual Saf Health Care* 16:135–139, Apr. 2007.
2. World Alliance for Patient Safety: *The Second Global Patient Safety Challenge: Safe Surgery Saves Lives.* Geneva: World Health Organization, 2008.
3. Mhyre J., et al.: A series of anesthesia-related maternal deaths in Michigan 1985–2003. *Anesthesiology* 106:1096–1104, Jun. 2007.
4. Phipps D., et al.: Human factors in anesthetic practice: Insights from a task analysis. *Br J Anaesth* 100:333–343, Mar. 2008.
5. Merali R., et al.: Medication safety in the operating room: Teaming up to improve patient safety. *Healthc Q* 11(suppl.):54–57, 2008.
6. Smith J.: *Building a Safer NHS for Patients: Improving Medication Safety.* National Health Service, UK Department of Health, Jan. 22, 2004. http://www.dh.gov.uk/en/Publicationsandstatistics/Publications/PublicationsPolicyAndGuidance/DH_4071443 (accessed Jul. 24, 2010).
7. Llewellyn R., et al.: Drug administration errors: A prospective survey from three South African teaching hospitals. *Anaesth Intensive Care* 37:93–98, Jan. 2009.
8. Mascia M., Koch M., Medicis J.: Pharmacoeconomic impact of rational use guidelines on the provision of analgesia, sedation, and neuromuscular blockade in critical care. *Crit Care Med* 28:2300–2306, Jul. 2000.
9. Bair N., et al.: Introduction of sedative, analgesic, and neuromuscular blocking agent guidelines in a medical intensive care unit: Physician and nurse adherence. *Crit Care Med* 28:707–713, Mar. 2000.
10. Jacobi J., et al.: Clinical practice guidelines for the sustained use of sedatives and analgesics in the critically ill adult. *Crit Care Med* 30:119–141, Jan. 2002.
11. Loubert C., et al.: Complication during ultrasound-guided regional block: Accidental intravascular injection of local anesthetic. *Anesthesiology* 108:759–760, Apr. 2008.
12. Sandberg W., et al.: Real-time checking of electronic anesthesia records for documentation errors and automatically text messaging clinicians improves quality of documentation. *Anesth Analg* 106:192–201, Jan. 2008.
13. Epstein R., Dexter F., Piotrowski E.: Automated correction of room location errors in anesthesia information management systems. *Anesth Analg* 107:965–971, Sep. 2008.
14. Australian Patient Safety Foundation: *Crisis Management Manual.* http://www.apsf.com.au/crisis_management/crisis_management_manual.htm (accessed Jul. 24, 2010).
15. Ghoneim M.: Awareness during anesthesia. *Anesthesiology* 92:597–602, Feb. 2000.
16. American Association of Nurse Anesthetists: *Anesthesia Awareness Fact Sheet.* http://www.anesthesiapatientsafety.com/patients/ss/aware_factsheet.asp (accessed Jul. 24, 2010).
17. Myles P., Symons J., Leslie K.: Anaesthetists' attitudes towards awareness and depth-of-anaesthesia monitoring. *Anaesthesia* 58:11–16, Jan. 2003.
18. Sebel P., et al.: The incidence of awareness during anesthesia: A multicenter United States study *Anesth Analg* 99:833–839, Sep. 2004.
19. Eger E., Sonner J.: How likely is awareness during anesthesia? *Anesth Analg* 100:1544, May 2005.
20. Cutting errors out of the operating room. *ISMP Medication Safety Alert.* Mar. 6, 2002. http://www.ismp.org/Newsletters/acutecare/archives/Mar02.asp (accessed Jul. 29, 2010).
21. AORN guidance statement—Safe medication practices in perioperative practice settings. *AORN J* 79:674–676, Mar. 2004.
22. Hendrickson T.: Verbal medication orders in the OR. *AORN J* 86:626–629, Oct. 2007.

23. Wanzer L.: Perioperative initiatives for medication safety. *AORN J* 82:663, 665–666, Oct. 2005.
24. Cohen M.: Verbal orders in the O.R.: Masking the truth? *Nursing* 32:30, Jun. 2002.
25. Institute for Safe Medication Practices: *ISMP's List of High-Alert Medications.* 2008. http://www.ismp.org/Tools/highalertmedications.pdf (accessed Jul. 24, 2010).
26. Beyea S.: Patient safety first alert—Epinephrine and phenylephrine in surgical settings. *AORN J* 77:743–747, Apr. 2003.
27. Dronge A., et al.: Long-term glycemic control and postoperative infectious complications. *Arch Surg* 141:375–380, Apr. 2006.
28. Allen G.: Continuous blood glucose monitoring during surgery. *AORN J,* May 2008. http://findarticles.com/p/articles/mi_m0FSL/is_5_87/ai_n25429379/ (accessed Jul. 24, 2010).
29. Yamashita K., et al.: The accuracy of a continuous blood glucose monitor during surgery. *Anesth Analg* 106:160–163, Jan. 2008.
30. Shine T., et al.: Importance of perioperative blood glucose management in cardiac surgical patients. *Asian Cardiovasc Thorac Ann* 15:534–538, Dec. 2007.
31. Odom-Forren J.: Preventing surgical site infections. *Nursing* 36:58–63, Jun. 2006.
32. Frank S., et al.: Temperature monitoring practices during regional anesthesia. *Anesth Analg* 88, Feb. 1999. http://www.anesthesia-analgesia.org/content/88/2/373.full (accessed Jul. 24, 2010).
33. Pear S.: Patient risk factors and best practices for surgical site infection prevention. *Managing Infection Control* pp. 56–64, Mar. 2007.
34. Griffin F.: Best-practice protocols: Preventing surgical site infection. *Nurs Manage* 36:20–26, Nov. 2005.
35. Scott B.: Blood transfusion in cardiac surgery: Is it appropriate? *Ann Card Anaesth* 10:108–112, Jul. 2007.

Chapter 8

Avoiding Problems in the Operating Room

An open wound, an unconscious individual, several experts performing complex procedures—often at the same time—sharp instruments, multiple distractions, and combustible materials. All these factors are present in a typical operating room setting. It is no wonder that in this environment there are risks present for adverse events, which can negatively affect both patients and health care providers. This chapter discusses some of the problems that could occur in the surgical setting—including distractions, sharps injury, objects left in a patient's body after surgery, mishandling of specimens, and surgical fires—and provides suggestions on how to avoid these problems.

Minimizing Distractions

In one hour, the typical operating room can experience an average of 17 interruptions.[1] The duration of these interruptions can range from seconds to minutes.[2] Common interruptions include phones ringing, overhead pages, equipment and monitor alarms, conversations, and external staff visiting the operating room.[1,2] Although in certain instances an interruption can communicate new information that is valuable to a situation, at other times it can lead to distraction and medical error, such as blood transfusion errors or medication errors. Distractions and interruptions can negatively influence a provider's ability to stay focused on an activity or procedure, such as preparing medication, operating equipment, or assisting other providers.[3] One study showed that even if a provider is interrupted for as few as 10 seconds, it can result in the individual forgetting to carry out his or her task.[4]

Although distractions often have been considered an acceptable part of the surgical environment, they can present risks. Human beings have a limited capacity to manage interruptions and distractions in a safe manner, and so consequently every effort to minimize unnecessary distractions and interruptions should be considered.[3]

One effective way to minimize interruptions during critical phases of a procedure is to call for a "sterile" team environment. Within such an environment, all discussion and outside interruptions cease. Flight crews have used this technique during takeoffs and landings. The purpose is to avoid distractions that may lead to errors.[5] Fundamentally, calling for a sterile team environment can help refocus teams and maintain situational awareness (*see* Sidebar 8-1 on page 122). Evoking a sterile team environment may be appropriate during opening, closing, and sponge, sharp, or instrument counts; when verifying the surgical site, procedure, and patient; or whenever the full attention of the surgical team is needed.

To further minimize distractions in the surgical setting, organizations should make a close examination of processes and practices and eliminate any unnecessary distractions. As with other risk reduction activities discussed in this book, a systematic improvement process—such as Robust Process Improvement™ (RPI)—may be beneficial in this effort. Such a process could help pinpoint inefficiencies that cause distraction and make steps in a process as streamlined as possible. By eliminating unnecessary actions, providing tools at convenient locations, or engaging in other targeted interventions, organizations can systematically reduce the presence and impact of distractions.

Sidebar 8-1: Signs of a Loss in Situational Awareness

Distractions can pull people off task, add confusion, and derail communication, all of which can lead to a loss in situational awareness. As discussed in Chapter 1, *situational awareness* occurs when all team members agree about a procedure or process under way, recognize potential problem areas, and know the plans to address those areas. Within a complicated and hectic surgical procedure, situational awareness is easily lost, and the risk of accidents and problems goes up dramatically when this happens. Certain "red flags," or warning signs, can indicate the loss or potential loss of situational awareness, and the presence of any of the following red flags should alert team members that risk is increasing. Their presence should trigger a prompt discussion, such as a quick briefing or the call for a sterile team environment.

- *Something does not feel right.* This is probably the most important indicator of a problem. Individuals pattern-match against previous experience. If intuition is telling an individual there is a problem, then the chances are quite good that the team is getting into trouble. When someone feels this way during a procedure, that person should be empowered to verbalize any concerns to other team members so any problems can be addressed.
- *Ambiguity.* If it is becoming less clear what the plan is, then the team needs to talk to make sure all team members are in agreement. It is difficult to monitor the plan if team members are not sure what is supposed to be happening.
- *Reduced/poor communication.* Faced with a problem, effective teams and leaders should consciously enhance and increase communication. Raising concerns, gathering input, agreeing on how to approach problems, and having team members verify the results all should increase during problematic situations.
- *Confusion.* This is often a symptom of a lack of communication. Stopping and reconnecting as a team can help alter this state.
- *Trying something new under pressure.* Doing so reflects the sense that the practitioner does not have a workable approach to the problem at hand. In general, staying with the tried-and-true approach, used many times before, is far more successful than launching into novel approaches under duress.
- *Deviating from established norms.* Norms have been established because they often reflect safe approaches to care. Unless there is a clear and compelling benefit, discussed and clarified by the team, a deviation from the norm can be an indicator of a problem.
- *Verbal violence.* This is a sign of frustration. Effective communication becomes difficult when someone is being verbally unpleasant. It also affects people's comfort level in speaking up or questioning the current approach.
- *Fixation.* When people become task fixated, they lose the ability to see the context of the situation.
- *Boredom.* It takes conscious effort to maintain vigilance and attention. When people are bored, it is easy for their mind to wander from the task at hand. Being "on autopilot" can cause people to miss critical information.
- *Task saturation.* Being busy and feeling overwhelmed indicate a need to ask for help and communicate with other team members. Lagging behind and struggling to keep up can narrow an individual's ability to process important information.
- *Being rushed/behind schedule.* In today's busy world of medical practice, everyone feels rushed or behind at some point. The danger with this situation is that it is human nature to take shortcuts when behind, and when that happens, something important may be missed.

Source: Leonard M., Frankel A., Simmonds T.: Effective teamwork and communication. In Frankel A., et al. (eds): *The Essential Guide for Patient Safety Officers*, Oak Brook, IL: Joint Commission Resources, 2009, pp. 49–60.

Preventing Sharps Injuries

Sharps injuries are one of the most common dangers to health care workers. Needlestick injuries—wounds caused by needles that accidently puncture the skin—are the most common, with some organizations reporting one third of nursing and laboratory staff suffering such injuries each year.[6] Other sharps injuries, including scalpel injuries, also occur more often than they should, with studies indicating 6% to 16% of sharps injuries occur during hand-to-hand passing of sharp instruments, suture needles, and other sharp devices; the most commonly injured area is the nondominant hand.[7] Such injuries can also occur when loading or repositioning a needle, during suturing, when retracting or stretching tissue, when loading a disposable scalpel blade, during disposal, during waste removal, or if the sharp is left unattended.[7]

Sharps injuries can expose health care providers to many bloodborne pathogens, including diphtheria, Ebola, herpes, malaria, tuberculosis, and syphilis. Although there are reports of these bacteria, viruses, and fungi transferring through sharps injuries, the most commonly transmitted pathogens are human immunodeficiency virus (HIV), hepatitis B virus (HBV), and hepatitis C virus (HCV).[8] The risk of infection from a sharps injury depends on the pathogen involved, the severity of the injury, and the availability and use of appropriate prophylactic treatment.

Although most sharps injuries occur among nurses, other health care providers can be susceptible, including surgeons, anesthesiologists, surgical technologists, nurse anesthetists, surgery attendants, housekeeping staff, and students.

The operating room is ripe for sharps injuries, and more injuries may occur in this setting of an organization than in any other.[9] As with other types of events, the unique operating room environment affects the nature of sharps injuries. Within the operating room, surgeons, scrub nurses, and other surgical team members work closely together, handling the same instruments in a confined space. Health care providers can be rushed and inadvertently injure themselves or one another. Unfortunately, despite the risks, operating rooms are lagging behind other areas of the health care organization in implementing safety devices to reduce the risks of these types of injuries.[10]

To address the issue of sharps safety in the operating room and other procedure areas, health care organizations should consider convening a multidisciplinary group to examine the issue of sharps injuries, specifically as they relate to the operating room setting, and develop a comprehensive and integrated approach to addressing them. Such an approach requires more than just a few safety devices and one training seminar. It requires a coordinated, multidisciplinary effort in which perioperative team members communicate effectively, actively use engineering controls, and engage in safe practices. It requires constant vigilance, regular education, and consistent monitoring. The following sections discuss key elements in such a coordinated approach.

Safety Devices That Prevent Injury

An important aspect of sharps safety involves using safety devices in the operating room. Safety devices are engineering controls that prevent surgical team members from sticking, stabbing, or cutting themselves with sharps. Although there are many sharps safety devices that exist to prevent injury across organizations, following is a discussion of some of the more common safety devices applicable to the surgical area.

- *Protective scalpels.* Injuries from scalpel blades pose not only an infection risk for providers but also a risk for structural damage to the body, generally the hand.[11] Traditional scalpels can cause more serious injuries than needlesticks because of their size, sharpness, and propensity to be slippery because of blood or other fluids with which they come in contact. Protective scalpels—sometimes called *safety scalpels*—resemble traditional scalpels but have a mechanism that allows the user to either retract the blade into the handle or cover the blade with a protective sheath before and after use. Protective scalpels are available in both disposable and reusable varieties. These scalpels can prevent injury if used appropriately.

  Although protective scalpels can help reduce the likelihood of some types of sharps injuries, such as those that occur before use, during transfers, and between uses, they cannot prevent injuries during use. Also, health care providers must manually engage the safety mechanism for the protective scalpel to be effective in preventing sharps injuries.[11] Some users consider these instruments safer, but others contend that they make little difference in protecting health care providers. In fact, many surgeons believe that these scalpels compromise the care they give their patients. To them, these scalpels feel too light or too clumsy or do not accommodate their grip. According to others, the retractable shields and other safety mechanisms interfere with their view of the blade and make the devices a bad choice for a deep incision.

- *Blunt-tipped suture needles.* Suture needles are a primary cause of injury in the surgical setting.[10] Surgical staff can be injured by a suture needle before, during, and after use. The typical suture needle is sharp and can easily pierce the skin. Blunt-tipped suture needles are curved and have a tip that is less sharp than a conventional tapered needle. Although the blunt tip can still be used for suturing, it does not penetrate the skin as easily and is therefore less likely to cause injury. In fact, these needles have been shown to reduce sharps injuries by nearly a third, and the cost is comparable to other suture needles.[10] Significant decreases in glove perforation can be realized with this type of device as well.[12] While shown to be effective, blunt-tipped suture needles have not gained acceptance among most surgeons. Complaints regarding the "feel" of the needle have persisted.[13] However, in recent years, manufacturers have improved these needles and provide a wider range of options.[10] According to one surgeon, "the new generation of blunt needles have a different taper which makes them easier to use."[13] Health care organizations that choose to use the blunt-tipped devices should engage in an education program targeted at gaining approval and acceptance from the surgical staff. When possible, the selection process should involve surgeons and others who will be using the needles. It can be helpful to identify champions among these populations to help select, educate other providers on, and influence the acceptance of this equipment.

In addition to needles and scalpels, other equipment in the operating room can present a risk for injury. For example, manual tissue retraction devices can present a risk for injury. There are mechanical alternatives to these devices that can help reduce the risk.[14] Towel clips have also been identified as a cause for sharps-related accidents. There are blunt towel clips available that do not cause injury and are adequate for securing surgical towels and drapes. Other examples of equipment with safety features include surgical scissors, surgical wire, and pickups or forceps.[11]

Although safety devices have been shown to reduce the likelihood of sharps injuries, some health care organizations cite the cost of buying these devices as an issue. Cost concerns may indeed be a factor, but it is important to note that it is significantly less expensive to prevent a sharps injury than to treat it. Costs of treatment include the direct costs associated with the initial and follow-up treatment of exposed health care personnel, which are estimated to range from $500 to $3,000, depending on the treatment provided.[15] In addition, there are the psychological and emotional costs to the injured provider. This stress can affect performance and attitude; it may even cause someone to rethink his or her career choice.

Safe Practices to Reduce Sharps Injuries

Although the use of safety equipment can go a long way toward preventing sharps injuries, such equipment cannot eliminate the possibility of such injuries. Organizations can further reduce the risks associated with sharps by encouraging safe practices among perioperative team members. Some of these practices include the following:

- *Use a neutral zone.* Approximately one third of scalpel injuries occur when providers are passing the device, and many of these injuries are sustained by the person on the receiving end of the pass.[10] A "neutral zone" can help limit the potential for this type of injury. A neutral zone is a previously agreed on location on the sterile field, where sharps are placed and whence the surgeon, scrub nurse, or surgical technologist can retrieve items without hand-to-hand contact.[16] Organizations should encourage surgical team members to define such neutral zones before the start of a procedure. A neutral zone should also be conveniently located, puncture-resistant, and sized to accommodate sharps but not so big as to risk injury. Users should not have to reach across others to access this area. Raised sides can also limit inadvertent use of the zone for a purpose other than hands-free passing.[17] The use of a neutral zone is recommended by several professional organizations, including the American College of Surgeons (ACS) and the Association of periOperative Registered Nurses (AORN).
- *Use a hands-free passing technique.* In a hands-free passing technique, health care providers never pass the scalpel from hand to hand. Instead, the scrub

> **TIP Announce Items in the Neutral Zone**
>
> In addition to using a neutral zone, organizations should consider requiring health care providers to verbally announce when they are placing items in the neutral zone. This verbal announcement can alert other health care providers to the presence of a sharp instrument so that they can proceed with caution.

nurse places it on a passing tray or in a neutral zone and removes his or her hand from the area. The surgeon then picks up the item. The process is reversed for the surgeon to return the item to the scrub nurse. This process can reduce the likelihood that surgical team members could inadvertently jab or cut one another. Hands-free passing is not a new concept, and many surgical suites have now prohibited hand-to-hand passing of scalpels in favor of such a technique. This move is supported by the U.S. Occupational Safety and Health Administration (OSHA), AORN, ACS,[18] and the International Sharps Injury Prevention Society.[19] (*See* Sidebars 8-2 and 8-3 on page 126.)

- *Practice double gloving.* As discussed in Chapter 5, the practice of double gloving involves wearing two pairs of surgical gloves to prevent and mitigate the effects of *barrier failure*—the ripping, tearing, or puncturing of a glove.[20] Recent research shows that wearing double gloves reduces needle penetration from 69% with single gloves to 19% with double.[10] Significant reduction in the quantity of blood transferred during needlestick is also possible.[21]
- *Consider cut-resistant gloves or glove liners.* These can be used in addition to or as an alternative to double gloving techniques. Although this approach is still being tested, a recent analysis of literature on the topic noted that in both clinical and laboratory conditions, the use of a cut-resistant glove or glove liner reduced the number of inner latex glove perforations as compared to double latex.[22]
- *Regularly change surgical gloves.* As discussed in Chapter 5, changing gloves at regular intervals during surgery can reduce the amount of time that a perforated glove is in use. Also, fresh gloves may be less likely to perforate than ones that have been in use for a period of time.
- *Use a suturing technique that prevents injury.* Although the use of blunt-tipped suture needles is recommended, sometimes a straight needle is used in the surgical setting. When this occurs, providers should consider a technique that reduces the risk for injury. One such technique uses another object besides the finger to guide the needle as it emerges from the skin. Bret P. Nelson, M.D., developed a technique that uses a needle cap from the central venous access kit to "receive" the sharp needle after it penetrates the skin. In other words, the plastic needle sheath acts as a thimble and offers counterpressure without having fingers near the sharp end of the suture.[23]
- *Stay out of the way.* Although this advice may seem like common sense, it is important to note that health care providers can reduce the likelihood of experiencing a sharps injury by remaining clear of the suture area while the surgeon is suturing and remaining clear of the incision area when the surgeon is cutting.
- *Wear appropriate footwear.* Although most discussion about sharps injuries centers on or around the hands and upper body, it sometimes happens that scalpels, needles, and other sharp instruments fall to the floor and injure the feet. For this reason, it is important to consider the type of shoes worn in the operating room. As mentioned in Chapter 5, certain shoes are better at preventing injury than others. Rubber shoes and those with an inner lining offer the greatest amount of protection. Steel-toed work boots also can be effective.

An Exposure Control Plan

An exposure control plan is a health care organization's written program to reduce or eliminate health care provider exposure to bloodborne pathogens, such as via sharps injury. Such a plan should include a list of all jobs and tasks with potential for bloodborne pathogen exposure.[14] This plan must be available to all employees and should be reviewed and updated as often as necessary, but at least annually. Revisions must reflect any changes in technology that have occurred in the interim that may eliminate or reduce bloodborne pathogen exposure. Revisions must

Sidebar 8-2: Scalpel Safety

Several physician leaders in the emergency department at Princess Alexandra Hospital in Brisbane, Australia, coined the term *scalpel safety* (as opposed to *safety scalpel*) to emphasize the choice of techniques to reduce the risk of health care worker injury from scalpel blades. The scalpel safety technique—which involves using a single-handed scalpel blade remover and hands-free passing technique—avoids potential patient safety concerns by allowing the surgeon to continue to use a traditional reusable scalpel handle.

Although this practice can present a potential point of danger for operating room personnel when a disposable blade is detached from the scalpel handle, providers can use a method in which the scalpel blade remover is held in a single-handed fashion and the top half of the scalpel blade is placed into the remover. The handle is withdrawn, leaving the blade inside the remover cartridge. Although there are different types of removers, organizations should consider using ones that give the user an audible signal as the blade drops into the remover cartridge.

Source: Fuentes H., et al.: "Scalpel safety": Modeling the effectiveness of different safety devices' ability to reduce scalpel blade injuries. *International Journal of Risk & Safety in Medicine* 20:83–89, 2008.

Sidebar 8-3: Using Technology to Reduce the Use of Sharp Instruments

As technology advances, so does an organization's ability to prevent sharps injuries. There are several technologies that virtually eliminate the need to use sharp instruments, such as scalpels or needles. These technologies include the following:

- *Catheter securement devices.* Traditionally, catheters have been attached to a patient with sutures or surgical tape. Catheter securement devices do not use sutures and consequently do not require the use of suture needles, thereby reducing the risk of needlesticks.
- *Laser technologies.* Some lasers can be used as an alternative to a scalpel for cutting. Certain electrocautery equipment can be used for this purpose as well. When using laser or electrosurgical equipment, organizations should be aware of the components of the "fire triangle" and reduce means of fuel, oxidation, and ignition. (*See* page 137 for more information about the fire triangle.)
- *Needleless infusion devices.* The majority of U.S. hospitals have eliminated unnecessary use of needles through the implementation of intravenous delivery systems that do not require (and in some instances do not permit) needle access. This strategy has largely removed needles attached to intravenous tubing, such as that for intermittent infusion, and other needles used to connect and access parts of the intravenous delivery system.
- *Drug delivery systems.* These systems deliver medication without the use of a needle. One example is a device that delivers insulin to diabetics via a pressurized, microthin stream of medication that penetrates the skin.
- *Wound closure technologies.* Organizations can close small wounds with surgical glue, which eliminates the need for sutures and suture needles for these kinds of wounds.

Organizations should stay abreast of new technology and consider implementing systems that would benefit the organization.

Sources:

Centers for Disease Control and Prevention: *Workbook for Designing, Implementing, and Evaluating a Sharps Injury Prevention Program.* Updated 2008. http://www.cdc.gov/sharpssafety (accessed Jul. 22, 2010).

International Health Care Worker Safety Center, University of Virginia: *Checklist for Sharps Injury Prevention.* http://www.healthsystem.virginia.edu/internet/EPINet/chcklst2.pdf (accessed Jul. 22, 2010).

National Alliance for the Primary Prevention of Sharps Injuries: *Primary Prevention Devices.* http://www.nappsi.org/whynappsi6.shtml (accessed Jul. 22, 2010).

also include any safer medical devices that have been evaluated and considered.

As part of an exposure control plan, organizations must maintain a sharps injury log that ensures employee privacy and contains, at a minimum, the type and brand of device involved in an incident, if known; the location of the incident; and a description of the incident. Consensus among experts is that sharps injuries are often unreported so it is important that organizations encourage health care providers to report such injuries in order for organizations to quickly respond to those injuries and obtain a true picture of the problem within the organization.[13,24]

TIP Workbook Available

The U.S. Centers for Disease Control and Prevention (CDC) offers a comprehensive prevention workbook that includes tools and worksheets to assist organization leaders in managing their entire sharps safety program. The CDC's *Workbook for Designing, Implementing and Evaluating a Sharps Injury Prevention Program* can be accessed online at http://www.cdc.gov/sharpssafety/.

A critical component in the exposure control plan is the process for evaluating and responding to exposures. Health care providers who are exposed to bloodborne pathogens via sharps injuries face a daunting array of short- and long-term consequences. U.S. OSHA standards require exposed workers to go through a postexposure prophylaxis procedure, which involves a meeting with a health care practitioner who has experience in sharps injuries. The exposed worker will be asked about the injury, what type of device was used, and whether he or she knows the health status of the patient in relation to hepatitis and/or HIV/AIDS. If the patient's health status is unknown, the organization must obtain the patient's consent for a blood draw. The blood of the source individual should be tested as soon as possible and the results made available to the exposed employee. The exposed employee's blood should also be tested, if the employee consents, followed by postexposure prophylaxis (if indicated), counseling, and evaluation of the reported illness.

To promptly address exposure risks, health care providers should be aware of signs, symptoms, and potential exposures that should prompt a call to occupational health or infection prevention and control personnel. Health care organizations should also have an easy, accessible, and consistent way of reporting these incidents. (Figure 8-1 on page 128 shows a standardized report form for needlestick and other sharps injuries.) Some organizations choose to include sharps injury reporting as part of an organization-wide reporting system. (*See* Sidebar 8-4 on page 129.)

In addition to the physical effects of the exposure, the mental well-being of the health care provider needs to be evaluated and treated. Counseling and support should be provided following an exposure to an infectious disease. Counseling should involve understandable, objective information about the risk of infection associated with the type of exposure and also include the risks and benefits of the possible treatment options. Depending on the type of exposure, it can be a frightening experience for a health care provider. Organizations should respond accordingly and express empathy and reassurance. Because of the stress some exposures put on members of the exposed individual's family, organizations should consider providing the family members with counseling and support along with the health care provider.

An Education Program

Despite recent introduction of safety devices in many health care organizations, sharps injuries continue to occur. One of the reasons is that many health care providers are not knowledgeable about the risks of sharps injuries and the consequences of those injuries. Each provider should be trained about the risks associated with bloodborne pathogen exposure at the time of initial assignment and at least annually thereafter. Training should include an explanation of the epidemiology and symptoms of bloodborne diseases, modes of transmission, information about the exposure control plan, decontamination and disposal processes for personal protective equipment, procedures following emergencies, and postexposure information. Providers should be aware of the requirements associated with U.S. OSHA's bloodborne pathogens standard and how their organization complies with that standard. Organizations outside the United States should be aware of the specific standards and regulations

Figure 8-1: Occupational Exposure Report Form

Name:

Phone number and e-mail address:

Date:

Time of exposure:

Description of the exposure event:
- Where did it occur?
- How did it occur?
- What sharp was involved?
- How severe was the exposure? Was blood drawn?

Details of the exposure source
- Is there known HIV, HBV, or HCV? If so, which one(s)?
- What is the status of the patient's disease?

Details of the exposed individual
- Has the individual had an HBV vaccination?
- Does the individual have HIV, HBV, or HCV?

Details of follow-up
- Has the exposed individual received counseling?
- Has the exposed individual received postexposure management?
- What further work needs to be done?
- Who is responsible for managing the follow-up with the individual?

This form can be adapted for use in helping health care providers consistently report needlestick or other sharps injuries. (HBV=hepatitus B virus; HCV=hepatitus C virus)

required by their own country or locality, such as those of the European Agency for Safety and Health at Work for European countries.

As with other safety education, training efforts can take a variety of forms, including in-services, posters, tent cards, and role-playing exercises. Whenever possible, organizations should craft a training program that illustrates actual exposures within their facility (without identifying the name of the exposed individual), including (1) type of device, (2) job title of employee, (3) description of event, including location, and (4) suggestions for preventing a similar exposure. Such tailored training reinforces the message that all providers are at risk for such exposures and that prevention is the key.

Avoiding Leaving Objects Behind

Retained foreign objects are a rare—yet often unreported—problem in the operating room.[25] Although difficult to estimate, it is thought that such errors occur about 3,000 times a year in the United States.[26] In most cases, fabric items, such as sponges and gauze, are left behind, although metal items—such as surgical instruments—may also be inadvertently retained.[26]

Sidebar 8-4: Reporting System for Sharps Injuries and Other Medical Mishaps

One critical source of information about sharps injuries, medication mishaps, or other near misses (close calls) and errors is a spontaneous reporting system. This is a system in which any individual in the organization can report an issue, concern, or problem. Such a system should be designed to capture all issues from all persons, whether employed or independent—both global and unit specific—in an organization. Reporting systems can generate information about actual errors, near misses, injuries, or general concerns. They also provide a way for staff to be heard by leadership. Organizations that have a reporting system in place can capture information on events for use in proactive risk reduction efforts.

To be effective, reporting systems must be easy to use, be part of a safety culture, and elicit a leadership response. If health care providers find a reporting system difficult to use, they will not use it. To help make reporting easy, it may be helpful to have multiple avenues that providers may take to report issues. There are a variety of mechanisms for spontaneous reporting, including via telephone, a Web-based form, an e-mail, or a paper form. Of all the mechanisms, the electronic formats may be the most helpful because of the speed of reporting and ease of analysis.

Data from reporting systems should be tracked over time and trended. Doing so can help identify underlying issues that may be concealed in day-to-day operations. Examining reported issues in aggregate and looking for trends, themes, or patterns can help discover problems during shift changes, in particular surgical areas, or with particular types of procedures. From those patterns, organizations can develop interventions to address issues.

As individuals report events, leadership must acknowledge these reports and communicate how management will address the systems responsible for the events. Employee newsletters, staff meetings—including medical staff meetings—posters, and personal contact are all avenues through which an organization can acknowledge error reporting.

In theory, a spontaneous reporting system captures all areas of risk in an organization; however, in reality, such a system becomes just one perspective on risk because not every event that occurs in an organization is reported. Reporting systems tend to be utilized preferentially by some disciplines, such as nursing, and very little by others, such as physicians.

Source: Frankel A., Grillo S.: Systematic flow of information. In Frankel A., et al. (eds): *The Essential Guide for Patient Safety Officers.* Oak Brook, IL: Joint Commission Resources, 2009, pp. 39–47.

In many cases of such errors, the offending item is removed, and the patient recovers; however, unintentionally retained foreign objects can lead to severe illness and sometimes death. Delays in diagnosis and treatment may increase the likelihood for these severe consequences.[27] Retained foreign objects can cause bowel perforations, organ damage, fistula formation, infection and sepsis, intestinal blockage, and acute pain.[28] Gossypiboma—a mass lesion due to a retained surgical sponge surrounded by a foreign body reaction—is one of the more common consequences of this type of error and can sometimes be difficult to diagnose.[29] It can present itself as an intra-abdominal mass and can lead to unnecessary biopsy attempts and manipulations.[30]

Typically, metal items will cause more acute clinical symptoms faster, while fabric items will tend to induce more chronic symptoms over several years.[26] Diagnosis of a retained foreign object is typically made through an x-ray, ultrasound, or computed tomography (CT) scan, with the latter being the most promising tool to diagnose fabric foreign bodies.[31]

From the organization's perspective, retained foreign object errors can lead to lawsuits, financial losses, and disciplinary actions, not to mention the time and resources required to remove the foreign body and address any possible infections that may have resulted from the incident. It is estimated the costs of retrieving a sponge can be upward of $50,000 or more.[32] Also, a retained foreign object is considered by the U.S. Centers for Medicare & Medicaid Services as a health care–associated condition and thus does not qualify for reimbursement.

Why Does It Happen?

There are many reasons why objects are left behind in a patient, but these reasons can be categorized into the following three groups:

1. **Surgical factors.** The sheer number of tools and equipment used in a surgical procedure—estimated to be between 200 and 500—creates an environment in which losing or misplacing something is not surprising.[26] Certain procedures present a further risk for retained foreign objects. For example, emergency surgeries, complex procedures, surgeries that include unplanned changes or additional procedures, cases in which sponges are used as packing and/or for retraction, and surgeries that involve multiple surgical teams can all present higher risk for retained foreign objects.[25] Risk is present any time there is a change in surgical teams during a procedure or any time the pace and speed of the procedure is fast.
2. **Patient factors.** Certain patients can present a greater risk for foreign body retention. For example, surgeries involving patients with a higher body-mass index are more prone to retained foreign objects.
3. **Human factors.** During a complex surgical procedure, staff members can be rushed or distracted and may need to introduce new equipment. In these cases, the counting process can become confusing and complicated. In addition, fatigue, stress, interruptions, ineffective communication between surgical team members, and level of surgeon experience can all play a role.[33]

Strategies for Preventing the Retention of Foreign Objects

Retaining objects in a patient after surgery is considered a preventable occurrence and can be virtually eliminated if organizations take a systematic and proactive approach to the issue. The following sections offer some strategies organizations should consider.

Review the Counting Policy

Counting policies that require the staff to count equipment before, during, and after surgery have long been an effective way to prevent the retention of foreign objects. However, these policies are effective only if they are followed, and even then, sometimes something can be missed. Studies have shown that even with correct counts, foreign objects can still be left behind.[34]

Although effective, counting is subject to human error.[25] Counting errors can occur when unpacking items during surgery preparation, when reconciling items at the end of the procedure, or at any point in between.

Despite the possibility for error, a well-considered, well-followed count policy can identify more than 80% of possible retained objects.[35] One study performed at Columbia University Medical Center in New York City showed that surgical counting was off in less than 1% of cases, but when it was off, the rate of a foreign body being left in the patient was more than 100 times higher than in cases in which the count was correct.[36]

An organization's counting policy should be standardized for all procedures and be clear and concise. Effective policies should outline what needs to be counted, when it needs to be counted, how it should be counted, and by whom it should be counted. They should also outline what to do when the count is incorrect. Organizations should consider convening a multidisciplinary group to conduct a review of the current counting policy and determine what, if any, revisions are necessary. Team members could include surgeons as well as representatives from nursing, the biomedical department, organization leadership, and purchasing. Along with the World Health Organization, several United States–based, safety-focused organizations have developed guidelines addressing counting policies. These organizations include the Agency for Healthcare Research and Quality, the Association for Surgical Technologists, the American College of Surgeons, the U.S. Food and Drug Administration, and AORN. When creating a policy, organizations should consider these recommendations because they are based on evidence-based best practice.

An effective policy addresses the who, what, where, and when of prevention and response efforts. Following are some points to consider about these aspects.

- *Determine what to count.* Ideally, perioperative staff should count all items that enter the sterile field. However, depending on the procedure, doing so may not be practical or cost-effective. Organizations should work with surgical team members to determine what needs to be counted for each different type of procedure. This may include sponges, needles, other sharps, and bags. Sponges should be counted in every operation, including labor and delivery. Instruments, such as forceps and retractors, should also be counted for all procedures in which there is a likelihood that an instrument could be retained.

- *Determine when to count.* The appropriate time to count items will vary depending on the type of procedure and the type of equipment; however, recommended practice dictates the following times[37]:
  — Prior to procedure to establish a baseline
  — Before closure of a cavity within a cavity
  — Before wound closure begins
  — At skin closure or end of procedure and
  — At the time of permanent relief of either the scrub person or the circulating nurse

To help minimize confusion and miscounts, organizations should consider requiring a consistent order for counting. For example, providers could start counting items in the surgical field and move out. A scripted order may be helpful. The staff should not disperse instruments to another area of the surgical field, such as a Mayo tray, until an initial count is complete. The risk of forgetting to count an item increases when an instrument is put in two locations.[38]

- *Decide how to count.* When counting, AORN recommends that sponges, sharps, and instruments be counted audibly and viewed concurrently by two individuals, one of whom should be a registered nurse. Interruptions should be minimized so as not to distract the individuals who are counting. The surgeon should verbally acknowledge the count and should never be allowed to waive the counting process.[39] If a sponge is soiled, it should be removed from the surgical field and placed in a previously identified location, such as an impervious drape on the floor. If a sponge is added to the surgical field, it should be counted and recorded.

TIP Consider Sponge Counting Bags

To help systematize the counting process for sponges, some organizations are using "sponge counters." These are bags that include several rows and slots. After using a sponge, a nurse inserts it into a designated slot within the bag.[39] The sponge counter allows nurses to verify sponge counts visually as they proceed through a surgical event.

TIP Numbered Sponges Facilitate Counting

One option for helping with sponge counts is to use sequentially numbered sponges. These sponges have a number sewn into the corner with suture material approved by the U.S. Food and Drug Administration. Each sponge is individually numbered so that it can be identified specifically. A recent survey of staff using this type of sponge reported that staff found the sponges easy to use and said using the sponges did not lengthen or affect the flow of the surgical procedure.[40]

- *Determine how to document the count.* Surgical teams should consistently document all sponge, sharps, and instrument counts. Some organizations use a whiteboard located in the operating room as the primary count recorder. (*See* Sidebar 8-5 on page 132.) Counts should also be recorded in the patient's intraoperative record. According to the American College of Surgeons, this documentation should include at least the following [41]:
  — Results of surgical item counts
  — Notifications of the surgical team members
  — Instruments or items intentionally left as packing
  — Actions taken if count discrepancies occur
  Individuals should document only what they personally count. If someone documents for someone else, the risk of double counting can be present.
- *Outline how to respond to a count discrepancy.* In the event that there is a discrepancy in a count, the

surgical team should know what steps to follow to locate the missing item. Following are several steps organizations should consider in developing a protocol for responding to a count discrepancy[42]:

1. Report the discrepancy to the surgeon. This reporting is typically done by the circulating nurse, and the surgeon should verbally acknowledge the count discrepancy.
2. Suspend the procedure if the patient's condition permits.
3. Inspect the operative site.
4. Visually inspect the area surrounding the surgical field, including the floor, kick buckets, and linen and trash containers. No trash or linens should be removed until the patient leaves the room.
5. If the patient's condition permits, take an intraoperative x-ray and read it before the patient leaves the operating room.

TIP Use Preprinted Forms to Help Document the Count

To help with documentation, organizations may wish to create a preprinted sheet that lists the contents of surgical trays and any necessary instruments for a particular procedure. Providers can use the sheet as a checklist for packing, for unpacking, and before closure. Each time a count is done, it can be documented in a column on the sheet. Providers can easily see when the count is off because the columns do not match. These count sheets should group like instruments, such as retractors or needle holders, together under their specific names. Instrument names should be standardized and consistent, and those names should be used on any count sheets.[43]

TIP Slow Down

One of the risk factors for retaining objects after surgery arises when providers are rushed. Although the speed of a procedure sometimes cannot be helped—such as during an emergency—organizations can help minimize this risk factor by smoothing the operating room schedule, avoiding back-to-back surgeries if possible, appropriately staffing the operating room, effectively coordinating vacation schedules, and reducing staff turnover.

Sidebar 8-5: Minnesota's Retained Object Protocol

A multidisciplinary work group, including nurses, surgeons, radiologists, physicians, and patient safety and quality professionals from several of Minnesota's hospitals and health systems, has developed a step-by-step protocol for preventing retained foreign objects. The protocol includes a detailed flow sheet with recommendations for each step. Items addressed within the protocol include performing and recording counts and addressing human factors.

Based on guidelines from the Association for periOperative Registered Nurses (AORN), the American College of Surgeons, and others, the protocol recommends the following actions to prevent retained foreign objects:

- Record counts on a whiteboard in each operating room. Doing so helps ensure that every team member is aware of the count. The board serves as a memory aid and documentation tool.
- Conduct a room survey before the base count. Performed by the nurse, this activity ensures that no supplies have been left in the room from the previous patient. The nurse also verifies that the whiteboard and other recordkeeping documents are clean and free of previous information.
- Keep distractions and interruptions to a minimum during the count.
- Establish Red Rules regarding counting sponges and sharps, baseline counts, and imaging if the count cannot be reconciled. As mentioned in Chapter 1, Red Rules are nonnegotiable rules that, except in rare, urgent situations, should always be followed. These rules ensure that a critical activity—such as counting sponges—is always done.

Sources:

Minnesota's retained object protocol. *OR Manager* 24:14, 16, Dec. 2008.

Yates G., et al.: Sentara Norfolk General Hospital: Accelerating improvement by focusing on building a culture of safety. *Jt Comm J Qual Saf* 30:534–542, Oct. 2004.

6. Document all measures taken on the patient's record.
7. Report the incident using the organization's reporting system.
8. Review the incident for cause, effect, and prevention.

As with other initiatives to reduce retained foreign objects, organizations should solicit multidisciplinary involvement in developing protocols that outline the proper response to a count discrepancy.

Perform X-rays on All High-Risk Patients

To help verify the count in high-risk patients, organizations may want to consider establishing a policy that requires all high-risk patients to receive an x-ray to verify the absence of foreign bodies. High-risk patients to consider x-raying include the following[44,45]:

- Patients with a high body-mass index
- Patients in cases that involve multiple surgeons or multiple surgical fields, such as abdominal or thoracic surgeries or procedures that take a particularly long time
- Patients in emergency cases in which the pace of the surgery is fast, such as ruptured aortic aneurysms or emergency caesarean sections

The use of x-rays to identify possible retained foreign objects can prevent error; however, x-rays are not foolproof. Health care providers must review the x-rays prior to the patient leaving the surgical suite to ensure that the x-ray has captured all the anatomic areas that were operated on. An x-ray is not effective if it misses areas in which equipment may be "hiding."

To effectively use x-rays in capturing retained foreign objects, organizations must use equipment and supplies with radiopaque markers that will be visible during the x-ray. An x-ray cannot capture foreign objects without such markers. In addition, size can affect the ability to capture foreign objects on an x-ray. Smaller needles, scalpels, and other instruments may not be clearly visible.

It is important to note that postsurgical dressings and external towels should not be radiopaque because they can obstruct views within the x-ray.[39]

Consider Technology

New technology is emerging that can help organizations reduce the risk of retained foreign objects. For example, bar-coding systems can help nurses and technicians keep track of sponges and other items.[32] Within such systems, each sponge has a unique bar code attached and heat-sealed to the sponge. A counter keeps a running total of the sponges scanned in and out, along with the times of scanning. The system rejects double counts, and the surgery cannot end until all sponges are accounted for.[39] A study by Greenberg et al. showed that the use of bar-coded surgical sponges improved detection of miscounted and misplaced sponges.[46]

Similar to bar coding, electronic or radio frequency identification (RFID) tagging marks supplies and equipment with an electronic or radio frequency marker, which can be detected by a wand that passes over the patient or by passing the patient under an RFID reader. Such a system alerts health care workers that items are still inside a patient before the surgeon closes.[32] This type of technology is used every day by commercial couriers who are able to deliver millions of packages a day at a low cost and track all of them at the same time. Although this technology may make tracking equipment easier, organizations will still need a culture that promotes effective communication and procedures that prevent human error to eliminate the retention of foreign bodies after surgery.

TIP Make Sure Equipment Is Sound

When equipment is broken or damaged, it can leave particles or pieces behind in a patient. To prevent this from happening, surgical team members should inspect devices prior to use for damage that might increase the likelihood of breakage or fragmentation.[39]

Educate Surgical Team Members

Education efforts should discuss the importance of preventing retained foreign objects and describe the consequences if an object is retained. Case studies can be particularly helpful in communicating the seriousness of the issue (*see* Case Study 8-1 on pages 134–135). Education efforts should also familiarize providers with

Case Study 8-1: Mayo Clinic Rochester

About the Organization: At the Mayo Clinic Rochester (MCR) in Rochester, Minnesota, surgeons, anesthesia providers, residents, nurses, and allied health professionals perform approximately 50,000 operations each year. The organization's 98 main operating rooms, 3 obstetrical operating rooms, and 8 labor and delivery birthing rooms are distributed between two acute care hospitals.

Purpose of the Project: To reduce the incidence of retained foreign objects within the surgical setting, MCR used a multifaceted, multidisciplinary approach that involved assessing current efforts, revising current policy and procedure, providing education and training, and monitoring performance.

In 2005 the Mayo Clinic Rochester (MCR) was experiencing a retained foreign object incident nearly every two weeks on average. To improve the safety of patients undergoing surgery within the organization, MCR embarked that year on a multidisciplinary effort that consisted of the following three phases:

Phase 1: Analyzing Events and Reviewing Policy
Phase 2: Building Awareness and Enhancing Communication
Phase 3: Monitoring and Sustaining Success

Phase 1: Analyzing Events and Reviewing Policy
As a first step in its improvement project, MCR performed a detailed analysis of all retained foreign object incidents—both true and near-misses—to identify patterns of failures. The review showed that out of nearly 200,000 operations, there were 34 near-miss events and 34 true retained foreign object events. The 34 items retained in the true events included 23 sponges, 1 instrument, 3 needles, and 7 miscellaneous items. None of these incidents occurred in high-risk cases, and in 62% of the cases, the "counts" at the end of the procedure were thought to be correct. Root cause analysis performed on each actual retained foreign object event demonstrated that a failure of communication among operating room team members was the most frequent contributor to the event.

After the defect analysis, nursing and surgeon leadership performed a review of all relevant institutional policies, including policies governing the who, what, where, when, and how of the counting process. Within this review process, team members discovered that many of the policies had been amended or altered over time in response to specific events without a complete revision of the entire policy or consideration of how it related to other policies, which resulted in long, confusing policies that often had intra- and interpolicy contradictions.

In response to this comprehensive review, a leadership team—comprised of nurses and physicians—developed a single operational definition of what was considered a retained foreign object and revised all relevant polices. The group also created a new policy and an education tool to assist operating room staff on how to respond to a miscount or concern about the instance of a retained foreign object. Both new and revised policies were aligned with external standards and internal best practices and restructured to ensure intrapolicy and interpolicy consistency. This leadership group garnered feedback on the new and revised policies from organization staff before finalizing the procedures.

Phase 2: Building Awareness and Enhancing Communication
The second phase of the retained foreign object project involved increasing awareness and communication among all operating room personnel, including surgeons, residents, nursing, and allied health staff. As a first step in this effort, the organization convened a mandatory all-staff meeting for all operating room personnel. In total, more than 3,500 staff members either attended the meeting or viewed delayed video recordings. During this meeting, institutional, surgical, and nursing leadership discussed the data and findings from the systematic defect analysis as well as provided a review of all the new policies to be implemented to address the surgical retained foreign objects. Misconceptions about risk factors and staff concerns about retained foreign object investigations were addressed in this open forum.

After the all-staff meeting, the organization launched a campaign to further educate nurses, certified surgical technicians, and surgical assistants on the proper counting techniques and revised count policies. This effort involved the creation of a video documenting the correct counting process, which was reviewed at surgical services staff meetings. Additional education included team training in the Mayo Simulation Center and in-room audits with immediate feedback provided by frontline nurse managers. Daily "reminders" of appropriate counting technique, policies, and procedures were included in staff morning reports.

In addition to building awareness about retained foreign objects, MCR implemented a standardized counting process across all surgical specialties and surgical units, including labor and delivery. To facilitate this counting process, MCR

(continued on page 135)

Case Study 8-1: Mayo Clinic Rochester (continued)

installed whiteboards in every operating room, which allowed for standardized documentation. In recognition that each specialty may have unique counting needs, magnetic labels for specialty-specific items were manufactured and placed on the whiteboards to track these unique items.

MCR also implemented a "Red Rule" related to instrument and sponge counting. The rule requires that all counts of instruments and sponges be performed by two team members in the standardized manner. During a pause before closing, the surgeon and residents are to stop all activity other than performing the required appropriate local wound exploration, thus avoiding any interruptions of the count process. Any violation of the rule would be considered reckless behavior and would immediately be passed forward to the leadership team.

Phase 3: Monitoring and Sustaining Success

The final phase of the project aimed to effectively monitor and sustain improvements through a rapid leadership response to any events, enhanced staff communication, and policy reviews. A leadership response team was informed of any near miss or true retained foreign object event in the operating room and within 24 hours of the event convened a meeting that included the event response team and all operating room personnel involved in the incident. The purpose of the meeting was to debrief all team members about the event. This process was not designed as a replacement for the formal sentinel event root cause analysis or to assign responsibility for the event. Rather, it was intended to quickly inform operating room leadership of the circumstances to determine areas of potential system weakness. After the leadership team performed the analysis of the event, a memo describing the circumstances of the event and findings was prepared and shared with all operating room personnel within 48 hours of the event.

Another tactic to keep the operating room staff aware of the retained foreign object initiative was the use of posters tracking the number of days since the last retained foreign object incident. These posters were placed at the entrances to the operating rooms. Finally, quarterly all-staff meetings were held that focused on operating room safety, team communication, and retained foreign object performance updates.

Results of the Effort

The retained foreign object reduction effort resulted in a significant and sustained reduction in the frequency and types of surgical retained foreign object incidents within the organization. When the program started, the Mayo Clinic Rochester was averaging a surgical retained foreign object event every 16 days. After the intervention, the average interval between retained foreign object events increased to 69 days, a level of performance that has been sustained.

Additional Source:

Cima R., et al.: A multidisciplinary team approach to retained foreign objects. *Jt Comm J Qual Patient Saf* 35:123–132, Mar. 2009.

the organization's policies relating to retained foreign objects and outline the ways compliance and competency will be measured. Health care providers should know for a particular procedure what needs to be counted, when, how, and by whom. Role-playing exercises, demonstrations, and in-services may be helpful in this effort.

Handling Specimens Properly

One aspect of surgery that presents risk for error is the care and handling of specimens—tissue, blood, body fluids, or foreign bodies removed from a patient during surgery or other invasive procedure. A lost or mislabeled specimen is problematic in the operative setting and can significantly—and negatively—impact patient outcomes because of delays in treatment, errors in diagnosis or treatment, or the need for additional procedures.[47]

To ensure safe and appropriate handling of specimens, organizations should develop comprehensive, written policies and procedures related to specimen management. These policies and procedures should be created with input from all the disciplines involved in collecting, handling, examining, storing, transporting, and disposing of these materials. The policies should emphasize a proactive approach to specimen handling that minimizes the time required for specimen collection during a procedure and reduces the potential for mishandling, mislabeling, or losing specimens.

When creating policies and procedures for specimen management, it is important to consider both law and regulation and the recommendations and requirements of safety-focused organizations, such as The Joint

Commission, Joint Commission International (JCI), and the U.S. Association for periOperative Registered Nurses (AORN). Standards and recommendations from these organizations address a variety of topics related to specimen management but focus mainly on the following aspects.[47] (*Note: The following list is not meant to be all-inclusive but rather to give an idea of the areas to address in specimen-related policies. For a more complete list of regulations and requirements, see the relevant Joint Commission and JCI standards and the AORN guidelines addressing this topic.*)

- *Containers and collection devices.* These should be of appropriate size and type to safely secure the specimen and prevent leakage or unnecessary exposure to those handling the specimen. Surgical team members should determine which containers and what preservatives are necessary before the start of a procedure and have these present in the procedural area before the procedure begins.
- *Patient and specimen identification.* The Joint Commission, JCI, and AORN all require organizations to identify patients before taking specimens. This confirmation should be done with two unique identifiers to minimize the possibility of misidentification. After the specimen is taken, surgical team members should confirm the identity of the specimen using both verbal and written communication. Structured communication techniques, such as a *repeat-back*—in which the information receiver repeats back what the information sender says and the sender then confirms the accuracy of the statement—can help ensure accurate identification. Written documentation of the identification process can also help ensure accuracy. Organizations may find printed tools helpful with such documentation.
- *Specimen labeling.* To prevent confusion and possible misidentification, specimen containers should be clearly labeled, and information about the specimen should be documented in the operative record and pathology documents. The label should include the patient's name and other identifier, originating source of the specimen, type of tissue, current date and time, and other pertinent information. If the specimen is considered biohazardous, that information should be documented on the label as well. In addition, any chemical preservatives found in the specimen container should also be noted.
- *Transportation of specimens.* When removing a specimen off the sterile field, surgical team members should use standard precautions. The integrity and sterility—if appropriate—of the specimen should be maintained. Containers for tissue transport should be available before the start of a procedure and be able to transport the sample safely without leaking.
- *Communication about specimens.* After a specimen has left the procedural area, organizations should have specific processes in place that address how members of the procedural team will communicate about the specimen with members of the pathology department. This communication may involve written documentation as well as verbal communication. Any communication between surgeons and pathologists should be direct and not through an intermediary. Organizations should have a process in place for communicating about test results and other information related to the specimen.
- *Disposal of specimens.* All specimens should be disposed of according to law and regulation. Organizations should consult their local, regional, and national regulations to determine the most appropriate methods of specimen disposal.

Surgical team members should be educated on any policies and procedures related to specimen management and be competent to perform these activities. Competency should be assessed at the time of employment, following education activities, and periodically to ensure that appropriately qualified individuals are performing specimen collection, transport, and disposal activities at all times.

Specimen management is a complex issue. Applying a systematic process improvement technique, such as RPI, can be beneficial in streamlining this effort and ensuring accuracy, effectiveness, and proactive error prevention.

An offshoot of specimen management is transplant safety. Although the scope of this publication does not allow an in-depth discussion of this topic, readers can access further information online (*see* Online Extras).

online extras

To see Joint Commission and Joint Commission International requirements related to specimen management and transplant safety, visit http://www.jcrinc.com/SSW10/Extras/.

Preventing Surgical Fires

Although there are no worldwide statistics on the number of operating room fires that occur every year, data from studies in the United States indicate that there are 650 such fires annually in U.S. hospitals, and there may be three to four times as many near misses.[48] Statistics show that the most common ignition sources of surgical fires are electrosurgical units and lasers, and the most common locations of surgical fires are in the airway, on the head, and near the face.[49,50] In fact, almost 80% of fires in the health care environment occur during facial, neck, or tonsil surgery.[51] Head and neck surgeries carry high risk because of the proximity of the electrosurgical equipment to the oxygen used on the patient.[48]

Although they do not happen often, surgical fires can have severe consequences, including injury to patients and providers as well as significant damage to surgical equipment. As described by The Joint Commission in a 2003 *Sentinel Event Alert* on preventing surgical fires,[52] the operating room is at particular risk for fires because of the concept of a "fire triangle" (*see* Figure 8-2). The three sides, or "legs," of a fire triangle are a fuel source, an oxygen source, and an ignition source. When these three elements interact, a fire starts. For example, if a patient is having facial surgery and receiving supplementary oxygen (oxygen source) at the same time that an active electrode (ignition source) is being used, the heat from the active electrode tip could ignite the oxygen and cause an explosion. If this explosion were to touch the patient's drape (fuel source), a fire could occur.

Figure 8-2: The Fire Triangle

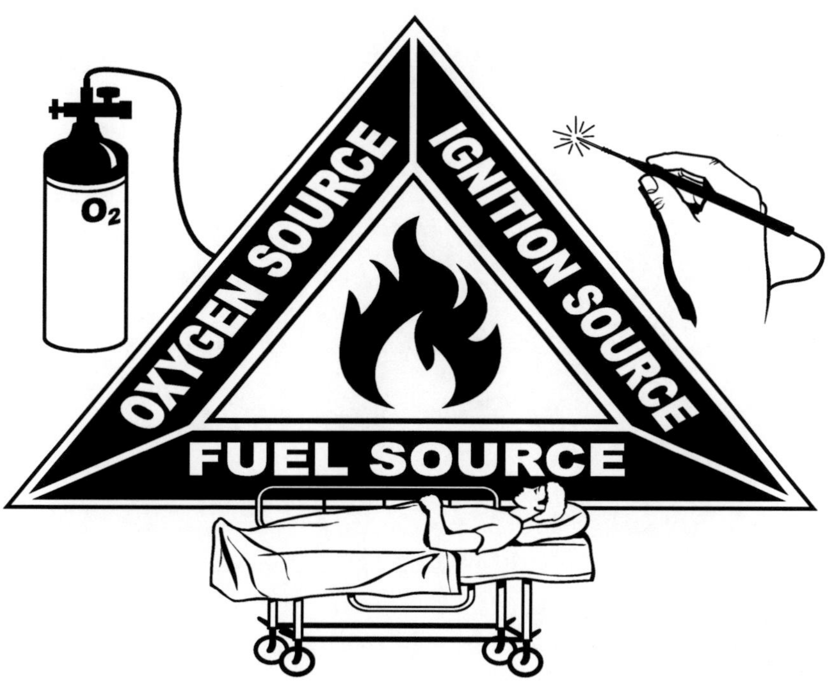

The "fire triangle" illustrates how a surgical fire may occur when a fuel source, an oxygen source, and an ignition source converge.

The surgical setting is rife with components of the fire triangle. For example, fuel sources in this environment may include alcohol-based prepping agents; linens such as drapes, towels, gowns, hoods, and masks; or surgical equipment and supplies. Ignition sources, which typically give off heat and must get hot enough to ignite any fuel material, may include electrosurgical units or electrocautery units, fiber-optic light sources and cables, or lasers. The oxygen "leg" of the triangle is present because many surgical procedures are performed in what is labeled an "oxygen-enriched environment." In the United States, the National Fire Protection Association defines this type of environment as having an atmospheric oxygen concentration greater than 23.5%.[53]

The higher the concentration of oxygen, the more serious a potential fire is likely to be. Medical-grade oxygen is the most obvious source of additional oxygen in the operating room; however, nitrous oxide can also cause combustion and can result in fires as serious as those resulting from 100% oxygen.[54] Other oxidizers include medically compressed air and ambient air. Because of the fire risk associated with oxygen, it is easy to see why the risk for intraoperative fires is greatest during induction of anesthesia when the highest concentration of oxygen is present.[50]

TIP Know the Law

A U.S. law that went into effect in 2009 requires outpatient surgery centers to submit data on a number of quality and safety measures or face a 2% reduction in Medicare payments. In the United States, he National Quality Forum has identified burn prevention as one of the top five safety measures for surgery centers. If they have not already, outpatient surgery centers in the United States should familiarize themselves with this law and respond accordingly.[48]

Strategies to Reduce Fire Risk

The components of the fire triangle are always present to some degree in a surgical setting, yet most surgical fires can be prevented if health care providers understand how fires occur and take the proper precautions to avoid risky situations. Following are some strategies organizations can use to help eliminate the risks of surgical fires and enhance patient safety.

Prepare Patients Appropriately

How a patient is prepared for surgery or other invasive procedure can have a significant impact on whether he or she is at risk for experiencing a surgical fire. When preparing a patient for a procedure, all areas of the patient's body that could become fuel sources during a fire should be appropriately prepped. This may involve coating all exposed facial hair in a water-soluble jelly to make it nonflammable; covering the patient's eyes with swabs soaked in sodium chloride; and letting a prepped area dry completely before covering the site with a nonflammable or fire retardant drape. Ideally, surgical preparation should not use alcohol-based solutions because such solutions generate volatile vapors that can ignite easily.[55] If an alcohol-based prep has been used when readying the surgical site, preparing materials—such as sponges—should be removed from the surgical site before the start of a procedure. The surgical site should be allowed to thoroughly dry before starting the procedure. When arranging surgical drapes, team members should configure them to prevent oxygen from accumulating under the drapes or from flowing into the surgical site.[55] When placing sponges near an ignition source, surgical team members should moisten the sponges with either water or saline.

In surgeries that require an endotracheal tube, team members should ensure that there are no leaks present around the tube because leaking oxygen can present a fire risk. When an endotracheal tube filled with oxygen or nitrous oxide is ignited, it becomes like a blowtorch, sending flames and heat down the trachea to combust and char tissues throughout the airway.[56] Studies have shown that conventional endotracheal tubes are more likely to ignite when exposed to a laser, so using laser-resistant tubes may be warranted during surgeries involving a laser.[55]

Use Equipment Safely

Some surgical equipment can serve as an ignition source to a potential fire. To prevent this, organizations should make sure that the surgical team uses any equipment properly and "engages" the equipment only when working on the patient. (*See* Sidebar 8-6 on pages 140–141.)

Maintain Equipment

Faulty equipment can wreak havoc during surgery. For example, equipment that shorts out or sparks during surgery can cause a fire. All electrical equipment that is used in the operating room should be calibrated and inspected frequently. In addition, organizations should have a maintenance plan for all equipment and document regular and preventive maintenance to ensure that equipment is safe to operate. Installing safety features on electrical equipment, such as over-current protection, can also be helpful.[57]

> **TIP Ensure Appropriate Maintenance**
>
> Before beginning surgery, perioperative team members should ensure that any electrosurgical equipment or other equipment that could act as an ignition source has had the appropriate maintenance. Easy verification can take place through stickers placed on the equipment. In addition, perioperative staff should inspect all electrical cords for fraying before plugging them in to an outlet or using them on a patient.

Limit Flammable Chemicals

Organizations should carefully monitor the amount of potentially explosive chemicals that are brought into the operating room. For example, 10% buffered formalin is explosive, and therefore organizations should consider prohibiting large volumes of it in the operating room.[58]

Control Excess Oxygen

Surgical settings have higher-than-average concentrations of oxygen. Most health care providers are aware of the fire risks associated with lights, lasers, and electrocautery devices, but they may be less aware of the fact that supplemental oxygen delivered during facial surgery performed under conscious sedation poses a significant risk.[52] Providers should understand that the use of oxygen in any form offers an opportunity for fire. Anesthesiologists in particular should be aware of the amount of oxygen given to patients. Because oxygen and nitrous oxide are colorless and odorless, surgical team members will not know what quantity of gases are present in the operating field unless the anesthesiologist tells them.[59] Anesthesiologists should be particularly mindful of the potential of closed draping techniques to foster the accumulation of oxygen when supplemental oxygen is being used.[56]

Not all surgeries require 100% oxygen. In fact, organizations are encouraged to use the lowest possible concentration of inspired oxygen that ensures adequate oxygen saturation.

New recommendations from the Anesthesia Patient Safety Foundation and ECRI Institute suggest that organizations use only air for open delivery on the face for spontaneously breathing sedated patients who can maintain a safe blood oxygen saturation without supplemental oxygen. If the patient does need extra oxygen, providers should secure the airway with a laryngeal mask or tracheal tube, except for procedures in which an open oxygen delivery is required, such as carotid artery surgery, neurosurgery, and some pacemaker implementations. Securing the airway prevents oxygen-enriched gases from accumulating under the surgical drape.[60]

Engage Providers in the Fire Prevention Process

Each member of the surgical team—surgeon, anesthesiologist, nurse, and others— should play a role in preventing surgical fires. It may be helpful to assign each team member a side of the fire triangle that he or she is responsible for managing. For example, the nurse may be responsible for limiting and properly addressing fuel sources; the surgeon may be responsible for ensuring that surgical equipment is used properly, thus limiting ignition possibilities; and the anesthesiologist may be responsible for limiting the presence of excess oxygen. Tailoring the education process to the relevant specialty—for example, gynecologic or orthopedic—will make the process more effective and successful.

Foster Effective Communication and Teamwork

The primary cause of surgical fires is poor communication.[48] As with other risks in the operating room, conducting a preprocedure briefing that includes a discussion of any fire risks, particularly for high-risk procedures, may be beneficial. This briefing could include a short discussion of a strategy to reduce the likelihood of fire and manage one if it occurs. Christiana Care—a U.S. health system based in Newark, Delaware—is incorporating a fire risk assessment within its performance of the

Sidebar 8-6: Laser Safety

Today, lasers are not just the technology behind barcode scanners and optical storage devices, such as CDs and DVDs, but also the technology for a host of powerful medical tools. Among the scores of uses for lasers in health care are applications as diverse as dental procedures, eye surgery, facial resurfacing, removal of facial port wine stains, and pulverization of kidney stones. Lasers are also used in treating esophageal tumors and in a type of coronary surgery called transmyocardial revascularization, in which a laser drills holes into the heart to allow blood flow to the ischemic heart muscle.

Lasers offer convenience, accuracy, and precision, allowing surgeons to get up close and target a small area of tissue without having to disrupt anything around it. A large amount of energy can travel through a fiber-optic device to the surgical target without requiring more invasive surgery. All this is done simply by selecting the appropriate wavelength and adjusting the parameters of the laser beam according to the surgeon's needs.

Like many tools in health care, lasers are both powerful and potentially dangerous if not handled appropriately. Some of the potential hazards associated with lasers include the following:

- *Burns to eyes and skin.* Although any burns to the skin are usually minor, burns to the eyes can damage the retina, the cornea, or the lens—and even cause total blindness. These types of burns can happen when a laser beam bounces off a shiny surface, such as an instrument or a stainless-steel tray or cart.

  To prevent burns to their skin, providers should wear long-sleeved gowns made of flame-resistant fabric.

  The American National Standards Institute standard ANSI Z136.3 (2005) for the safe use of lasers in health care facilities recommends that, to protect against eye injury, hospitals and surgical center personnel use laser protective eyewear, such as goggles or glasses with side shields, during laser operations. This eye protection will attenuate laser light to safe levels and help protect wearers. When selecting appropriate laser protective eyewear, U.S. organizations should consider laser wavelength and optical density, visual transmittance, impact resistance, and the user's comfort level. To ensure proper protection, it is important to verify both the wavelength and optical density imprinted on all laser eyewear in use, particularly when more than one laser is located in the same room. The wavelength marked on the eyewear should match the wavelength of the laser being used. In addition, the optical density should be appropriate for the power of the laser being used. If either of these parameters is incorrect, a user will not be protected from the laser beam.

  In Europe, organizations should consider similar recommendations regarding laser eye protection. There are three legal requirements regarding such eye protection that are enforceable. These requirements pertain to direct hit testing and labeling, eyewear for laser alignment, and optical density for eyewear.

  Further suggestions regarding eyewear include the following:

  — Laser eyewear should not be moved from one laser room to another; the eyewear should remain with the laser.

  — Users should not carry eyewear in the pocket of their lab coat in between use.

  — Inspecting laser eyewear periodically can help proactively identify small cracks or loose-fitting filters, which could permit hazardous levels of laser light to pass through directly to the eye.

- *Fire in the surgical suite.* When lasers are in use, the risk for a fire goes up. The first step in avoiding a fire in the surgical suite is to minimize or remove one side of the "fire triangle." For example, all alcohol- and petroleum-based products should be removed, and the use of inhalation gases, such as oxygen, nitrous oxide, and anesthetic gases, should be controlled to reduce combustion. The buildup of oxygen and nitrous oxide beneath surgical drapes should be minimized. The laser assistant should place the laser in standby mode when it is not in active use and activate it only when the tip is under the surgeon's direct control. Only the person delivering the laser energy should be allowed to operate the foot pedal, and before removing the laser from the surgical site, the laser assistant should put it in standby mode.
- *Smoke plume.* Surgical procedures that use a laser unit can produce a smoke byproduct that may contain toxic gases and vapors. At high

(continued on page 141)

Sidebar 8-6: Laser Safety *(continued)*

concentrations, that byproduct causes ocular and upper respiratory tract irritation among health care personnel. Other hazards of the smoke plume include eye, nose, and throat irritation; nausea; fatigue; nasal congestion; vomiting; and flulike symptoms. Smoke evacuators can help remove surgical smoke from most operating rooms.

Lasers can be an important and effective part of today's health care, and a laser safety program is necessary to help protect patients and providers alike. If an organization works regularly with lasers, such a program should be created, implemented, and enforced.

Source: The Joint Commission: *2010 Environment of Care Essentials for Health Care*. Oak Brook, IL: Joint Commission Resources, 2010.

Universal Protocol.[60] This assessment scores fire risk using a three-point scale for each of the following:

1. Procedure site
2. Open oxygen source (face mask/nasal cannula)
3. Ignition source (cautery, laser, fiberoptic light source)

A score of 3 indicates a high risk for fire and triggers the activation of a high-risk fire protocol.

In addition to preprocedure briefing, surgical teams should consider other communication techniques, such as callouts and repeat-backs, so team members can be aware of what is going on around them and avoid dangerous situations.

Responding to a Surgical Fire

Although fire prevention is critical to safety in the operating room, health care providers should be prepared to fight a fire and treat a patient if a fire does occur. It is important to note that fire response in the operating room is very different from the response that occurs in other areas of a health care organization. RACE—rescue, alarm, contain, extinguish—is the acronym that describes the fire response in which all health care staff members have been drilled, and this approach makes sense in other fire situations. For example, response to a fire that starts in a supply closet would involve staff members first rescuing patients, sounding the fire alarm, containing the fire, and then extinguishing it, if possible. But in the case of an operating room fire (unless it is out of control enough that evacuation is necessary), health care providers should take the following steps:

1. Halt the procedure. This should be done at any early signs of fire, including a flame, a flash, unusual sounds, odors, smoke, or heat.[55]
2. Extinguish the fire by disconnecting the patient's oxygen and ventilating the patient with air.
3. Contain the fire by removing any burning materials from the patient.
4. Follow an evacuation protocol when medically appropriate.

Different types of surgery might require slight alterations in the response plan. For example, in the case of fires in the airway or breathing circuit, the tracheal tube should be removed immediately as well as any and all flammable and burning materials. Delivery of airway gases should stop, and saline should be poured into the airway to extinguish any remaining fire and cool tissues.[55]

After the fire has been extinguished, team members should assess the patient and develop a plan for his or her ongoing treatment. Organizations may want to have instructions on how to care for a burn patient in the operating room. This could include instructions regarding fluid control, pain management, and wound care. Providers can refer to these as they prepare the patient for transport to a burn unit or other area of the health care organization.[61]

To ensure an effective fire response, leadership responsible for an operating room should develop a fire plan that is specific to its location, risks, and types of procedures. The fire plan should establish what everyone on the team will do in the process of extinguishing the fire and ensuring the safety of the patient. The fire plan should also assume that the patient is in the middle of a surgical procedure when the fire breaks out and therefore is at extreme risk. The plan should determine exactly how the perioperative team will manage the fire quickly and address the interrupted procedure. Surgical teams should be trained on this plan and participate in drills to reinforce learning.

> **TIP Do Not Stomp on Burning Materials**
>
> When extinguishing burning materials, it is important to refrain from stomping on them, because the materials could stick to shoe covers and ignite surgical scrubs.[62] Providers should drop burning materials to the floor and extinguish them with water or a fire suppressant.

> **TIP Keep Water Handy**
>
> It can be helpful to keep a bowl of water or saline in the operating room. In some cases, this may be enough to extinguish a small fire. If providers douse part of the surgical drapes, all drapes covering the patient should be removed and the patient should be redraped.

Education Is the Key

To lessen the risk of surgical fires, surgical team members should be educated on surgical fire prevention strategies and any organization protocols for minimizing fire risk. Every member of the surgical team should receive this education, including surgeons, anesthesiologists, and nurses. Areas to emphasize in training efforts include the following:

- How to minimize fire ignition risks, such as proper equipment use and care
- How to minimize oxidizer risks, including reducing oxygen concentration
- How to minimize fuel risks, such as properly preparing the patient for surgery
- Specific risks for the types of surgery conducted in the organization

Education for perioperative team members should review flammability levels of the materials and substances with which they work. This review includes not just surgical site prepping agents but also drapes, towels, gowns, hoods, and masks, as well as the dressings, ointments, equipment, and supplies used during surgery.

Health care providers should also be educated on how to effectively respond to a fire. Each surgical team member must know his or her role during a fire and be able to execute that role. Fire response education should include the following:

- How to quickly extinguish the fire
- How to treat the patient
- How to safely remove the patient if necessary
- How to safely evacuate the operating room if necessary
- How to activate the fire safety systems
- How to prevent the spread of smoke
- How to locate and use fire extinguishers
- The role of outside firefighting personnel, such as the organization's fire response team or the community fire department

It may be helpful to educate nurses and physicians together and encourage them to discuss the best strategies for surgical fire prevention. By involving all surgical team members in the development of surgical fire protocols, an organization can ensure surgical team buy-in and participation.

Organizations should conduct surgical fire drills to make sure surgical team members understand their role during a fire. Participation in a fire drill can provide more in-depth instruction than learning about fire response in a meeting. As with any activity, the more one practices, the better one becomes. Regular drills of the operating room team members help them function appropriately when a real emergency occurs. Organizations are conducting drills that teach how to fight fires that break out on a patient's surgical drapes, gown, or skin and to extinguish flames inside a patient's airway or tracheal tube.[49] When conducting operating room–related fire drills, organizations should consider focusing on the following:

- Properly using operating room firefighting equipment
- Dealing with patient rescue and escape
- Identifying and locating medical gas, ventilation, and surgical systems and controls

- Knowing when, where, and how to shut off key systems
- Using the organization's alarm system and its procedure for contacting the local fire department

After completing drills, organizations may want to conduct a debriefing session to evaluate the fire response, highlight what went well, and identify areas that need improvement. Drill debriefings can determine the need for more training, the need to revamp response procedures, or the need to tweak certain aspects of fire response, such as the most appropriate door from which to evacuate or the most effective way to extinguish a fire.

TIP Turn to the Experts

When designing education programs, organizations should consider guidelines from several safety-focused organizations, including the Anesthesia Patient Safety Foundation and ECRI Institute. To remind perioperative staff members of what they can do to help prevent surgical fires, safety managers at ambulatory care and office-based surgical centers can download, print, and mount a fire safety poster in each surgical suite. The free poster is available online from ECRI at http://mdsr.ecri.org. Click on "Surgical Fire Poster."

References

1. Healey A., Sevdalis N., Vincent C.: Measuring intra-operative interference from distraction and interruption observed in the operating theatre. *Ergonomics* 39:589–604, Apr. 15–May 15, 2006.
2. Healey A., Primus C., Koutantji M.: Quantifying distraction and interruption in urological surgery. *Qual Saf Health Care* 16:135–139, Apr. 2007.
3. Beyea S.: Distractions, interruptions, and patient safety. *AORN J* 86:109–112, Jul. 2007.
4. Parker J., Coiera E.: Improving clinical communication: A view from psychology. *J Am Med Inform Assoc* 7:453–461, Sep.–Oct. 2000.
5. Air Force's 11 patient safety tools build better team communication. *OR Manager* 19:1, 12–13, Feb. 2003.
6. Canadian Centre for Occupational Health and Safety: *Needlestick Injuries.* http://www.ccohs.ca/oshanswers/diseases/needlestick_injuries.html (accessed Jul. 24, 2010).
7. Association of periOperative Registered Nurses (AORN): *AORN Guidance Statement: Sharps Injury Prevention in the Perioperative Setting.* 2005. http://www.aorn.org/docs/assets/A33331A5-17A4-49A8-866909AF7F01B91D/AGS_Sharps_Injury_Prevention_in_the_Perioperative_Setting.pdf (accessed Jul. 24, 2010).
8. Stoker R.: Zero sharps injuries—A goal we can live with! *Managing Infection Control,* Dec. 2008. http://www.isips.org/reports/Articles/december2008zeroneedlestick.pdf (accessed Jul. 24, 2010).
9. Perry J., Parker G., Jagger J.: EPINet report: 2007 percutaneous injury rates. *International Healthcare Worker Safety Center,* Aug. 2009. http://www.healthsystem.virginia.edu/internet/epinet/EPINet-2007-rates.pdf (accessed Jul. 24, 2010).
10. Saver C.: Blunting sharps injuries in the OR continues to be a work in progress. *OR Manager* 26:1, 7–11, Jan. 2010.
11. Fuentes H., et al.: "Scalpel safety": Modeling the effectiveness of different safety devices' ability to reduce scalpel blade injuries. *International Journal of Risk & Safety in Medicine* 20:83–89, 2008.
12. Sullivan S., et al.: Blunt needles for the reduction of needlestick injuries during cesarean delivery: A randomized controlled trial. *Obstet Gynecol* 114:211–216, Aug. 2009.
13. Blunt assessment: Surgeons stuck by suture needles endanger themselves and patients. *Hospital Infection Control & Prevention* 37:1, 3, Jan. 2010.
14. International Health Care Worker Safety Center, University of Virginia: *Checklist for Sharps Injury Prevention.* http://www.healthsystem.virginia.edu/internet/EPINet/chcklst2.pdf (accessed Jul. 24, 2010).
15. Centers for Disease Control and Prevention: *Workbook for Designing, Implementing, and Evaluating a Sharps Injury Prevention Program.* Revised 2008. http://www.cdc.gov/sharpssafety (accessed Jul. 29, 2010).
16. Stringer B., Infante-Rivard C., Hanley J.: Effectiveness of the hands-free technique in reducing operating theatre injuries. *Occup Environ Med* 39:703–707, Oct. 2002.
17. Stoker R.: Sharps injuries: Just part of the job…right? *Managing Infection Control,* Nov. 2008. http://www.isips.org/reports/Articles/November2008.pdf (accessed Jul. 24, 2010).
18. American College of Surgeons: [ST-58] *Statement on Sharps Safety.* http://www.facs.org/fellows_info/statements/st-58.html (accessed Jul. 24, 2010).
19. Stoker R.: Scalpel safety: Protecting patients and clinicians. *Managing Infection Control,* May 2008. http://www.isips.org/reports/Articles/mic0508r24.pdf (accessed Jul. 24, 2010).
20. Twomey C.: Double gloving: A risk reduction strategy. *Jt Comm J Qual Saf* 29:369–378, Jul. 2003.
21. Wittmann A., et al.: Study of blood contact in simulated surgical needlestick injuries with single or double latex gloving. *Infect Control Hosp Epidemiol* 30:53–56, Jan. 2009.
22. Watt A, et al.: *Scalpel Safety in the Operative Setting.* ASERNIP-S Report no. 59. Stepney, Australia: Royal Australasian College of Surgeons, Australian Safety and Efficacy Register of New Interventional Procedures (ASERNIP)–Surgical, 2007.
23. Nelson B.: Making straight suture needles a little safer: A technique to keep fingers from harm's way. *J Emerg Med* 34:195–197, Feb. 2008.

24. Makary M., et al.: Needlestick injuries among surgeons in training. *N Engl J Med* 356:2693–2699, Jun. 28, 2007.
25. Godara R., et al.: Retained forceps: An unusual cause of intestinal obstruction. *Asian J Surg* 31:148–150, Jul. 2008.
26. DiConsiglio J.: Count on a backup: Technology can help cut risk of retained items in surgical patients. *Mater Manag Health Care,* Nov. 2008. http://www.matmanmag.com/matmanmag_app/jsp/articledisplay.jsp?dcrpath=MATMANMAG/Article/data/11NOV2008/0811MMH_FEA_CoverStory&domain=MATMANMAG (accessed Jul. 24, 2010).
27. Alis H., et al.: Surgical intervention may not always be required in gossypiboma with intraluminal migration. *World J Gastroenterol* 13:6605–6607, Dec. 2007.
28. Jackson S., Brady S.: Counting difficulties: Retained instruments, sponges, and needles. *AORN J* 87:315–321, Feb. 2008.
29. Aminian A.: Gossypiboma: A case report. *Cases J* 1:220, Oct. 7, 2008.
30. Is M., et al.: A retained surgical sponge (gossypiboma) mimicking a paraspinal abscess. *Br J Neurosurg* 21:307–308, Jun. 2007.
31. Lincourt A., et al.: Retained foreign bodies after surgery. *J Surg Res* 138:170–174, Apr. 2007.
32. Japsen B.: Technology cuts risk of surgical sponges: Objects left in patients expensive to remove. *Chicago Tribune,* Jan. 2, 2008.
33. McLeod R., et al.: Risk factors for retained foreign bodies after surgery. *Can J Surg* 47:57–59, Feb. 2004.
34. Cima R., et al.: Incidence and characteristics of potential and actual retained foreign object events in surgical patients. *J Am Coll Surg* 207:80–87, Jul. 2008.
35. Regenbogen S., et al.: Prevention of retained surgical sponges: A decision-analytic model predicting relative cost-effectiveness. *Surgery* 145:527–535, May 2009.
36. Egorova N., et al.: Managing the prevention of retained surgical instruments: What is the value of counting? *Ann Surg* 247:13–18, Jan. 2008.
37. Beyond the count: Preventing retention of foreign objects. *Pennsylvania Patient Safety Advisory* 6:39–45, Jun. 2009.
38. Porteous J.: Surgical counts can be risky business! *Can Oper Room Nurs J,* Dec. 2004. http://findarticles.com/p/articles/mi_qa4130/is_200412/ai_n9466871/ (accessed Jul. 24, 2010).
39. Berger P., Sanders G.: Objects retained during surgery: Human diligence meets systems solutions. *Patient Safety & Quality Healthcare*, Sep.–Oct. 2008. http://www.psqh.com/sepoct08/objects.html (accessed Jul. 24, 2010).
40. Pelter M., Stephens K., Loranger D.: An evaluation of a numbered surgical sponge product. *AORN J* 85:931–936, 938–940, May 2007.
41. American College of Surgeons: Statement on the prevention of retained foreign bodies after surgery. *Bull Am Coll Surg* 90:15–16, Oct. 2005.
42. AORN's recommended practices for sponge, sharp, and instrument counts is up for review. *Infection Control Today,* Apr. 1, 2005. http://www.infectioncontroltoday.com/news/2005/04/aorn-s-recommended-practices-for-sponge-sharp-and.aspx (accessed Jul. 24, 2010).
43. Erickson S.: Left behind: Counting surgical instruments reduces medical errors. *Mater Manag Health Care* 12:32–34, Jul. 2003.
44. Minnesota's retained object protocol. *OR Manager* 24:14, 16, Dec. 2008.
45. Minnesota takes extra steps on wrong surgery, retained items. *OR Manager* 21:1, 18–20, Apr. 2005.
46. Greenberg C., et al.: Bar-coding surgical sponges to improve safety: A randomized controlled trial. *Ann Surg* 247:612–616, Apr. 2008.
47. Association of periOperative Registered Nurses (AORN): Recommended practices for the care and handling of specimens in the perioperative environment. In *Perioperative Standards and Recommended Practices*, 2010 ed. Denver: AORN, 2010.
48. Landro L.: In just a flash, simple surgery can turn deadly. *Wall Street Journal,* Feb. 18, 2009.
49. ECRI: A clinician's guide to surgical fires: How they occur, how to prevent them, how to put them out. *Heath Devices* 32:5–24, Jan. 2003.
50. Wang K., Advincula A.: "Current thoughts" in electrosurgery. *Int J Gynaecol Obstet* 97:245–250, Jun. 2007.
51. Meneghetti S., et al.: Operating room fires: Optimizing safety. *Plast Reconstr Surg* 120:1701–1708, Nov. 2007.
52. The Joint Commission: Preventing surgical fires. *Sentinel Event Alert* 29, Jun. 24, 2003. http://www.jointcommission.org/SentinelEvents/SentinelEventAlert/sea_29.htm.
53. Rodgers L., Kulwicki A.: Safety in the use of compressed air versus oxygen for the ophthalmic patient. *AANA J* 70:41–46, Feb. 2002.
54. Pollock G.: Eliminating surgical fires: A team approach. *AANA J* 72:293–298, Aug. 2004.
55. American Society of Anesthesiologists Task Force on Operating Room Fires: Practice advisory for the prevention and management of operating room fires. *Anesthesiology* 108:786–801, May 2008.
56. Rinder C.: Fire safety in the operating room. *Curr Opin Anaesthesiol* 21:790–795, Dec. 2008.
57. Spigelman A., Swan J.: Skin antiseptics and the risk of operating theatre fires. *ANZ J Surg* 7:556–558, Jul. 2005.
58. Salmon L.: Fire in the OR—Prevention and preparedness. *AORN J* 80:42–48, 51–54, Jul. 2004.
59. Sosis M.: Anesthesiologists must do a better job of preventing operating room fires. *J Clin Anesth* 18:81–82, Mar. 2006.
60. Fire prevention: Avoid oxygen to face. *OR Manager* 26:19–21, Jan. 2010.
61. Bales L., et al.: Be aware of fuel sources, ignition to reduce fire risk. *Same Day Surgery* (suppl.):1–3, Apr. 2005.
62. McCarthy P., Gaucher K.: Fire in the OR—Developing a fire safety plan. *AORN J* 79:588–597, 600, Mar. 2004.

PART 3

After the Procedure

This part of the book examines what must be done after a surgical or other invasive procedure is finished to maintain a high level of patient safety and quality. Chapter 9 discusses proper cleanup of the operating environment. Chapter 10 focuses on the health care organization's postoperative care of the patient. Chapter 11 explains how to effectively handle the patient's discharge from the organization, including appropriate follow-up.

Chapter 9

Cleanup of the Operating Environment

The process of surgery or other invasive procedures can generate a lot of mess. Soiled linens, contaminated surfaces, dirty instruments, and medical waste are all present after an invasive procedure. Organizations should take the time to make sure their cleanup procedures are effective to prevent hazards for subsequent patients and providers who enter the surgical area. Such cleanup procedures should involve the following:

- Disposing of medical waste properly
- Gathering soiled linens and equipment and transporting them out of the procedure area for cleaning
- Cleaning the procedure area

This chapter provides a brief look at these activities.

Disposing of Medical Waste

There is no universal definition of *medical waste,* and it is known by many names—regulated medical waste, biomedical waste, infectious waste, and health care waste, to name just a few.[1] Different criteria are used by different organizations and agencies. However, all medical waste originates from a patient's care, treatment, or immunization.

In the United States, the Occupational Safety and Health Administration (OSHA) defines *regulated medical waste* under its Bloodborne Pathogens Standard as "liquid or semi-liquid blood or other potentially infectious materials; contaminated items that would release blood or other potentially infectious materials in a liquid or semi-liquid state if compressed; items that are caked with dried blood or other potentially infectious materials and are capable of releasing these materials during handling; contaminated sharps; and pathological and microbiological wastes containing blood or other potentially infectious materials."[2]

The U.S. Environmental Protection Agency (EPA) uses a slightly different classification system for medical waste that incorporates a broader range of items. Following are some of the U.S. EPA's categories of waste often found in the surgical setting.[3]

- *Pathological waste.* Human pathological waste, including tissues, organs, body parts, and fluids that are removed during surgery, autopsy, or other medical procedures and specimens of body fluids and their containers.
- *Human blood and blood products.* These include liquid waste, human blood, blood products, items saturated and/or dripping with human blood, and previously saturated items that are now caked with dried human blood. These divisions include serum, plasma, and other blood components and their containers that were used or intended for use in patient care, testing, and laboratory analysis, or the development of pharmaceuticals. Intravenous bags are also included in this category.
- *Sharps.* These include sharps that have been used in patient care, including hypodermic needles, syringes (with and without the attached needle), Pasteur pipettes, scalpel blades, blood vials, needles with attached tubing, and culture dishes (regardless of the presence of infectious agents). Also included are other types of broken or unbroken glassware that were in contact with infectious agents, such as used slides and cover slips.

- *Isolation waste.* Includes biological waste and discarded materials contaminated with blood, excretions, exudates, or secretions from humans who are isolated to protect others from certain highly communicable diseases.
- *Unused sharps.* These include unused hypodermic needles, suture needles, syringes, and scalpel blades that have been discarded.

Organizations around the world that are focused on improving worker safety—such as the European Agency for Safety and Health at Work—are also concerned with ensuring safety when handling regulated medical waste, including sharps and needles.[4]

Medical waste can house dangerous pathogens, which can lead to infection and so must be disposed of carefully. (*See* Sidebar 9-1 on page 149.) Organizations should have procedures that outline how to appropriately identify, handle, and dispose of medical waste, and all surgical team members should be aware of these procedures.

One specific type of waste that must be disposed of properly is sharps—needles, blades, and other sharp equipment. As mentioned in Chapter 8, sharps have the potential to not only transmit infection but also cause serious injury if handled improperly. Because these implements pose a danger of puncturing or cutting the skin, special care must be taken to dispose of sharps into specially designated sharps boxes. Sharps disposal containers must be puncture resistant, leakproof, and closable. And they should be kept in a secure location within the procedural area that decreases the risk of injury to patients and health care providers. When boxes are three quarters full, they should be closed securely and placed at a designated collection point. It is important for health care providers not to overfill sharps boxes.[1]

When handling medical waste, those individuals who collect the waste, including environmental services personnel, should wear appropriate personal protective equipment to prevent exposure to medical waste and sharps injuries. For example, gloves should be worn when it is anticipated that a health care provider may have contact with blood or other potentially infectious materials. Masks, eye protection, and face shields should be worn by providers whenever contact with splashes, spray, splatter, or droplets of blood or other infectious materials is anticipated.[2,5]

After medical waste has been collected, health care providers—often environmental services staff—must transport it to an appropriate storage area. Health care organizations should consider the travel paths of waste and sterile or clean supplies within the building so that the two do not come into regular contact. Integrity must also be maintained during transportation. Leakproof carts lined with plastic can be used to transport infectious waste from the point of origin to the storage area where it is picked up and transported out of the organization.[3] To prevent the potential spread of infection, carts must be cleaned according to a cleaning and disinfection schedule.[1]

TIP Separate Regular Trash from Medical Waste

It should be noted that many forms of waste generated in the process of providing health care are noninfectious. Miscellaneous waste—such as slightly soiled dressings, sponges, and disposable gloves—does not need to be classified as infectious and can be placed in the regular trash. In addition, waste generated by support functions—such as paper, cardboard, and glass products—does not fit into the regulated medical waste category and does not require special handling or disposal methods. In fact, from a financial perspective, it is extremely important to separate regular trash from medical waste because disposal of medical waste typically costs more.

Transporting Contaminated Laundry

Dirty linens are present after any procedure and must be removed from the operating environment before cleaning can begin. Special care should be taken when collecting and transporting laundry that is visibly soiled with blood or bodily fluids. According to U.S. OSHA, laundry and/or housekeeping personnel should handle contaminated textiles and fabrics with a minimum of agitation to avoid contaminating the air, environmental surfaces, and persons in the room where the contaminated laundry is located.[2]

Sidebar 9-1: The Potential of Medical Waste to Spread Disease

Although medical waste has the potential to spread infection to those who handle it, such waste can cause an infection only if the following five conditions are met:

1. *A pathogen must be present.* Such pathogens may include hepatitis A, hepatitis B, human immunodeficiency virus (HIV), *Clostridium difficile,* and methicillin-resistant *Staphylococcus aureus* (MRSA).
2. *The pathogen must be of sufficient virulence.* Virulence is the disease-evoking power of a microorganism. Not all pathogens are equally capable of causing infectious disease.
3. *The pathogen must be present in sufficient quantities.* There must be a sufficient number of microorganisms present for infection to occur. This number varies according to several factors, including but not limited to organism type, susceptibility, and portal of exit.
4. *The organisms must have a portal of entry,* or a way to get into the body, such as a puncture, cut, surgical incision, or other type of wound.
5. *There must be a susceptible host.* Not all persons are equally susceptible to infectious diseases. For example, immunosuppressed patients or those with significant comorbid diseases, such as coronary artery disease and diabetes, may be more susceptible to infection.

It is important to note that all five of these conditions must be met for disease transmission to occur.

Sources:

United States Environmental Protection Agency (EPA): *Infectious Waste Management Guidelines.* Washington, DC: EPA, 1986.

Wideman J.: Waste Management. In *APIC Text of Infection Control and Epidemiology,* 3rd ed. Washington, DC: APIC, 2009, pp. 102-1–102-11.

Before removing laundry from any surface in the operating environment, health care providers should remove any sharps, equipment, or other nonlaundry items from the contaminated laundry to ensure safe transport and avoid sharps injuries. Doing so can also increase the efficiency of the laundering process. If objects are not removed and the laundry is sorted and washed with the items inside, it can result in extensive damage to laundry equipment.

When removing laundry, it may be helpful to follow a procedure that incorporates a folding or rolling technique that places the most soiled areas of the textile in the center of the bundle. In other words, health care providers fold up the heavily soiled area or item into the lightly soiled, or comparatively clean, area or item, so that the cleaner part of the textile serves as a barrier to the dirtier part.[6]

U.S. OSHA recommends placing contaminated laundry —such as laundry contaminated with blood or bodily fluids—in a red bag or putting it in containers that are labeled with a biohazard symbol. Contaminated laundry that is wet and presents a risk of soaking through the bag or leaking should be placed or transported in bags or containers that prevent leakage. When transporting contaminated laundry in bags, laundry personnel for their own safety should not hold the bags close to their body or squeeze the bags. This precaution will help avoid punctures from improperly discarded syringes or other sharps.

After it has been collected, contaminated laundry can be transported by cart or chute. If a health care organization uses a chute for transport, the U.S. Centers for Disease Control and Prevention (U.S. CDC) recommends bagging the linen because improperly designed chutes can offer a way for transmitting pathogens throughout a health care organization.[7]

During transport from the operating room or procedure area, soiled items should be covered. These supplies should travel through a semirestricted zone to a decontamination area to be stored before reprocessing. This storage area should be for only soiled items; clean or sterile items should not be stored in the same area with soiled items.[8]

Disposable linens that are contaminated with blood or other potentially infectious materials should be handled as medical waste. Disposable linens that are not soiled with infectious materials may be placed in the regular trash.[5]

Cleaning the Operating Area

The operating room or other invasive procedure rooms should be thoroughly cleaned before the first patient of the day arrives and recleaned after each subsequent patient.[9] The U.S. CDC recommends thorough cleaning of operating rooms once every 24 hours even if no procedure has been performed in the room.[10] This regular cleaning can help decrease microorganisms and contamination risks (particularly contamination of bacteria that are resistant to antibiotics) and may help control the spread of infection to patients. Regular cleaning is critical for the safety of all patients and staff in a health care organization, not just surgical patients, because such cleaning can cut down on the transmission and subsequent transmission of infection throughout an organization.

To ensure appropriate and effective cleaning in the operating environment, health care organizations should have cleaning and disinfecting protocols that outline activities to effectively reduce the bioburden on environmental surfaces and lessen the likelihood that they could serve as a source for pathogenic agents.[11] Such policies should address cleaning activities in surgical procedure areas and scrub and utility areas. These cleaning activities should involve a wet vacuum or a single-use mop and a U.S. EPA–registered hospital disinfectant/detergent. The following equipment should be cleaned during cleaning procedures[12]:

- Surgical lights and external tracks
- Fixed and ceiling-mounted equipment
- All furniture, including wheels and casters
- Medical equipment
- Handles of cabinets and push plates
- Ventilation faceplates
- Horizontal surfaces, including countertops, autoclaves, and fixed shelving
- The entire floor
- Kick buckets and scrub sinks

To help ensure effective cleaning in the operating room or procedure area, some health care organizations use a checklist that lists all the surfaces that need to be cleaned. Surgical team members can use this form to document areas where cleaning is below acceptable levels. Information obtained from the checklist can be used to identify and correct problem areas. In addition, environmental services personnel can use the checklist to verify they have cleaned all the appropriate parts of the operating environment.[12]

When Blood and Body Fluids Are Present in the Environment

Routine cleaning is the first step in removing blood and body fluids from environmental surfaces. Routine cleaning involves the use of a detergent or a germicidal detergent. Because organic materials, such as blood or body fluids, inactivate many disinfectants, they should be removed from any surfaces before disinfectant is applied.[9]

If a blood or blood product spill is small, housekeeping personnel can clean and decontaminate the area with a disinfectant in one step.[10] The U.S. CDC's 2003 guidelines for environmental infection control, which are still in use today, recommend removal of visible organic matter with absorbent material, followed by cleaning and disinfection of the area/surface. If the spill is larger and involves a higher concentration of bacteria, absorbent material should be placed over the spill and then disinfectant should be poured over the spill and the absorbent material until both are thoroughly soaked. For these types of spills, absorbent powders that solidify liquids can be particularly helpful.[10]

U.S. OSHA's *Occupational Exposure to Bloodborne Pathogens: Final Rule* states that "all equipment and environmental and working surfaces shall be cleaned and decontaminated after contact with blood or other potentially infectious materials."[2] U.S. OSHA requires hospitals to use one of the following types of decontaminants when cleaning up a blood or body fluid spill[9]:

- A U.S. EPA–registered hospital disinfectant that is effective against hepatitis B virus and the human immunodeficiency virus (HIV)
- A chemical germicide that is a tuberculocidal germocide
- An appropriate dilution of household bleach. Dilutions will vary depending on quantity of blood as well as the type of surface (for example, whether the environmental surface is porous or nonporous).

TIP Anticipate Evaporation

Because chlorine can evaporate from an open container, the solution must be mixed fresh daily or stored in a bottle or closed brown opaque container. Bleach stored in this manner will retain 50% of its initial value and remain stable for 30 days.

Addressing the Issue of Dust

Controlling and reducing dust in the operating environment is an important aspect of the cleaning process. Dust can be a vehicle to transport human skin and hair, fibers, pollen, spores, and a variety of microorganisms, including bacteria, mold, and fungi. Dust, circulating on air currents, can settle into open wounds, either directly or via contaminated equipment in contact with the wound. Dust can also present problems for patients with compromised respiratory or immune systems.

Regular and thorough cleaning can address the issue of dust control. During this cleaning, environmental services personnel should use a chemically treated dust cloth or mop to prevent dispersal of any dust. For areas above shoulder height, housekeeping personnel should use a specially designed mop that can reach high surfaces. Dust cloths and mops should never be shaken because fungal spores can be released into the air as a result.[9]

Avoiding Slips, Trips, and Falls

Liquids spilled on the floor of the operating room or procedure area can transform that surface from slip-resistant to slippery, which, coupled with the equipment present in the operating room or procedure area and the fast-paced nature of the surgical procedure, can present opportunity for slips, trips, and falls. Although these events can happen anywhere in a health care facility, slips, trips, and falls in the operating room or procedure area are particularly risky because they can harm patients as well as health care providers.

When cleaning the operating environment after a procedure, environmental services personnel should promptly remove any spills that could present a risk for slips, trips, and falls. Fluid solidifiers can soak up liquids and prevent them from spreading across the floor. Sprinkling a solidifier into the medical waste container may prevent a liquid spill in the first place and thus lessen the chance of a slipping, tripping, or falling incident.

Following are some guidelines for the environmental services staff to follow in cleaning the operating room or procedure area and making it safe from slips, trips, and falls:

- Clear the area of all employees except members of the cleaning crew.
- Wall off the areas to be cleaned, block the doors, and post signs prohibiting entry.
- Start with the cleanest area of the floor of the operating room or procedure area and then move to the areas that are less clean, saving the least-clean areas for last.
- Use no-skid waxes and grit coatings to create nonslip surfaces in the operating room or procedure area.
- Remove the barriers and warning signs only when the floors are completely dry.

In addition to these cleaning procedures, surgical team members should be instructed to use slip-resistant footwear in the surgical suite. Floor mats should also be slip resistant. When these mats become saturated with fluids, they should be replaced.

Health care providers should also make sure any cords or cables do not extend across the walking path in the operating room or procedure area. Cords should be bundled wherever possible or suspended from the ceiling. Providers should also watch out for step stools, buckets, equipment stands, and boxes of supplies and equipment.

Another common cause of slips, trips, and falls in the operating room or procedure area is obstructed views of the surroundings. Surgical team members should keep monitors and equipment out of the way so that everyone on the procedure team can see the floor clearly. Organizations should also make sure there is plenty of light in the operating environment so that providers can avoid tripping and slipping hazards.

Cleaning Up Effectively Is Everyone's Concern

Although responsibility for cleaning the operating environment typically falls to environmental services staff, all team members should be familiar with the various aspects of the process—disposing of waste, gathering linens, and cleaning environmental surfaces—so they do not inadvertently violate procedure and put themselves or their patients at risk. Incorporating information about appropriate cleaning and disposal procedures may be helpful within team member orientation and training efforts.

Organization leadership can help ensure appropriate cleanup of the operating environment by doing the following[5]:

- Establishing written policies and procedures for environmental cleaning and disinfection
- Reviewing the policies and procedures annually
- Making the policies and procedures readily available in surgical practice settings
- Establishing a quality management program to evaluate products, processes, and outcomes of the environmental cleaning and disinfection program
- Monitoring staff performance on an ongoing basis

Concern for the cleanliness of the operating environment should be an integral part of an organization's safety culture.

References

1. Wideman J.: Waste management. In *APIC Text of Infection Control and Epidemiology,* 3rd ed. Washington, DC: Association for Professionals in Infection Control and Epidemiology, 2009, pp. 102-1–102-11.
2. Occupational Safety and Health Administration: *Bloodborne Pathogens.* Standard 1910.130, 29 CFR. http://www.osha.gov/pls/oshaweb/owadisp.show_document?p_table=STANDARDS&p_id=10051 (accessed Jul. 24, 2010).
3. Environmental Protection Agency (EPA): *Infectious Waste Management Guidelines.* Washington, DC: EPA, 1986.
4. European Agency for Safety and Health at Work: *Risk Assessment and Needlestick Injuries.* E-Facts 40. http://osha.europa.eu/en/publications/e-facts/en_efact40.pdf (accessed Jul. 24, 2010).
5. Association of periOperative Registered Nurses (AORN): Recommended practices for environmental cleaning in the perioperative setting. In *Perioperative Standards and Recommended Practices,* 2010 ed. Denver: AORN, 2010, pp. 241–256.
6. McDonald L., Pugliese G.: Textile processing service. In Mayhall C.: *Hospital Epidemiology and Infection Control,* 2nd ed. Philadelphia: Lippincott Williams & Wilkins, 1999, pp. 1031–1033.
7. Pyrek K.: Lessons in linen: Following aseptic technique in the laundry department. *Infection Control Today,* Feb. 1, 2003. http://www.infectioncontroltoday.com/articles/399/399_321feat1.html (accessed Jul. 24, 2010).
8. Church N., Bjerke N.: Surgical services. In *APIC Text of Infection Control and Epidemiology,* 3rd ed. Washington, DC: Association for Professionals in Infection Control and Epidemiology, 2009, pp. 45-1–45-14.
9. Chou T.: Environmental services. In *APIC Text of Infection Control and Epidemiology,* 3rd ed. Washington, DC: Association for Professionals in Infection Control and Epidemiology, 2009, pp. 100-1–100-13.
10. Centers for Disease Control and Prevention: *Guidelines for Environmental Infection Control in Health-Care Facilities.* 2003. http://www.cdc.gov/hicpac/pdf/guidelines/eic_in_HCF_03.pdf (accessed Jul. 24, 2010).
11. Arias K., Soule B.: The environment of care and infection prevention and control. In Arias K., Soule B. (eds.): *The APIC/JCR Infection Prevention and Control Workbook,* 2nd ed. Oak Brook, IL: Joint Commission Resources, 2009, pp. 95–105.
12. Neil J., Nye P., Toven A.: Environmental surveillance in the operating room. *AORN J* 82:43–49, Jul. 2005.

Chapter 10

Postoperative Care

After patients leave the procedure room, they typically go to a postoperative care area for monitoring. During this time, health care providers—usually nurses—observe several aspects of the patients' response to the surgery or other invasive procedure and address patient care needs. Outpatient, inpatient, and same-day admit surgical patients all receive postoperative monitoring. A consistent policy should be in place throughout an organization for postoperative monitoring. This policy should address any differences in monitoring appropriate to each patient's condition, anesthesia, and procedure. This chapter discusses some of the activities that take place during the critical postprocedure period.

Assessing and Responding to Mental Status

Within the postprocedure setting, health care providers must assess the patient's mental status, including the presence of delirium. Postoperative delirium can have negative effects, such as delaying postoperative movement, prolonging treatment, extending length of stay, and preventing early rehabilitation.[1] There are several diagnostic tools available to help providers assess patients effectively and consistently (*see* Sidebar 10-1 at right). Organizations should consider using such a tool.

Based on the results of the assessment, perioperative team members will decide next steps for the patient, which may include altered medication, a longer stay in the postoperative area, or transfer out of the postoperative area.

Assessing and Responding to Physiological Status

Just as mental functioning must be assessed, so should a patient's physiological status after surgery or other invasive procedure. Depending on the procedure, this assessment should include vital signs, the presence and degree of pain, presence of any unanticipated swelling, respiratory function, or perhaps wound drainage. If a patient shows an adverse reaction to anesthesia during postprocedure monitoring, such as nausea, vomiting, dizziness, or excessive bleeding, or if the patient has abnormal vital signs or impaired respiratory effort, then he or she will need a longer stay in the recovery area.[2] For particular types of surgeries, perioperative staff should monitor for potential adverse events, such as deep vein thrombosis (*see* Sidebar 10-2 on page 154), which more commonly develops after discharge but can sometimes present symptoms before the patient has left the organization. Deep vein thrombosis must be treated immediately to prevent the

Sidebar 10-1: The Short Portable Mental Status Questionnaire

To help assess postoperative mental status and delirium, health care organizations may want to use a diagnostic tool, such as the short portable mental status questionnaire. This questionnaire is easy to use and does not require training for successful administration. The tool involves asking the patient a series of questions, such as the following:

1. What is the date today?
2. What day of the week is it?
3. What is the name of this place?
4. What is your telephone number?
5. What is your street address?
6. How old are you?
7. When were you born?
8. What is your mother's maiden name?
9. What number do you get if you subtract 3 from 20? And what do you get if you subtract 3 from that number? (Repeat last question several times.)

Sidebar 10-2: Preventing Deep Vein Thrombosis

Total knee replacement and hip replacement surgeries have been commonplace for decades. Currently, nearly a half-million total knee replacements and nearly a quarter-million primary total hip replacements are performed each year in the United States.

Although surgical techniques have improved and recovery times have shortened, these procedures still come with a high risk of deep vein thrombosis. Deep vein thrombosis originates in the calf or thigh due to a combination of venous stasis, vessel wall damage, and hypercoagulability. Blood clots can then form and travel to the lungs, causing fatal pulmonary embolism.

Certain factors exacerbate the risk for deep vein thrombosis. For example, it can be clinically silent, in some cases presenting no symptoms until long after the surgery. Other factors have to do with the patient's demographics, such as his or her age. Older patients can be at a higher risk of deep vein thrombosis or pulmonary embolism than younger patients. Unfortunately, older patients are also more likely to need knee or hip replacement surgeries. The average age for knee replacements is 67.1 years, and the average age for hip replacement is 65.4 years. Gender can be a factor as well. Research indicates that women are more likely than men to undergo total hip and knee surgeries. Along with the age and gender of the patient, the likelihood of deep vein thrombosis is higher among those who have other health problems, including obesity, history of smoking, family history of thrombosis, or the presence of another condition such as cancer.

Because deep vein thrombosis and pulmonary embolism are serious but preventable, the U.S. National Quality Forum has designated these conditions after total knee replacement or hip replacement surgery to be serious reportable events, commonly called "never events."

Although pulmonary embolism is a common and sometimes fatal complication associated with knee and hip replacement surgery, preventive measures exist that health care providers can use to protect patients. One such measure is the use of regional anesthesia, such as spinal or epidural anesthesia, instead of general anesthesia. Use of regional anesthesia has been shown to reduce the rate of deep vein thrombosis by allowing more blood flow to the lower extremities.

Ensuring that the patient walks as soon as possible after surgery is also beneficial. Patients who are sedentary are more likely to develop deep vein thrombosis than those who are mobilized earlier and more often.

Chief among preventive measures that have proven effective is thromboprophylaxis—administration of anticoagulation medication prior to or during surgery. An estimated 40% to 60% of patients undergoing total hip and knee replacements without pharmacological prophylaxis experience deep vein thrombosis. Conversely, evidence shows that the correct use of thromboprophylaxis could prevent an estimated 20,000 to 30,000 deaths in the United States alone.

Despite extensive research, no individual agent has been determined to be the ideal medication in deep vein thrombosis prevention. The type of medication that should be used will depend on a number of factors, from the use of regional anesthesia to a patient's propensity to bleed to his or her age, among other factors. Ultimately, the physician and/or surgical team determines which prophylactic regimen to use after weighing the risk of potential bleeding and the effectiveness for deep vein thrombosis and pulmonary embolism prevention.

The duration of postoperative anticoagulant therapy can be just as important as the type of medication used. For knee surgeries, for example, the anticoagulant must be taken for at least 10 to 14 days. Patients who have undergone hip replacements should receive anticoagulant therapy for at least 30 days and perhaps more.

When deep vein thrombosis does occur, diagnosis and treatment are critical to stopping it from progressing to pulmonary embolism, which can, if left undetected, cause a fatality within as little as one hour. During a health care organization stay, knee and hip replacement patients are regularly checked for any unusual swelling, redness, or pain. Rapid screening measures may be used if swelling is found; venography, magnetic resonance imaging, and ultrasonography may also be used to diagnose deep vein thrombosis.

Because deep vein thrombosis can develop after discharge, patients are also monitored by home health professionals and can check in for additional testing and follow-ups with their physicians following discharge. Although many cases of deep vein thrombosis present within a few days after surgery, the risk can extend for three months or longer, especially for patients who have undergone hip surgery.

(continued on page 155)

Sidebar 10-2: Preventing Deep Vein Thrombosis *(continued)*

Patient education, which begins at the health care organization, can also lead to the identification of complications and to a medical diagnosis of deep vein thrombosis. Patients who are instructed on what symptoms to look for and when and how often to return for monitoring can play a role in their own care. (*See* Chapter 11 for more information about educating patients before discharge.)

Sources:

American Academy of Orthopaedic Surgeons (AAOS): *Clinical Guideline on Prevention of Pulmonary Embolism in Patients Undergoing Total Hip or Knee Arthoplasty.* Rosemont, IL: AAOS, 2007.

American Academy of Orthopaedic Surgeons: *Deep Vein Thrombosis.* http://orthoinfo.aaos.org/topic.cfm?topic=a00219 (accessed Jul. 21, 2010).

Centers for Disease Control and Prevention: *National Hospital Discharge Survey.* http://www.cdc.gov/nchs/nhds.htm (accessed Jul. 21, 2010).

Ennis R.: *Deep Venous Thrombosis Prophylaxis in Orthopedic Surgery.* Updated Jun. 12, 2009. http://emedicine.medscape.com/article/1268573-overview (accessed Jul. 21, 2010).

Lieberman J., Hsu W.: Prevention of venous thromboembolic disease after total hip and knee arthroplasty. *J Bone Joint Surg Am* 87:2097–2112, Sep. 2005.

Ponticello M., Steinberg J.: Pertinent pointers on DVT prophylaxis. *Podiatry Today* 20, Apr. 1, 2007. http://www.podiatrytoday.com/article/6955 (accessed Jul. 21, 2010).

Yen D., Weiss W.: Results of adjusted-dose heparin for thromboembolism prophylaxis in knee replacement compared to those found for its use in hip fracture surgery and elective hip replacement. *Iowa Orthop J*: 27:47–51, 2007.

creation of blood clots that can travel into the lungs and cause death from a pulmonary embolism in less than an hour.[3] Organizations should have standardized processes in place for monitoring a patient's physiological health and responding to worrisome physiological assessments.

Assessing the Need for Medications

The postoperative period is a time for ceasing certain medications, such as preoperative antibiotics, and starting new medications, such as those to address pain. Providers verify that any intravenous fluids and medications administered during the surgery or other invasive procedure need to be continued, including blood and blood components. If these fluids and medications do not need to be continued, providers then stop them.

As with other aspects of medication management discussed in this book, the prescribing and administering of medication in the postoperative period should involve clearly written orders, repeat-backs of any verbal orders, and appropriately labeled medications. Technology, such as computerized provider order entry systems, can be particularly helpful in this setting. Such systems not only can help ensure clearly written orders but also can provide automated prompts that remind perioperative staff to discontinue antibiotics within 24 hours of the completion of the procedure. It is important that providers follow through with appropriate preparation, administration, and evaluation of medications while the patient remains in the organization.

Preventing Infection

Infections are the major source of morbidity and mortality following surgical care. These infections can be divided into two categories: those that occur at the surgical site and those that occur away from the surgical site, such as within the urinary tract or at the site of intravenous lines.[4] The following sections take a brief look at how to prevent these types of infections.

Surgical Site Infections

As mentioned in Chapter 4, surgical site infections (SSIs) are a significant problem in the surgical setting and can yield both high human costs and financial costs. In the United States alone, 22% of health care–associated infections are related to the surgical site.[5]

TIP Helpful Resources for Infection Prevention and Control

To help health care organizations with their infection prevention and control efforts, the Society for Healthcare Epidemiology of America and the Infectious Diseases Society of America have partnered with The Joint Commission, the American Hospital Association, and the Association for Professionals in Infection Control and Epidemiology to create a *Compendium of Strategies to Prevent Healthcare-Associated Infections in Acute Care Hospitals.* This tool organizes evidence-based strategies that have been found to prevent infection into a set of easy-to-understand, practical guidelines. The compendium provides information on all the infections discussed here and would be a good source of further information when planning infection prevention and control efforts. Organizations can access the compendium at http://www.preventinghais.com.

Organizations can also turn to the World Health Organization and the International Federation of Infection Control for information about infection prevention and control. These two agencies provide myriad resources on a variety of topics and can be quite helpful when designing an infection prevention and control program. Organizations can access these two entities at http://www.who.int/en/ and http://www.theific.org/, respectively.

Certain individuals are more at risk for SSIs than others. Older patients, diabetics, smokers, patients with pre-existing infections, and patients with colonization of *Staphylococcus aureus* are particularly at risk. Procedure-related risks include improper surgical technique, the duration of the operation, the quality of surgical site preparation, and inadequate cleaning, disinfection, and sterilization of medical instruments.[6] Also, the nature of the wound can be a predictor of surgical site infection. (*See* Sidebar 10-3 for a classification of types of wounds.)

Sidebar 10-3: Wound Classifications

Although there are several factors that can contribute to the likelihood of a surgical site infection (SSI), the type of wound can be a significant factor. Following is a description of four types of surgical wounds.

1. *Clean wounds.* These are uninfected, operative wounds, where the operative procedure does not enter viscous, respiratory, alimentary, or genital or urinary tracts. Examples of procedures that cause a clean wound include breast biopsies and open-heart surgeries. SSI rates for this type of wound tend to be less than 2%.
2. *Clean-contaminated wounds.* These are operative wounds where respiratory, alimentary, or genital/urinary tracts are entered but under elective and controlled circumstances. Examples of procedures that cause this type of wound include gynecological procedures, head/neck procedures that involve the mouth, and pulmonary resection. SSI rates for this type of wound tend to range from 4% to 10%.
3. *Contaminated wounds.* These are wounds where gross contamination is present but no obvious infection is present. They include operations in which major breaks in aseptic technique have occurred. Examples include gunshot wounds to the abdomen or accidental bowel perforations. SSI rates for these wounds are greater than 10%, even with preventive antibiotics and other strategies.
4. *Dirty wounds.* These are wounds that involve an active infection which is already present. Procedures that lead to these kinds of wounds include abdominal exploration of peritonitis and the exploration and draining of abscesses. Like contaminated wounds, the SSI rates for dirty wounds are greater than 10%, even with preventive antibiotics and other strategies.

Source: Odem-Forren J.: Watch that incision! *Nurs Manage* 35(suppl.):16–21, Nov. 2004.

Many of the ways to reduce the risk of surgical site infections in patients have been discussed earlier in this book. Actions such as preoperative scrubbing of health care providers' hands, administering prophylactic antibiotics, and preparing the surgical site on the patient before surgery can help reduce the risk of postoperative infection. Monitoring temperature and blood glucose levels during surgery also can help reduce that risk.

In the postoperative setting, if there is a wound, wound care is critical to ensure that the surgical site remains free of contamination. Wound dressings assist with healing by acting as a physical barrier to bacteria, protecting the wound from injury, and minimizing pain.[7]

To help prevent surgical site infections in the postoperative setting, health care providers should protect incisions that have sutures in place with sterile dressings for 24 to 48 hours. Whenever dressings are changed, health care providers should use sterile technique, which involves appropriate hand hygiene, use of personal protective equipment,[6] and asepsis practices.

Providers should also give education to patients about how to care for their incision to further prevent the likelihood of surgical site infection. More information about patient education before discharge can be found in Chapter 11.

> **TIP Consider Using a Tool for Predicting SSIs**
>
> There are several tools surgical teams can use to predict whether a patient is going to contract a surgical site infection. In the United States, for example, the National Noscomial Infections Surveillance System (NNIS) created a risk index that helps providers assess a patient's likelihood of developing a surgical site infection (SSI). The index takes into consideration an anesthesia score, wound class, and operative duration and classifies surgical procedures into four categories of increasing risk.[8] Similarly, the Australian Clinical Risk Index (ACRI) was developed as an alternative to the NNIS tool. The ACRI helps stratify risk after coronary artery bypass surgery. This risk index considers the diagnosis of diabetes mellitus and body mass index.[8] The Department of Veterans Affairs (VA) in the United States created a 14-variable tool that assesses patient factors, preoperative laboratory values, and operative characteristics. A study by the VA showed that its scoring tool was more effective then the NNIS instrument.[9]
>
> By using an SSI-predictive tool, providers can identify patients at high risk for surgical site infection and closely monitor those patients in the postoperative period.

Preventing Infections Associated with Urinary Catheters

Infections of the urinary tract are the most common health care–associated infection, accounting for more than 30% of all health care–associated infections reported by acute care hospitals.[10] A urinary tract infection occurs when bacteria enter and proliferate in the normally sterile urinary tract and cause infection.

Although urinary tract infections arise from multiple sources, indwelling urinary catheters account for 80% of these infections in hospitals.[11] More than 30 million Foley catheters—the catheter used in urinary tract catheterization—are inserted each year in the United States, contributing to about 1 million catheter-associated urinary tract infections (CAUTIs).[12]

Other risk factors for CAUTIs include being female, being older, having a compromised immune system, and having comorbid conditions such as diabetes, renal dysfunction, and incontinence.[13] Clinical risk factors include unnecessarily long duration of catheter use, improper insertion and care of urinary catheters, insertion of catheters outside of the operating room or procedure area, use of urinary catheters for urine monitoring beyond surgery, and failure to maintain a closed drainage system.[14]

There are many reasons why a patient would need a urinary catheter during surgery. For example, a urinary catheter is warranted during selected surgical procedures, such as urologic surgery, surgery on contiguous structures, prolonged surgery, surgeries in which large-volume infusions or diuretics are administered, and surgeries involving patients who are incontinent. Such catheters can also be used for urine output monitoring during surgery.[14]

CAUTIs occur when bacteria can gain access to the urinary tract during catheterization or from the catheter itself. For example, bacteria can infiltrate the urinary tract when a catheter is first inserted from the external or internal surfaces of the catheter; at the drainage port or outlet of the collection bag; at junctions such as the catheter–drainage tube connection and drainage tube–collection bag connection; or when microorganisms from contaminated drainage tubes or collection bags enter the bladder through reflux.

Not every CAUTI causes a problem for patients. In fact, many such infections in otherwise healthy patients are often asymptomatic and resolve spontaneously when the catheter is removed. Occasionally, infection continues and leads to complications, such as prostatitis, epididymitis, or cystitis.[14]

Although not all CAUTIs can be prevented, there are many strategies health care organizations can take to significantly reduce the rate of these infections. A description of best practices to prevent CAUTIs is detailed as follows:

- *Use urinary catheters only when necessary.* For patients who need them, urinary catheters are an essential part of medical treatment. However, inappropriate catheter use can be detrimental to patient health, and unfortunately this problem occurs frequently in health care organizations. It is estimated that more than 50% of patients are catheterized inappropriately.[15,16] Catheterization should never occur for mere convenience or because a patient requests it. Catheters should be used only in specific circumstances in which their use is beneficial to the patient's health and recovery. Organizations should have clear guidelines that list and describe the approved uses for urinary catheters and educate physicians, nurses, and other health care providers about these guidelines. Health care organizations can create an indication sheet that lists the specific reasons for ordering a urinary catheter and require physicians to fill out the sheet prior to catheter insertion. This process can also be incorporated into the facility's electronic order entry system, if it has one.
- *Decrease the amount of time for catheterization.* One of the most significant risk factors for developing a CAUTI is the duration of catheterization.[14] Because of this risk, health care organizations that reduce the length of time catheters remain in place can reduce the rate of CAUTIs occurring in their facilities. To reduce catheterization duration, health care organizations should institute an organizationwide program that involves reminders for physicians to review the need for continued catheterization and remove catheters promptly when they are no longer medically necessary. Such reminders should take place frequently—ideally on a daily basis. Health care organizations can use a variety of strategies to help with reminders. For example, stickers on medical charts can serve as reminders, as can preprinted indication forms housed in the medical records of catheterized patients that physicians must fill out to continue the use of the catheter. To systemize reminders and rely less on human memory, health care organizations can also use computerized provider order entry systems in which reminders or stop orders are automatically generated at set intervals.

TIP Monitor Postoperative Urinary Retention

For surgical patients who receive urinary catheters, health care organizations need to have specific guidelines in place to monitor postoperative urinary retention. In addition, health care organizations need to implement procedure-specific guidelines for postoperative catheter removal, including the use of bladder scanners.

- *Use appropriate catheter insertion, care, and maintenance techniques.* Many cases of CAUTI result when aseptic techniques are not followed during catheter insertion and improper care procedures are not followed after a catheter is in place. Therefore, health care organizations need to have written guidelines for urinary catheter insertion and maintenance; ensure that all health care providers involved with urinary catheters are properly educated and trained on these guidelines; and monitor compliance with the guidelines. Only health care providers who have been thoroughly educated and trained on proper insertion, maintenance, and removal procedures should perform urinary catheter insertions and maintenance activities. These individuals also need to be knowledgeable about alternatives to indwelling urinary catheters and CAUTI prevention strategies. It is also important to teach the patient and family about proper catheter care.
- *Document catheter use.* For patient safety, it is essential that all information related to the insertion, care, and maintenance of urinary catheters be documented. Information can be documented in the patient record as well as on the nursing flow sheet, nursing notes, or physician orders. If possible, data and information should be documented using

a standardized format and, ideally, an electronic format; this facilitates data collection, analysis, and reporting as well as quality improvement projects. Documentation should include the indication sheet for urinary catheter insertion (if the health care organization uses one), date and time of catheter insertion, name of the individual who inserted the catheter, rationale for continued use, use of a procurement device, use of a bladder scanner, and date and time of catheter removal.[13]

In addition to documenting catheter use, health care organizations should also document any instances of adverse events associated with catheter use. Adverse events are not limited to CAUTI but also include catheter obstructions, accidental catheter removals, trauma caused by catheters, and the reinsertion of catheters within 24 hours after they were removed.

To aid analysis, data collected on catheter use and adverse events should be stratified according to important risk factors such as age, sex, unit, and duration. These data should be analyzed and reported to stakeholders in a timely fashion.

Preventing Infections Associated with Intravenous Lines

Each year, nearly 250,000 central line–associated bloodstream infections (CLABSIs) occur in U.S. health care organizations,[17] and many of these infections are associated with central venous catheters. Such infections can lead to increased hospital stays, elevated medical costs, and sometimes patient mortality. In fact, about 14,000 deaths occur annually due to central line infections, and some estimates put this figure as high as 28,000 deaths per year.[18] Concern over these levels of CLABSI occurrences and their consequences led The Joint Commission to establish a National Patient Safety Goal requiring organizations to implement evidence-based practices to prevent central line–associated bloodstream infections.

In the United States, the National Healthcare Safety Network defines a *central line* as a catheter whose tip terminates in a great vessel, such as the aorta, pulmonary artery, superior vena cava, inferior vena cava, brachiocephalic veins, internal jugular veins, subclavian veins, external iliac veins, and common femoral veins.[18] Such catheters are used for a variety of reasons, including the administration of fluids and electrolytes, blood products, medications, and nutritional support to patients.[19] Central lines disrupt skin integrity, making it possible for bacteria and fungi to enter the bloodstream and cause infection.[20]

As with CAUTIs, CLABSI risks are present when central lines are inserted and maintained. To help reduce the infection risks associated with central line insertion and care, health care organizations should have standardized protocols that govern these activities. Such protocols should include the following:

- A central venous catheter insertion checklist. This checklist outlines all the steps involved in effective central venous catheter insertion and can ensure that all required steps are completed, according to organization policy. (*See* Figure 10-1 on page 160.)
- Requirements for hand hygiene prior to central venous catheter insertion and manipulation
- Guidelines for optimal catheter site selection. The majority of CLABSIs develop at the insertion site,[21] and some sites present greater risks than others. To help prevent infection at the insertion site, health care organizations should establish guidelines that restrict the use of femoral and jugular veins unless other sites are not available.
- A standardized cart or kit that contains all of the supplies needed for central venous catheter insertion
- Requirements for maximal sterile barrier precautions for health care providers when inserting or caring for the central venous catheter. These precautions include the use of sterile gloves, sterile gowns, large sterile drapes, mask/face shields, and caps during insertion. As with other surgical procedures, the cap should cover all hair, and the mask should cover the nose and mouth tightly. Sterile precautions also apply to patients, who should be covered from head to toe with a sterile drape with a small opening for the insertion site.[18]
- Skin preparation guidelines. They should require the use of an antiseptic for skin preparation during central venous catheter insertion that is cited in scientific literature or endorsed by professional organizations.

Figure 10-1: Checklist for Central Line Insertion

PATIENT Label

Advancing Medicine Enhancing Health
Bloomington Hospital of Orange County

Central Line Procedural Checklist

Type of catheter (brand): ❐ Arrow
❐ Cook antibiotic coated

Is this a NEW line: ❐ YES ❐ NO

Is the procedure: ❐ Elective ❐ Emergent

Location of Line placement: ❐ER ❐OR ❐ NW room#______

Procedural Checklist		
Safety Practice	***YES***	***YES*** *(After Reminder)*
Before procedure, *did the provider:*		
PERFORM PROCEDURAL PAUSE Perform patient ID X 2 Announce the procedure to be performed Mark / assess site		
Cleanse hands? *(ASK, if unsure)*		
Prep procedure site with ChloraPrep? **30 seconds for dry site* ***2 minutes for moist site (esp. femoral)*		
Use large drape to cover patient in sterile fashion?		
During procedure, did the provider:		
Wear sterile gloves during catheter insertion?		
Wear hat, mask, and sterile gown?		
Maintain sterile field?		
Did assisting physician, anesthetist or nurse follow the same precautions? (hand washing, mask, gloves, gown)		
Did all staff and patient in the room wear a mask?		
After the procedure:		
Was sterile technique maintained when applying dressing?		
Was dressing dated?		

Name of physician placing Line: ______________________________

Name of assisting nurse: ______________________ Date: ___-___-___

PLEASE RETURN COMPLETED FORM TO INFECTION CONTROL

Bloomington Hospital of Orange County uses this checklist to ensure standardized central line insertion and care.

Source: Bloomington Hospital of Orange County, Paoli, Indiana. Used with permission.

- Catheters of particular material, which resist infection. These can include catheters made of Teflon, silicon, elastomer, or polyurethane.[22]
- Cleaning requirements associated with central venous catheters. These requirements should address disinfecting catheter hubs and injection ports, among other activities.
- Recommendations for the use of antimicrobial-impregnated catheters. The U.S. Centers for Disease Control and Prevention recommends the use of antimicrobial-impregnated catheters for adults in whom the catheter will remain for more than five days, assuming the organization has implemented a comprehensive strategy to reduce rates of CLABSI and that the CLABSI rate remains above the goal set by the individual institution based on benchmark rates and local factors.[23] Such catheters have been shown to reduce the incidence of central venous catheter–related bloodstream infections.[24] The disadvantage of using antimicrobial-impregnated catheters is that they are significantly more expensive than regular catheters. For this reason, health care organizations may want to consider using these types of catheters for specific high-risk patients. In these cases, the increased cost of the catheter would be less than the cost of treating such a patient who acquires a CLABSI.[25]

As with urinary catheters, central venous catheters are sometimes used unnecessarily or for too long. To address this issue, health care organizations should establish a mechanism for routinely evaluating all patients with a central venous catheter and removing nonessential catheters. One method to ensure that this occurs is to incorporate daily evaluation for need into the nursing care plan or medical staff rounds for all patients with central lines and include a follow-up mechanism to ensure prompt central venous catheter removal when the line is no longer needed.

After a health care organization has implemented its CLABSI protocols, it should make sure those protocols are being followed. This may involve having observers—health care providers who are familiar with central venous catheter insertion and care processes—watch the procedure and document appropriate completion. As part of the organization's culture of safety, all health care providers should be empowered to stop any process at any time if they believe it is unsafe or breaches protocols.

References

1. Zakriya K., et al.: Preoperative factors associated with postoperative change in confusion assessment method score in hip fracture patients. *Anesth Analg* 94:1628–1632, Jun. 2002.
2. Halliday A.: Shades of sedation: Learning about moderate sedation and analgesia. *Nursing* 36:37–41, Nov. 2006.
3. Rahme E., et al.: Postdischarge thromboprophylaxis and mortality risk after hip- or knee-replacement surgery. *CMAJ* 178:1545–1554, Jun. 2008.
4. Fry D.: A systems approach to the prevention of surgical infections. *Surg Clin North Am* 89:521–537, Apr. 2009.
5. Centers for Disease Control and Prevention: *Estimates of Healthcare-Associated Infections.* http://www.cdc.gov/ncidod/dhqp/hai.html (accessed Jul. 24, 2010).
6. Owens C., Stoessel K.: Surgical site infections: Epidemiology, microbiology, and prevention. *J Hosp Infect* 70(suppl. 2):3–10, Nov. 2008.
7. Fletcher N., et al.: Prevention of perioperative infection. *J Bone Joint Surg Am* 89:1605–1618, Jul. 2007.
8. Chen L., et al.: Validating a 3-point prediction rule for surgical site infection after coronary artery bypass surgery. *Infect Control Hosp Epidemiol* 31:64–68, Jan. 2010.
9. Neumayer L., et al.: Multivariable predictors of postoperative surgical site infection after general and vascular surgery: Results from the patient safety surgery study. *J Am Coll Surg* 204:1178–1187, Jun. 2007.
10. Klevens R., et al.: Estimating health care-associated infections and deaths in U.S. hospitals, 2002. *Public Health Rep* 122, Mar.–Apr. 2007. http://www.cdc.gov/ncidod/dhqp/pdf/hicpac/infections_deaths.pdf (accessed Jul. 29, 2010).
11. Saint S., Chenowith C.: Biofilms and catheter-associated urinary tract infections. *Infect Dis Clin North Am* 17:411–432, Jun. 2003.
12. *Infection Control Today* Editors: Expert discusses strategies to prevent CAUTIs (interview with Dr. Rabih Darouiche). *Infection Control Today* 9:74–82, 2005.
13. Lo E., et al.: Strategies to prevent catheter-associated urinary tract infections in acute care hospitals. *Infect Control Hosp Epidemiol* 29(suppl. 1):S41–S50, Oct. 2008.
14. Gould C., et al.: *Guideline for Prevention of Catheter-Associated Urinary Tract Infections, 2009.* Centers for Disease Control and Prevention, Dec. 29, 2009. http://www.cdc.gov/hicpac/cauti/001_cauti.html (accessed Jul. 24, 2010).
15. Hazelett S., et.al.: The association between indwelling urinary catheter use in the elderly and urinary tract infection in acute care. *BMC Geriatr* 6:15, Oct. 12, 2006.
16. Gokula R., Hickner J., Smith M.: Inappropriate use of urinary catheters in elderly patients at a midwestern community teaching hospital. *Am J Infect Control* 32:196–199, Jun. 2004.
17. Centers for Disease Control and Prevention: *Central Line-Associated Bloodstream Infection (CLABSI) Event.* Jun. 2010. www.cdc.gov/nhsn/PDFs/pscManual/4PSC_CLABScurrent.pdf (accessed Jul. 24, 2010).
18. 5 Million Lives Campaign: *Getting Started Kit: Prevent Central Line Infections How-to Guide.* Cambridge, MA: Institute for Healthcare Improvement, 2008.
19. Maki D., Leonard A.: Infections due to infusion therapy. In Jarvis W. (ed.): *Bennett & Brachman's Hospital Infections.* Philadelphia: Lippincott Williams & Wilkins, 2007, pp. 612–639.
20. Mermel L.: Prevention of intravascular catheter-related infections. *Ann Intern Med* 132:391–402, Mar. 7, 2000.
21. Mermel L., et al.: The pathogenesis and epidemiology of catheter-related infection with pulmonary artery Swan-Ganz catheters: A prospective study utilizing molecular subtyping. *Am J Med* 91(3B):197S–205S, Sep. 1991.
22. Kline A.: Pediatric catheter-related bloodstream infections: Latest strategies to decrease risk. *AACN Clin Issues* 16:185–198, Apr.–Jun. 2005.
23. O'Grady N., et al.: Guidelines for the prevention of intravascular catheter-related infections. Centers for Disease Control and Prevention. *MMWR Recomm Rep* 51(RR-10):1–29, Aug. 2002.
24. Veenstra D., et al.: Efficacy of antiseptic-impregnated central venous catheters in preventing catheter-related bloodstream infection: A meta-analysis. *JAMA* 281:261–276, Jan. 1999.
25. State of Victoria, Australia, Department of Human Services: *Preventing Central Venous Catheter-Related-Bloodstream Infections: Toolkit.* Melbourne, Australia: Rural and Regional Health and Aged Care Services Division, Victorian Government Department of Human Services, Dec. 2005.

Chapter 11

The Discharge Process

With the average length of stay for patients in hospitals around the world decreasing, effective and comprehensive discharge planning has become more important than ever. Anecdotal evidence indicates that patients are now leaving hospitals "quicker and sicker," with some patients being sent home in "unstable" condition.[1] The increasing number of outpatient and same-day procedures also results in patients going home before significant post-procedure monitoring can take place. These decreased lengths of stay make it more difficult to detect and treat complications associated with surgery or other invasive procedures before discharge.[2]

Organizations must commit to effective discharge planning to help patients make a smooth transition to the next level of care. Unfortunately, effective discharge planning does not always occur. Lack of effective patient transfer and unclear discharge responsibilities among health care providers are just two of the reasons why health care organizations struggle with this important responsibility. This chapter examines what discharge planning is and how it can be handled effectively. It also discusses postdischarge follow-up.

What Is Discharge Planning?

Discharge planning is a process made up of several key steps or phases. The immediate goal of discharge planning is to anticipate changes in patient care needs while the long-term goal is to ensure continuity of care.[3] The ultimate goals of discharge planning are to smooth the transition from one level of care to another and prevent or diminish the likelihood of problems after discharge.[4]

For some patients, effective discharge planning addresses how needs will be met as the patient moves to another organization for his or her next level of care, treatment, or services. For other patients, planning consists of educating the patient or family on how to continue recovery at home and access services in the future if necessary.

Returning home after surgery or another invasive procedure is not always a smooth transition. Individuals, particularly older adults, can encounter a variety of problems in their first few weeks at home, including lower levels of independence, reduced ability to care for themselves, difficulty with reading medication labels, and not being able to get the proper help when needed.[4] Some patients may be at risk for falls, infections, or other adverse events. In addition, anxiety, stress, and frustration may be apparent during this difficult time. One study suggests that nearly one in five patients experience adverse events during the transition from a hospital setting to the home and that one third of these events are preventable.[5]

Key Components of Effective Discharge

Comprehensive discharge planning can significantly improve patient outcomes. It can also limit the likelihood of postdischarge-related adverse events and rehospitalization.[6] A comprehensive discharge planning process takes into account the conditions under which transfer or discharge can occur and how responsibility will be shifted from one clinician, organization, or service to another.

Following are some key points that organizations must keep in mind when structuring the discharge planning process[7]:

- *Communicate early and often with patients.* Such communication should start at the first moment of contact and occur regularly throughout a patient's stay. By getting to know the patient and family early on, health care providers can identify potential discharge issues early and respond to those issues before the patient is discharged.

- *Coordinate discharge.* It is important to coordinate discharge planning and teaching so that it occurs throughout the patient's stay and does not all occur on the last day. In most cases, the nurse responsible for the patient's direct care will coordinate the discharge process. Some organizations have dedicated discharge planners who help lead the discharge planning process. Even in these cases, the discharge planner should work with the nurse responsible for the patient's direct care to make sure the plan adequately meets the patient's needs.

  Effective documentation can help streamline communication efforts between providers. For example, when the discharge plan is documented in the patient's plan of care, all members of the care team can see it and refer to it as discharge needs change. Information to include in discharge documentation includes the following:
  - Goals of discharge
  - All patient and family teaching
  - Assessment of the patient and family's ability to manage care after discharge
  - Community resources needed
  - Health care equipment, supplies, and medications needed

  Incorporating discharge discussions in interdisciplinary team meetings can also be helpful in enhancing team communication. By regularly discussing patient discharge needs, teams can identify potential issues early and address them before discharge.
- *Systematize the process.* To help coordinate discharge planning, an organization may want to create an interdisciplinary checklist that can help navigate the various points in the discharge process. As discussed throughout this book, checklists can be helpful in ensuring that certain steps in a process are accomplished and certain opportunities for communication take place. For example, a research group at Boston Medical Center developed an 11-point checklist that hospital staff can follow during discharge. The checklist begins with educating patients about their diagnoses and includes other activities such as confirming the medication plan and providing the patient with written discharge instructions. The checklist is used by hospitals throughout the country and has been shown to decrease readmission by 30% when all the steps on the checklist are followed.[8]
- *Involve the patient in the discharge planning process.* The patient and his or her family must be involved in the discharge planning process. Whenever possible, the patient's preferences should be considered, and he or she should feel empowered to speak up if he or she is unclear about aspects of the discharge plan or if he or she has any questions or concerns.
- *Educate the patient and family.* Education at discharge is critical to ensuring a successful transition to the next level of care. It is important to share information about wound care, symptoms to watch out for, medications, medical equipment, and when the individual can resume daily activities, such as driving, walking, lifting, and returning to work. Providers should also review the steps of what to do when a problem arises. This information should include what constitutes a problem, whom to contact when there is a problem, and how to contact that individual.

TIP Educate Patients on Proper Wound Care

The risk for surgical site infection continues after a patient leaves a health care organization. Providers must educate patients and families on proper wound care, how to recognize the signs of surgical site infection, and the importance of reporting symptoms to either the surgeon or the primary care physician.[9]

When educating the patient about discharge following surgery or an invasive procedure, providers should begin the education process before the procedure. Often patients come to a health care organization thinking they will be cured before going home. What they may not realize is that they are stabilized in one setting and may need to go to another level of care, such as a rehabilitation or long term care facility, before returning home. Providers should begin discussions with the patient as soon as the procedure is scheduled, or as soon as the patient arrives at the organization if the procedure is not elective, so that information does not come as a shock on the day of discharge.[10]

Any education provided should be tailored to the patient's needs and abilities. Providers should take into account a patient's cognitive and physical abilities as well as his or her literacy and cultural needs. Providers should also ensure that the patient understands the education provided. Sidebar 11-1 on page 166 provides a description of some tools providers can use to share information and confirm patient understanding.

To help reinforce any discharge education, providers should consider offering written information. This could include printed information on specific precautions related to the patient's surgery or invasive procedure and the patient's condition after discharge; which activities the patient should and should not perform, such as bathing, eating, and exercising; appropriate wound care to prevent infection; and appropriate equipment needed after discharge and how to use it. Information should also be provided on whom to contact in case of problems, including unanticipated symptoms, problems with equipment, or medication concerns.

- *Share resources with the patient.* When a patient is discharged home, he or she often needs to access critical community resources, such as meal services or transportation services. Providers should offer contact information for community resources when possible, explain why these resources may be necessary, and confirm the patient's understanding. If possible, providers should offer brochures or lists of contacts for specific services. If appropriate, a social worker, nurse, or other staff member could provide a list and description of the location of several home health agencies or nursing homes and include recommendations and guidelines on how to choose an appropriate one.
- *Make appointments, if possible.* Ideally, providers should make appointments for follow-up visits. Patients should be clear on why such appointments are necessary and the importance of keeping those appointments. Such appointments should be coordinated with the patient and family schedule. Staff should provide patients and their family with a written record of follow-up appointments that includes the names, addresses, and telephones numbers of the health care providers.
- *Reconcile medications.* Before discharging a patient, the organization should conduct a final medication reconciliation. Providers, usually nurses, should double-check whether the medications prescribed while in the health care facility should be continued and, if so, make sure they do not conflict with medications the patient was taking before he or she came in for the procedure. Appropriate prescriptions should be written for the patient when necessary. Nurses should also check whether any medications taken prior to the procedure should be discontinued and make sure the patient is aware that they should be stopped. After final reconciliation, providers should give the patient a complete list of medications that he or she will be taking after discharge. This information should include a description of each medication the patient is taking as well as its purpose, dosage, administration schedule, and possible adverse effects. Providers should confirm this information with the patient and ask the patient to state his or her understanding of the medication plan in his or her own words. Providers should also encourage the patient to carry the list with him or her and to share the list with all other providers of care, including primary care and specialist physicians, nurses, pharmacists, and other caregivers.[11]
- *Collaborate with the community.* It is important to communicate early with the community providers that may be needed to meet the patient's postdischarge needs. Some consideration should be given to the following:
  - The suitability and capacity of community providers to meet the needs of the patient
  - Timing of discharge to coincide with the operating hours and availability of community services
  - Notifying community providers of the patient's planned discharge, to ensure that services will be in place by the discharge date[12]

Establishing and building relationships with community providers can help foster interactive communication during discharge.

Sidebar 11-1: Tools for Educating Patients

Described here are a few of the many available tools that can be used during discharge education to help ensure and confirm patient understanding:

- **The Teach-Back Method.** This is a way of providing patient education that allows the provider who is teaching to confirm that the patient has understood the material. This approach involves providers asking patients to "teach back"—that is, to state in their own words—key concepts, decisions, or instructions just discussed. If a patient can restate instructions correctly, then the patient education provided was effective. If not, then the provider needs to explain the instructions again, using simple words and additional methods of education, such as pictures or brochures. The teach-back method can be repeated until a provider confirms that the patient understands the message. If after two or three tries the patient still does not understand, then providers should look for other explanations (beyond the provider's teaching) about why the message is not understood. For patients who do not understand the provider's message, the next step might be to give a referral to a patient educator or make an appointment for a follow-up visit or phone call.

  Providers need to be very careful when using the teach-back method and ensure that it is done in a respectful way. They should frame the approach as help for themselves and not imply that the patient did not understand. For example, saying "I want to confirm that I've done a good job teaching" may be helpful. Another approach may be to say, "I know you will see your family today; what do you plan to say to them about your recovery process?"
- **Repeat-Back.** When giving verbal directions, providers can use the repeat-back method and ask the patient to repeat the instructions back in his or her own words. A verbal "repeat-back" can help show that an individual, in this case the patient, understands the information given. Remember that a patient's response of "yes" or a simple nod might mean that the patient is being polite or is ashamed to admit that he or she does not understand the information given.
- **Return Demonstration.** Return demonstration, or "show-back," is another patient education method in which the patient is asked to demonstrate to the caregiver how he or she will do what is taught. This technique is used routinely in diabetic education and physical therapy. It can also be helpful in situations involving wound care and infection prevention.

When communicating with a patient, health care providers should be aware of their tone of voice (Is it measured and calm?), the pace of the conversation (Are pauses long enough to allow those receiving the information to take in what has just been said?), and the power of touch and a direct gaze (as culturally appropriate). Within the conversation, the speaker should give the impression that he or she has all the time needed to have this important conversation. Body language can make all the difference in the way patients and their families respond to what health care providers have to say.

Sources:

Leonard M., Frankel A., Simmonds T.: Effective teamwork and communication. In Frankel A., et al. (eds): *The Essential Guide for Patient Safety Officers.* Oak Brook, IL: Joint Commission Resources, 2009, pp. 49–60.

Nielsen G., Connor M., Leonard M.: Ensuring patient involvement. In Frankel A., et al. (eds.): *The Essential Guide for Patient Safety Officers.* Oak Brook, IL: Joint Commission Resources, 2009, pp. 79–87.

Nielsen G., et al.: *Transforming Care at the Bedside How-to Guide: Creating an Ideal Transition Home for Patients with Heart Failure*: Institute for Healthcare Improvement, 2008. http://www.ihi.org/IHI/Topics/MedicalSurgicalCare/MedicalSurgicalCareGeneral/Tools/TCABHowToGuideTransitionHomeforHF.htm (accessed Jul. 21, 2010).

Osborne H.: Confirming understanding with the teach-back technique. *Boston Globe,* Nov. 20, 2007. http://www.boston.com/jobs/healthcare/oncall/articles/2007/11/20/confirming_understanding_with_the_teach_back_technique/ (accessed Jul. 21, 2010).

The Discharge Summary

When patients are transferred or discharged, appropriate information about care, treatment, and services must be exchanged with other providers to facilitate continuity of care. It is common for patients not to receive recommended follow-up after a procedure. This is due in part to poor communication between providers, such as the surgeon and the patient's primary care physician. In fact, direct communication between hospital physicians and primary care physicians occurs only between 3% and 20% of the time.[13]

Complete discharge summaries can help improve communication between care providers. Ideally these summaries are written and include the following elements[14]:

- Primary and secondary diagnoses
- Relevant medical history and physical findings
- Dates of surgery or other invasive procedures and hospitalization, if appropriate
- Procedure performed
- Results of procedure and abnormal laboratory test results
- Recommendations of any subspecialty consultants
- Information given to the patient and family
- The patient's condition or functional status at discharge
- Reconciled discharge medication regimen
- Reasons for any changes to the medication regimen
- Follow-up appointments
- Tests pending at discharge
- Details about follow-up arrangements
- Name and contact information of the responsible surgeon

Preparation of the discharge summary should begin upon admission. Waiting until the last minute to prepare the discharge summary can lead to errors. The patient should be given a copy of the discharge summary in his or her primary or preferred language and at the appropriate literacy level.

Sometimes it takes an organization several days to complete a patient's discharge summary. By the time the summary is ready, the patient has already moved to the next level of care and possibly has been seen by the primary care provider. The primary care provider is relying on the patient to communicate what happened during the procedure and what the hospital's recommendations are. Many times patients have a hard time articulating anything that was communicated to them about their procedure. To communicate discharge information quickly, health care providers may wish to place a phone call to the primary care provider to give brief information about the patient. A formal written discharge summary can follow later. This preliminary phone call provides the opportunity to share critical information and ask questions. Other ways to speed the process may involve faxing or e-mailing discharge summaries.[14]

TIP Create a Discharge Summary Form

To facilitate discharge, an organization may want to create a discharge summary form. This form could include check boxes and prompts for information to ensure that information is complete and consistent. The form should be easy to complete yet provide all the relevant information needed for the next provider of care.

Postdischarge Follow-Up

A patient's departure from a health care organization does not always end the responsibility of meeting assessed needs. Ideally, health care providers should follow up with patients after discharge. This follow-up may involve a phone call or e-mail to check on the patient's recuperation and any emergency conditions or care needs. During the call, providers can also assess for potential surgical site infections, reinforce teaching, and answer any questions the patient may have. The follow-up call can be effective in preventing readmission to a health care facility.[8]

The expected outcomes identified on the care plan should form the basis for questions during the follow-up phone call. For example, if an exercise regimen was initiated for the patient while in the hospital, providers may want to ask the patient if he or she is exercising and if range of motion is improving. If the patient is at high risk for a surgical site infection, questions about pain, swelling, redness, and the presence of discharge from the surgical site can help identify potential infection. A German study showed that using a questionnaire during postdischarge communication helped identify patients with surgical site infections.[15]

As with other aspects of care, a checklist can be helpful to remind providers to ask patients about critical information and document the results of those conversations. Effective and comprehensive follow-up can help identify and resolve any issues a patient is having and prevent adverse events and readmission.

TIP Check Out the Center for Transforming Healthcare

As of July 2010, the Joint Commission Center for Transforming Healthcare is working on four projects to help make surgery and other invasive procedures safer:

- Hand hygiene
- Handoff communications
- Wrong-site surgery
- Surgical site infections

Organizations should consult the center's Web site (http://www.centerfortransforminghealthcare.org/) for more information on this work and how to get involved.

Conclusion

As seen throughout this book, surgery is a complex, intricate process. It should not be done without careful forethought about how all its intricacies relate to one another. There are many risks present in the surgical setting, and the consequences of those risks can be fatal.

The operating room is no place for pride, ego, or status. Nor is it conducive to complacency, fierce independence, or a need to always be right. Instead, it functions best when there is communication, collaboration, and teamwork.

Organizations that take a systematic approach to improving the continuum of surgery and infuse a culture of safety into the surgical setting not only make surgical procedures more efficient, rewarding, and financially lucrative for providers and organizations but also make procedures safer, which in turn allows providers to more reliably and consistently save, improve, and enhance patients' lives.

A systematic and teamwork-driven approach to surgery and other invasive procedures cannot be achieved overnight or with the commitment of only one or two individuals. It requires a conscious, focused, collaborative effort involving all members of the procedure team. And it is worth the effort.

References

1. Kosecoff J., et al.: Prospective payment system and impairment at discharge: The "quicker-and-sicker" story revisited. *JAMA* 264:1980–1983, Oct. 17, 1990.
2. Iezzoni L., et al.: Screening inpatient quality using post-discharge events. *Med Care* 37:384–398, Apr. 1999.
3. Rorden J., Taft E.: *Discharge Planning Guide for Nurses.* Philadelphia: W.B. Saunders, 1990.
4. Mistiaen P., Francke A., Poot E.: Interventions aimed at reducing problems in adult patients discharged from hospital to home: A systematic meta-review. *BMC Health Serv Res* 7:1–19, Apr. 4, 2007.
5. Forster A., et al.: The incidence and severity of adverse events affecting patients after discharge from the hospital. *Ann Intern Med* 138:161–167, Feb. 4, 2003.
6. Greenwald J., Denham C., Jack B.: The hospital discharge: A review of a high risk care transition with highlights of a reengineered discharge process. *J Patient Saf* 3:97–106, Jun. 2007.
7. Carroll A., Dowling M.: Discharge planning: Communication, education, and patient participation. *Br J Nurs* 16:882–886, Jul. 26–Aug. 8, 2007.
8. Streit M.: Checklist of checkout: Guidelines designed to lessen rehospitalizations. *Mod Healthc* 40:17, Feb. 8, 2010.
9. Pear S.: Patient risk factors and best practices for surgical site infection prevention. *Managing Infection Control* pp. 56–64, 2007.
10. Discharge planning advisor. Basics may be pushed aside in rush to trendier remedies. *Hosp Peer Rev* 31:139–141, Oct. 2006.
11. Reconciling Medications Collaborative: *Reconciling Medications: Safe Practice Recommendations and Implementation Tools.* Massachusetts Coalition for the Prevention of Medical Errors, Massachusetts Hospital Association, Jun. 27, 2005. http://www.macoalition.org/Initiatives/RecMeds/ProjectOverview.pdf (accessed Jul. 24, 2010).
12. Spath P.: Are your hospital's discharges really effective? *Hosp Peer Rev* 32:157–160, Nov. 2007.
13. Kripalani S., et al.: Deficits in communication and information transfer between hospital-based and primary care physicians: Implications for patient safety and continuity of care. *JAMA* 297:831–841, Feb. 28, 2007.
14. Patient satisfaction planner. Study shines light on poor transfer communications. *Hosp Peer Rev* 32:79–81, Jun. 2007.
15. Knaust A., et al.: Three questions to screen for postdischarge surgical site infections. *Am J Infect Control* 37:420–422, Jun. 2009.

Glossary

active communication A brief oral acknowledgment, a nod, or some other gesture that requires action on the part of an individual.

adverse event As defined by Joint Commission International, an unanticipated, undesirable, or potentially dangerous occurrence in a health care organization.

ambulatory care As defined by Joint Commission International, types of health care services provided to individuals on an outpatient basis. Ambulatory care services are provided in many settings ranging from freestanding surgical facilities to cardiac catheterization centers. *See also* outpatient.

anesthesia As defined by Joint Commission International, anesthesia consists of general anesthesia and spinal or major regional anesthesia. It does not include local anesthesia. General anesthesia is a drug-induced loss of consciousness during which patients are not arousable, even by painful stimulation. The ability to independently maintain ventilatory function is often impaired. Patients often require assistance in maintaining a patent airway, and positive pressure ventilation may be required because of depressed spontaneous ventilation or drug-induced depression of neuromuscular function. Cardiovascular function may be impaired.

blood component A fraction of separated whole blood (for example, red blood cells, plasma, platelets, granulocytes).

care The provision of accommodations, comfort, and treatment to an individual, implying responsibility for safety, including care, treatment, service, habilitation, rehabilitation, or other programs instituted by the organization for the individual served.

caregiver As defined by The Joint Commission, a family member, a significant other, a friend, a volunteer, or an individual employed by the patient or resident to provide services in the home.

cleaning As defined by Joint Commission International, removal of all visible dust, soil, and any other visible material that microorganisms might find favorable for continued life and growth. This is usually done by scrubbing with hot water and detergent.

code of conduct A document that outlines the core values of an organization and defines what behavior is expected and what behavior is not tolerated.

disinfection As defined by Joint Commission International, the use of a chemical procedure that eliminates most disease-producing organisms, but not all microbial forms.

failure mode and effects analysis (FMEA) **1.** *As defined by The Joint Commission:* An assessment that examines a process in detail, including sequencing of events; assesses actual and potential risk, failure, or points of vulnerability; and, through a logical process, prioritizes areas for improvement based on the actual or potential patient care impact (criticality). **2.** *As defined by Joint Commission International:* A systematic way of examining a design prospectively for possible ways in which failure can occur. It assumes that no matter how knowledgeable or careful people are, errors will occur in some situations and may even be likely to occur. Synonyms: *failure mode, effects, and criticality analysis (FMECA), proactive risk assessment.*

flowchart (flow diagram) A pictorial summary that shows with symbols and words the steps, sequence, and relationship of the various operations involved in the performance of a function or a process.

hand hygiene Hand washing or use of an alcohol-based hand rub.

health care–associated infection (HAI) **1.** *As defined by The Joint Commission:* An infection acquired concomitantly by an individual who is receiving or who has received care, treatment, or services from a health care organization. The infection may or may not have resulted from the care, treatment, or services. **2.** *As defined by Joint Commission International:* Any infection(s) acquired by an individual while receiving care or services in a health care organization. Common HAIs are urinary infections, surgical wound infections, pneumonia, and bloodstream infections.

health care organization As defined by Joint Commission International, a generic term used to describe many types of organizations that provide health care services. This includes ambulatory care centers, behavioral/mental health institutions, home care organizations, hospitals, laboratories, and long term care organizations. Also known as a *health care institution.*

health care professional As defined by Joint Commission International, any person who has completed a course of study and is skilled in a field of health care. This includes a physician, dentist, nurse, or allied health professional. Health care professionals are often licensed by a government agency or certified by a professional organization.

independent practitioner As defined by Joint Commission International, any individual permitted by law and by the organization to provide care and services, without direction or supervision, within the scope of the individual's license. In many countries, licensed independent practitioners include physicians, dentists, some categories of nurses, podiatrists, optometrists, and chiropractors. *See also* practitioner.

individual served The terms *individual served, patient,* and *care recipient* all describe the individual, client, consumer, or resident who actually receives health care, treatment, and/or services. *As defined by The Joint Commission for behavioral health care programs only:* An individual who receives care, treatment, or service; the individual can be a child, a youth, or an adult. When required for the well-being or age of the individual served, a legally responsible individual is also involved in the care, treatment, or service of the individual served.

invasive procedure As defined by Joint Commission International, a procedure involving puncture or incision of the skin or insertion of an instrument or foreign material into the body. *See also* invasive procedures.

invasive procedures As defined by The Joint Commission, invasive procedures involve the puncture or incision of the skin, insertion of an instrument, or insertion of foreign material into the body. Invasive procedures may be performed for diagnostic or treatment-related purposes. *See also* invasive procedure.

The Joint Commission An independent, not-for-profit organization, The Joint Commission is dedicated to improving the safety and quality of health care through standards development, public policy initiatives, accreditation, and certification. The Joint Commission accredits and certifies more than 18,000 health care organizations and programs in the United States.

Joint Commission Center for Transforming Healthcare An affiliate of The Joint Commission that aims to solve poor quality and unsafe health care and transform health care into a high-reliability industry. The Center's participants—the leading hospitals and health systems in the United States—use a proven systematic approach to analyze specific breakdowns in patient care and discover their underlying causes to develop targeted solutions that solve these complex problems.

Joint Commission International (JCI) JCI extends The Joint Commission's mission worldwide. Through both international consultation and accreditation, JCI helps to improve the quality and safety of patient care in many nations. JCI has extensive international experience working with public and private health care organizations and local governments in more than 40 countries.

Joint Commission Resources (JCR) Not-for-profit affiliate of The Joint Commission designated by The Joint Commission to publish publications and multimedia products. JCR reproduces and distributes these materials under license from The Joint Commission. *See also* www.jcrinc.org.

licensed independent practitioner As defined by The Joint Commission, an individual permitted by law and by the organization to provide care, treatment, and services without direct supervision. A licensed independent practitioner operates within the scope of his or her license, consistent with individually granted clinical privileges. When Joint Commission standards reference the term *licensed independent practitioner,* this language is not to be construed to limit the authority of a licensed independent practitioner to delegate tasks to other qualified health personnel (for example, physician assistants and advanced practice registered nurses) to the extent authorized by state law or a state's regulatory mechanism or federal guidelines and organizational policy. *See also* independent practitioner.

medical equipment Fixed and portable equipment used for the diagnosis, treatment, monitoring, and direct care of individuals.

medication Any prescription medications, sample medications, herbal remedies, vitamins, nutriceuticals, vaccines, or over-the-counter drugs; diagnostic and contrast agents used on or administered to persons to diagnose, treat, or prevent disease or other abnormal conditions; radioactive medications, respiratory therapy treatments, parenteral nutrition, blood derivatives, and intravenous solutions (plain, with electrolytes and/or drugs); and [as defined by The Joint Commission] any product designated by the U.S. Food and Drug Administration (FDA) as a drug. This definition of *medication* does not include enteral nutrition solutions (which are considered food products), oxygen, and other medical gases.

medication error **1.** *As defined by The Joint Commission:* A preventable event that may cause or lead to inappropriate medication use or patient harm while the medication is in the control of the health care professional, patient, or consumer. Such events may be related to professional practice, health care products, procedures, and systems, including prescribing; order communication; product labeling, packaging, and nomenclature; compounding; dispensing; distribution; administration; education; monitoring; and use. **2.** *As defined by Joint Commission International:* Any preventable event that may cause inappropriate medication use or jeopardize patient safety. *See also* sentinel event.

medication reconciliation The process of identifying the name, dosage, route, and frequency for each medication currently being taken and ordering medication based on reference to this list.

near miss (also known as *close call*) **1.** *As defined by The Joint Commission:* Any variation during the provision of care, treatment, or services that did not affect an outcome, but for which a recurrence carries a significant risk of an adverse outcome. A near miss is a sentinel event, by definition, but near misses are not subject to review by The Joint Commission under its Sentinel Event Policy. **2.** *As defined by Joint Commission International:* Any process variation that did not affect an outcome but for which a recurrence carries a significant chance of a serious adverse outcome. Such a "near miss" falls within the scope of the definition of an adverse event. **3.** *As defined by the World Health Organization International Classification for Patient Safety:* An incident that did not reach the patient.

outpatient As defined by Joint Commission International, generally, persons who do not need the level of care associated with the more structured environment of an inpatient or a residential program. In many countries, outpatient care is also known as *ambulatory care.* In some countries, outpatients are considered "admitted" to a health care organization; in others, outpatients are considered "registered." *See also* ambulatory care.

patient An individual who receives care, treatment, or services. (For JCI standards, the patient and family are considered a single unit of care.) Synonyms used by various health care fields include *resident, client, patient and family unit, individual served, consumer, health care consumer, customer,* or *beneficiary.*

plan-do-study-act (PDSA) cycle A four-part method for discovering and correcting assignable causes to improve the quality of processes. Synonyms: *plan-do-check-act (PDCA) cycle, Deming cycle, Shewhart cycle.*

policy A principle or method that is developed for the purpose of guiding decisions and activities related to governance, management, care, treatment, and services. A policy is developed by organization leadership, approved by the governing body of the organization, and maintained in writing.

practitioner **1.** *As defined by The Joint Commission:* Any individual who is licensed and qualified to practice a health care profession (for example, physician, nurse, social worker, clinical psychologist, or respiratory therapist) and is engaged in the provision of care, treatment, or services. **2.** *As defined by Joint Commission International:* Any person who has completed a course of study and is skilled in a field of health care. This includes a physician, dentist, nurse, pharmacist, respiratory therapist, among others. Practitioners are licensed by a government agency or certified by a professional organization. *See also* independent practitioner; licensed independent practioner.

prescribing or ordering The process of a licensed independent practitioner or prescriber transmitting a legal order or prescription to the organization directing the preparing, dispensing, and administering of a specific medication to a specific individual. It does not include requisitions for medication supplies.

procedure **1.** A series of steps taken to accomplish a desired end, as in a therapeutic, cosmetic, or surgical procedure. **2.** A unit of health care, as in services and procedures. A procedure is not necessarily developed by organization leadership, approved by the governing body of the organization, and maintained in writing.

process **1.** *As defined by The Joint Commission:* A goal-directed, interrelated series of actions, events, mechanisms, or steps that transform inputs into outputs. **2.** *As defined by Joint Commission International:* A series of actions (or activities) that transform the inputs (resources) into outputs (services).

quality improvement **1.** *As defined by The Joint Commission:* Continuous study and adjustment of an organization's operations and processes to better meet staff and customer needs. Also known as *continuous quality improvement, continuous improvement, organization-wide improvement,* and *total quality management.* **2.** *As defined by Joint Commission International:* An approach to the continuous study and improvement of the processes of providing health care services to meet the needs of patients and others. Synonyms include *continuous quality improvement, continuous improvement, organizationwide performance improvement,* and *total quality management.*

quality of care **1.** *As defined by The Joint Commission:* The degree to which care, treatment, or services for individuals and populations increases the likelihood of desired health or behavioral health outcomes. Considerations include the appropriateness, efficacy, efficiency, timeliness, accessibility, and continuity of care; the safety of the care environment; and the individual's personal values, practices, and beliefs. **2.** *As defined by Joint Commission International:* The degree to which health services for individuals and populations increase the likelihood of desired health outcomes and are consistent with current professional knowledge. Dimensions of performance include the following: patient perspective issues; safety of the care environment; and accessibility, appropriateness, continuity, effectiveness, efficacy, efficiency, and timeliness of care.

reviewable sentinel event As defined by The Joint Commission, a sentinel event that affects a recipient of care and that results in an unanticipated death or major permanent loss of function, not related to the natural course of the patient's illness or underlying condition. Such a sentinel event is subject to review by The Joint Commission and may be reported to The Joint Commission on a voluntary basis. *See also* sentinel event.

safety **1.** *As defined by The Joint Commission:* The degree to which the risk of an intervention (for example, use of a drug or a procedure) and risk in the care environment are reduced for a patient and other persons, including health care practitioners. Safety risks may arise from the performance of tasks, from the structure of the physical environment, or from situations beyond the organization's control (such as weather). **2.** *As defined by Joint*

Commission International: The degree that the organization's buildings, grounds, and equipment do not pose a hazard or risk to patients, staff, or visitors.

safety management Activities selected and implemented by the organization to assess and control the impact of environmental risk, and to improve general environmental safety.

sentinel event **1.** *As defined by The Joint Commission:* An unexpected occurrence involving death or serious physical or psychological injury or the risk thereof. The phrase *or the risk thereof* includes any process variation for which a recurrence would carry a significant chance of a serious adverse outcome. **2.** *As defined by Joint Commission International:* An unanticipated occurrence involving death or major permanent loss of function. *See also* medication error; reviewable sentinel event.

services Structural divisions of an organization, its medical staff, or its licensed independent practitioner staff.

staff **1.** *As defined by The Joint Commission:* As appropriate to their roles and responsibilities, all people who provide care, treatment, or services in the organization, including those receiving pay (for example, permanent, temporary, and part-time personnel, as well as contract employees), volunteers, and health profession students. The Joint Commission definition of *staff* does not include licensed independent practitioners who are not paid staff or who are not contract employees. **2.** *As defined by Joint Commission International:* According to their roles and responsibilities, all people who provide care, treatment, and services in the organization (for example, medical staff and nursing staff), including those receiving pay (permanent, temporary, and part-time personnel, as well as contract employees), volunteers, and health profession students. *Clinical staff* refers to those who provide direct patient care (physicians, dentists, nurses, among others). *Nonclinical staff* refers to those who provide indirect patient care (admissions, food service, among others).

standard **1.** *As defined by The Joint Commission:* A principle of patient safety and quality of care that a well-run organization meets. A standard defines the performance expectations, structures, or processes that must be substantially in place in an organization to enhance the quality of care, treatment, or services. **2.** *As defined by Joint Commission International:* A statement that defines the performance expectations, structures, or processes that must be in place for an organization to provide safe and high-quality care, treatment, and service.

sterile field A space in which select surfaces have been prepared, maintained, and segregated as sterile to minimize potential sources of contamination by nonsterile items.

sterilization The use of a physical or chemical procedure to destroy all microbial life, including highly resistant bacterial endospores.

survey A key component in the accreditation process, whereby a surveyor(s) conducts an on-site evaluation of an organization's compliance with Joint Commission or Joint Commission International accreditation requirements.

surveyor For purposes of Joint Commission accreditation, a licensed physician, surgeon, podiatrist, dentist, nurse, physician assistant, administrator, social worker, psychologist, behavioral health care professional, or any other health care professional who meets The Joint Commission's surveyor selection criteria, evaluates compliance with accreditation requirements, and provides education and consultation regarding compliance with accreditation requirements to surveyed organizations or systems.

time-out As defined by Joint Commission International, a pause, just prior to performing a surgical or other procedure, during which any unanswered questions or confusion about patient, procedure, or site are resolved by the entire surgical or procedural team. Even when there is only one person doing the procedure, a brief pause to confirm the correct patient, procedure, and site is appropriate. *See also* time-out, preoperative.

time-out, preoperative As defined by The Joint Commission, an immediate preoperative pause by the entire surgical team to confirm the correct patient, procedure, and procedure site. *See also* time-out.

Index

D

E

F

Q

R

S

T

U

V

W

X